Pediatric Oncology

Series Editors:

Gregory H. Reaman
Silver Spring, MD, USA

Franklin O. Smith
Cincinnati, OH, USA

More information about this series at http://www.springer.com/series/5421

Gary M. Kupfer • Gregory H. Reaman
Franklin O. Smith
Editors

Bone Marrow Failure

Springer

Editors
Gary M. Kupfer
Department of Pediatrics
Yale School of Medicine
New Haven, CT
USA

Gregory H. Reaman
Department of Pediatrics
George Washington University
Washington, DC
USA

Franklin O. Smith
Medpace
Cincinnati, OH
USA

ISSN 1613-5318 ISSN 2191-0812 (electronic)
Pediatric Oncology
ISBN 978-3-030-09662-5 ISBN 978-3-319-61421-2 (eBook)
https://doi.org/10.1007/978-3-319-61421-2

Printed on acid-free paper

This Springer imprint is published by the registered company Springer Nature Switzerland AG.
The registered company address is: Gewerbestrasse 11, 6330 Cham, Switzerland

Preface

For many years, bone marrow failure was a pathological entity, all thrown into the same bin without thought to pathogenesis, diagnosis, prognosis, and, certainly, treatment. Forward to the age of blood banking, advanced pharmacology, imaging, and other trappings of modern medicine, the full flower of the diversity of these diseases became apparent. Now, in 2018, with DNA sequencing occurring at the highest technical level, cheapest price, and overwhelming volume, a blizzard of genes that account for these varying syndromes has come into focus, with the science of investigating the function of these genes following close on the heels of this information.

In this volume we lay out a compendium of chapters outlining the bone marrow failure syndromes. Rather than proceeding in an encyclopedic way, importantly we have elected to follow the science. In particular, we start with a discussion of basic molecular hematopoiesis to obtain an understanding of the normal processes that go awry during development. In particular are genes that not surprisingly are mutated in some of the diseases are explored in these pages. Further we find threads of connection among seemingly disparate syndromes Diamond-Blackfan anemia, dyskeratosis congenita, and Shwachman-Diamond, all linked by the understanding of ribosome biology. While bone marrow failure classically invokes all three cell lines, the effects of genetic mutation in individual cell lines are apparent, as in the neutropenias and thrombocytopenias. The culmination of bone marrow failure is symbolized in the continuous shrinkage of the "idiopathic" aplastic anemias, as new genes are identified in the pathogenesis of bone marrow failure, and the joining of the circle with myelodysplasia, as inevitably entering into a Venn diagram together. Most compellingly is the emergence of GATA2 as the gene responsible for MDS. This is a reminder that, while our mission is certainly paramount to those patients afflicted with these rare diseases, these diseases are important and profound genetic models of normal biology. Perhaps no better example of this exists than Fanconi anemia, which not only lends insight into DNA repair but also into the genetics of common cancers, as 15–20% of all cancers in the cancer genome database contains mutations in FA genes or in related genes. Thus, rare has become mainstream.

Finally, as is recognized by many of us who care for these patients, the current state of the art of therapy remains hematopoietic stem cell transplant, with much research devoted to the safe and effective provision of such therapy. Current limitations and the promises of the future portend going further and suggest emerging therapies that will capitalize on new genomic technology.

May the efforts of all invested in scientific efforts to understand these diseases and those who care for the patients so afflicted, clinicians and families, be rewarded swiftly for their labor, perseverance, and devotion to good works.

New Haven, CT — Gary M. Kupfer
Washington, DC — Gregory H. Reaman
Cincinnati, OH — Franklin O. Smith

Acknowledgments

We would like to express our sincere appreciation to our colleagues who made such meaningful contributions in the writing of this book. We also thank the staff at Springer for their tireless efforts in support of this work.

To the authors, scientists, clinicians, families, and our patients, our appreciation and admiration for your sense of duty in your life's work.

Our love and appreciation to our spouses, Michele, Phyllis and Susan, and our children, Noa, Zev and Meital, Barrett and Ian, and Emily and Sarah.

Contents

The Cellular and Molecular Mechanisms of Hematopoiesis

1

Erinn B. Rankin and Kathleen M. Sakamoto

Contents

E. B. Rankin
Department of Radiation Oncology, Stanford University School of Medicine, Stanford, CA, USA

Department of Obstetrics and Gynecologic Oncology, Stanford University School of Medicine, Stanford, CA, USA

K. M. Sakamoto (✉)
Division of Hematology/Oncology, Department of Pediatrics, Stanford University School of Medicine, Stanford, CA, USA
e-mail: kmsakamo@stanford.edu

G. M. Kupfer et al. (eds.), *Bone Marrow Failure*, Pediatric Oncology,
https://doi.org/10.1007/978-3-319-61421-2_1

1.1 Hematopoiesis

Hematopoiesis is a complex and dynamic process where mature blood cells of the myeloid and lymphoid lineages are produced from a common hematopoietic progenitor cell. In adult mammals, this process occurs almost exclusively in the bone marrow under homeostatic conditions. This hierarchal process begins with a common hematopoietic stem cell (HSC) that is multipotential and capable of forming all blood lineages while maintaining their self-renewal capacity. In the classical model of hematopoiesis, it is thought that HSCs differentiate into a series of progenitor cell intermediates that undergo gradual fate restriction and commitment into mature blood lineages (Figs. 1.1 and 1.2, (Doulatov et al. 2012)). Recent advances in single-cell tracing, RNA sequencing, and transplantation have suggested an alternative model where lineage fate may be determined at an earlier stage than previously suggested. Single-cell RNA sequencing on myeloid progenitor cells revealed that very few

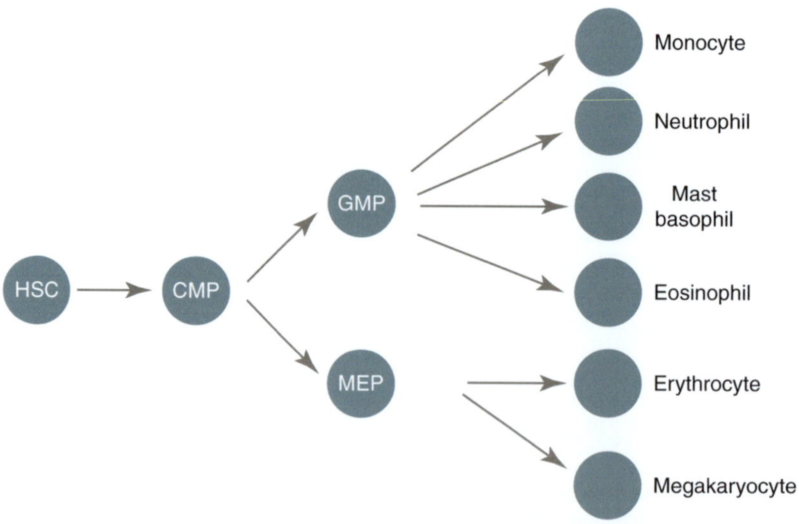

Fig. 1.1 Classical model of myeloid lineage commitment in the bone marrow. In the classical model of hematopoiesis, mature myeloid cells are generated through a series of myeloid progenitors including a common myeloid progenitor (CMP), granulocyte/macrophage precursor (GMP), and a myeloid/erythroid precursor. Recent studies indicate that myeloid specification may occur at an earlier stage where myeloid progenitors are a mix of committed progenitors rather than a homogenous population of cells with multilineage potential

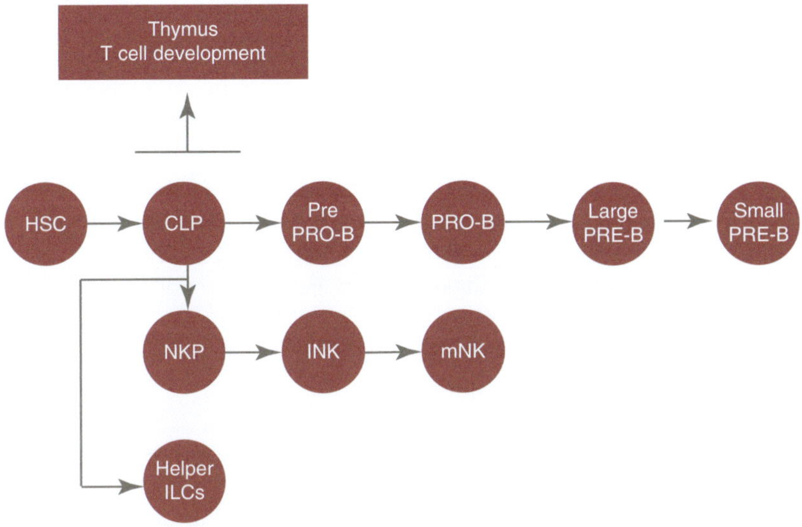

Fig. 1.2 Lymphoid lineage commitment in the bone marrow. During lymphoid develop, the common lymphoid progenitor is generated from hematopoietic progenitors that give rise to natural killer cell, B cell, and helper innate lymphocyte cell progenitors within the bone marrow. B cell and NK cell progenitors go through stages of maturation before leaving the bone marrow, whereas T cell progenitors mature within the thymus

progenitors expressed transcription factors that regulate multiple cell fates. Instead, individual cells clustered into lineage-specific differentiation programs (Paul et al. 2015). Additionally, single-cell lineage tracing through the transplantation of barcoded progenitor cells into mice suggested that very few myeloid progenitor cells have the ability to form erythroid and myeloid lineages suggesting that myeloid progenitors are a mixture of committed progenitors rather than a homogenous population of cells with multilineage potential (Perie et al. 2015). The regulation of HSC production, survival, self-renewal, and differentiation is a carefully orchestrated process that is dependent upon both systemic and local cues to produce approximately one trillion (10^{12}) cells daily. In this chapter, we will review the cellular intrinsic and extrinsic factors that control adult hematopoiesis in the bone marrow microenvironment.

1.2 HSCs

Hematopoietic stem cells (HSCs) are multipotent progenitors capable of forming all blood lineages while maintaining their self-renewal capacity. HSCs are extremely rare as only 1 in a million cells within human bone marrow is a transplantable stem cell (Doulatov et al. 2012). The isolation and purification of murine HSCs in combination with genetic approaches have been informative in revealing the molecular and biochemical pathways that control HSC function and differentiation.

1.2.1 Transcription Factors

There are a variety of transcriptional networks that control HSC production, survival, and self-renewal. Genetic inactivation of a number of these factors has identified important roles for Gata-2, Notch1, Erg, N-Myc and c-Myc, and Gfi-1 in the regulation of hematopoiesis in the bone marrow.

The zinc finger transcription factor GATA-2 is required for both primitive and definitive hematopoiesis. Germline inactivation of GATA-2 leads to embryonic lethality at E10.5 due to severe anemia (Tsai et al. 1994). The injection of GATA-2-deficient/wild-type ES cell clones into blastocysts revealed that GATA-2 is required for fetal liver and adult bone marrow hematopoiesis (Tsai et al. 1994). GATA-2 expression is decreased in CD34+ bone marrow cells in patients with aplastic anemia underscoring the importance of this transcription factor in the regulation of hematopoiesis (Fujimaki et al. 2001).

Notch1 is a membrane-bound receptor and transcription factor whose activity is regulated by interaction with its ligand Jagged. Upon ligand interaction, Notch1 is proteolytically cleaved to release the Notch-IC domain that translocates into the nucleus to regulate transcription. Notch1 is required for definitive hematopoiesis as Notch1-deficient ES cells fail to contribute to long-term definitive hematopoiesis (Hadland et al. 2004). A key mechanism by which Notch1 regulates hematopoiesis is through the regulation of Runx1 (Wilkinson and Gottgens 2013).

The E-twenty-six (ETS) transcription factor-related gene (ERG) plays an important role in the expansion and maintenance of HSCs during the early phases of definitive hematopoiesis. Conditional deletion of ERG in hematopoietic cells resulted in loss of myeloid cells associated with a defect in HSC numbers and function in transplantation assays (Knudsen et al. 2015). While HSC migration, homing, and adhesion are not dependent on ERG activity, ERG is required to maintain and prevent the differentiation of HSCs in the bone marrow. ERG-dependent regulation of HSCs is associated with the activation of HSC self-renewal genes and the repression of MYC target genes (Knudsen et al. 2015). The DNA-binding activity of ERG may be particularly important in the regulation of definitive hematopoiesis as $ERG^{Mld2/Mld2}$ DNA-binding mutant mice also fail to maintain HSCs in the bone marrow of adult mice (Taoudi et al. 2011).

The basic helix-loop-helix leucine zipper transcription factors N-Myc and c-Myc play an important role in controlling HSC proliferation, differentiation, and survival. Immature HSCs express both N-Myc and c-Myc. Conditional deletion of c-Myc in adult bone marrow cells results in the accumulation of HSCs that are impaired in differentiation (Wilson et al. 2004). While conditional inactivation of N-Myc did not affect steady-state hematopoiesis, the combined deletion of N-Myc and c-Myc resulted in severe pancytopenia in mice associated with a preferential loss of proliferating, but not quiescent HSCs (Laurenti et al. 2008).

The zinc finger repressor growth factor independent-1 (Gfi-1) restricts the proliferation and preserves the functional integrity of HSCs. Gfi-1-deficient HSCs display elevated proliferation rates but are functionally compromised in competitive repopulation and serial transplantation assays (Hock et al. 2004; Zeng et al. 2004).

1.2.2 Epigenetics

Epigenetic modification of chromatin and DNA plays an important role in the regulation of HSC function. A number of factors involved in DNA methylation, histone modification, and chromatin remodeling have been identified as key regulators of HSC development, self-renewal, and differentiation (for a recent review, see (Cullen et al. 2014)). Large-scale genetic screens in zebrafish have been utilized to identify multiple chromatin-modifying complexes important in hematopoietic development (Huang et al. 2013). Among these factors, the polycomb-group proteins (PRC1 and PRC2) mediate gene silencing through the methylation of histones. BMI1, a component of PRC1, maintains the self-renewal of adult stem cells through the repression of the Ink4a/Arf locus (Oguro et al. 2006). Moreover, BMI1 prevents premature lineage specification of HSCs by repression of developmental regulator genes Ebf1 and Pax5 (Oguro et al. 2010). Recent studies have identified a role for the histone deacetylase SIRT6 in the regulation of HSC homeostasis through the transcriptional repression of Wnt target genes (Wang et al. 2016). Sirt6 deletion in HSCs promoted proliferation and impaired self-renewal ability through the aberrant activation of Wnt signaling (Wang et al. 2016). Additionally, DNA methylation mediated by DNMT3A and TET2 plays an important role in repressing lineage-specific factors such as Klf1 in HSCs. Inactivation of DNMT3A and TET2 commonly occurs in hematological malignancies. In murine models, Tet2 and Dnmt3a inactivation leads to myeloid and lymphoid disease that is associated with Klf1- and Epor-enhanced HSC self-renewal (Zhang et al. 2016).

1.2.3 Microenvironment

The bone marrow is a complex and dynamic environment with multiple "niches" that control HSC quiescence, self-renewal, and proliferation. The niche provides a variety of signals including growth factors, cytokines, oxygen gradients, cell adhesion molecules, matrix proteins, and nutrients that control HSC function (Fig. 1.3). In particular, CXCL12 plays an important role in HSC retention and quiescence. Global deletion of CXCL12 or its receptor, CXCR4, results in HSC loss in the bone marrow. In addition to CXCL12, the Notch, Wnt/B-catenin, SCF/c-Kit, TPO/c-Mpl, TGF-B/Smad, and Ang-1/Tie2 signaling pathways have been implicated in the regulation of HSC function (for a recent review, see (Kosan and Godmann 2016; Seita and Weissman 2010)).

Research over the past decade has identified a number of cell types within the bone marrow microenvironment that support HSC function. Osteoblasts were the first cell population shown to support HSC frequency in the bone marrow (Calvi et al. 2003). Conditional expansion and deletion of osteoblasts were sufficient to modulate HSC numbers in the bone marrow (Calvi et al. 2003; Zhang et al. 2003). In addition to osteoblasts, endothelial cells, mesenchymal stromal cells, macrophages, osteoclasts, and non-myelinating Schwann cells have been shown to promote HSC maintenance in the bone marrow. The cells within the niche produce a variety of factors that regulate HSC function including SCF, CXCL12, pleiotrophin, Slit2, tenascin-C, osteopontin, and noncanonical Wnts (for a recent review, see (Morrison and Scadden 2014)). Recent technological advances in single-cell RNA sequencing are being employed to identify novel niche factors that contribute to HSC function in the bone marrow. Using these approaches, Silberstein et al. identified the secreted RNase angiogenin, the cytokine IL-18, and the adhesion molecule Embigin as novel factors produced by mesenchymal cells that regulate HSC quiescence (Silberstein et al. 2016). In summary, the bone marrow microenvironment contains many cellular and molecule factors that control HSC function (Fig. 1.3).

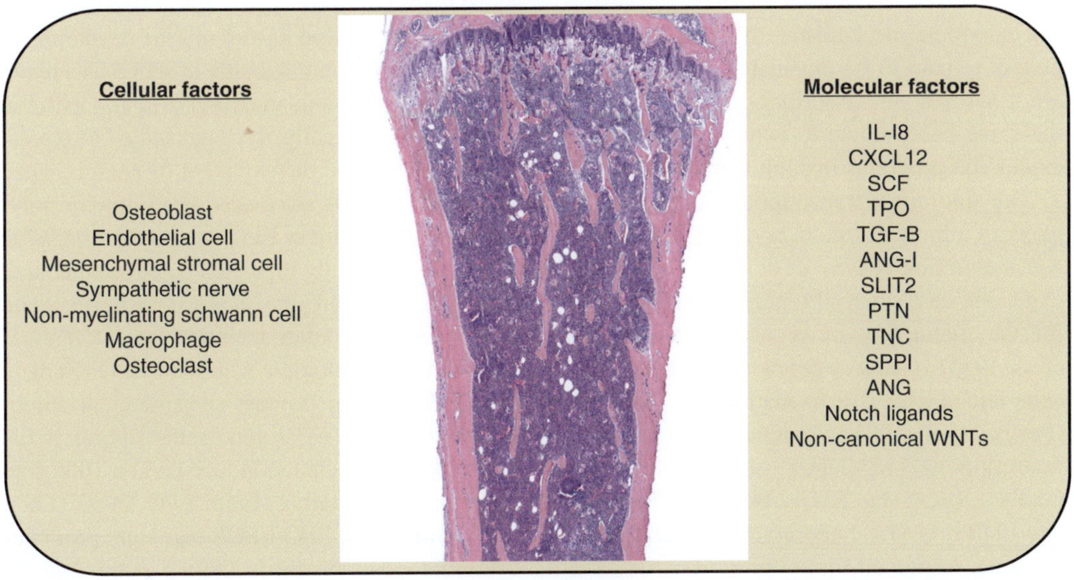

Fig. 1.3 Cellular and molecular factors within the HSC niche that control HSC function. Recent studies have demonstrated that the bone marrow microenvironment is highly complex and dynamic with multiple cellular and molecular factors contributing to the regulation of hematopoiesis

1.3 Erythrocyte

Erythropoiesis is the process by which mature red blood cells are produced from hematopoietic stem and progenitor cells in the bone marrow. Red blood cells are anucleate cells that play a critical role in carrying oxygen to tissues. Red blood cells are the most abundant cells in the blood (5 million/μL). In order to maintain RBC numbers in the blood, the bone marrow produces two million erythrocytes per second. At this level of production, intrinsic and extrinsic factors controlling erythropoiesis must be carefully coordinated (Palis 2014). In the bone marrow, erythroid precursors differentiate through a series of stages (proerythroblasts, basophilic and polychromatophilic erythroblasts, orthochromatophilic erythroblasts, and finally reticulocytes by enucleation) that have been defined morphologically, based on a gradual decrease in cell volume, increasing chromatin condensation and increasing hemoglobinization as well as by the expression of the cell surface molecules CD71 and Ter119 (Socolovsky et al. 2001).

1.3.1 Transcription Factors

The complete mechanisms that control erythropoiesis remain to be elucidated. However, there are a number of transcription factor complexes that have been shown to control erythroid gene expression programs in adult hematopoiesis.

The zinc finger transcription factor, GATA-1, plays an important role in erythroid development and maturation (Pevny et al. 1991). GATA-1 is expressed early in erythropoiesis and is required for the maturation of proerythroblasts (Pevny et al. 1995). GATA-1-deficient embryonic stem cells fail to give rise to mature red blood cells (Pevny et al. 1991). Together with additional transcriptional regulators including friend of GATA-1 (FOG-1), TAL1, IRF2, IRF8, LMO2, and LDB1, GATA-1 represses and activates target genes important for erythropoiesis.

In addition to GATA-1, the erythroid-specific Kruppel-like factor KLF1 is essential for erythropoiesis. KLF1 expression is restricted to erythroid cells where it plays an essential role in regulating erythroid-specific gene expression. Genetic inactivation of KLF1 in mice results in embryonic lethality associated with anemia and molecular features of B-globin deficiency (Perkins et al. 1995). In addition to regulating B-globin expression, KLF1 activates the expression of genes that control heme synthesis, globin chaperones, structural membrane and cytoskeletal proteins, ion and water channels, metabolic and antioxidant enzymes, and cell cycle regulators (Perkins et al. 2016). The importance of KLF1 in the regulation of erythropoiesis is underscored by recent identification of KLF1 variants in patients with red blood cell disorders (Perkins et al. 2016).

1.3.2 Growth Factor Signaling

The glycoprotein erythropoietin (EPO) is essential for the regulation of red blood cell mass in response to changes in tissue oxygenation. EPO induces erythropoiesis through the stimulation of the EPO receptor on erythroid precursor cells to stimulate survival, proliferation, and differentiation, thus enhancing the oxygen-carrying capacity of blood (review in ref. (Ebert and Bunn 1999)). Lack of Epo during murine development results in embryonic lethality at E13.5 as a result of cardiac failure and anemia (Wu et al. 1999; Wu et al. 1995). Clinically, dysregulated *EPO* expression results in the development of anemia when serum EPO levels are inadequately low or polycythemia as a result of EPO overproduction. *EPO* expression is tightly regulated by developmental, tissue-specific, and physiological cues (Ebert and Bunn 1999). In adult mammals, the kidney is the primary physiologic source of EPO (Zanjani et al. 1981). The primary physiological stimulus of increased *EPO* gene transcription is tissue hypoxia, which can induce up to a 1000-fold increase in circulating serum EPO levels (Ebert and Bunn 1999). EPO/EPOR signaling promotes erythroid development in large part through the activation JAK2 signaling. Inactivation of JAK2 results in the development of anemia, whereas constitutive JAK2 mutations lead to increased red blood cell mass and polycythemia (Neubauer et al. 1998; Levine et al. 2005).

1.3.3 Microenvironment

Within the bone marrow microenvironment, erythroblasts mature within erythroblastic islands where erythroblasts physically attach to a central macrophage. Macrophages are thought to promote erythroblast proliferation, supply iron for hemoglobin, promote enucleation, and clear nuclear debris (for a recent review, see (Giger and Kalfa 2015)). An important functional role for bone marrow macrophages in mediating erythroblast survival under stress has been described (Korolnek and Hamza 2015; Chow et al. 2013). Future studies are needed to determine the molecular mechanisms by which central macrophages support erythropoiesis.

1.4 Megakaryocyte

Platelets are the second most abundant cell type in the blood and play an important role in hemostasis, thrombosis, inflammation, and vascular biology. Platelets are anucleate cells that are derived from mature megakaryocytes in the bone marrow (Kaushansky 2008). A single megakaryocyte can give rise to 1000–3000 platelets (Kaushansky 2008). The adult human produces 10^{11} platelets daily at steady state (Kaushansky 2008). Platelets have an average lifespan of 9 days once they enter the circulation. Both cellular intrinsic and extrinsic factors control thrombopoiesis.

1.4.1 Transcription Factors

Platelets are generated in the bone marrow through a process of megakaryocyte differentiation and the fragmentation of the megakaryocyte cytoplasm. Megakaryocytes are derived from pluripotent HSCs that undergo differentiation to a common myeloid progenitor (CMP) and a bipotent megakaryocyte/erythroid progenitor (MEP) cell. There are a number of transcription factors that orchestrate megakaryocyte differentiation and platelet production within the bone marrow including GATA-1, friend of GATA-1 (FOG), NF-E2, Fli-1, PU.1, and RUNX1.

The zinc finger transcription factor GATA-1 is a key regulator of erythroid and megakaryocyte differentiation and maturation. In megakaryocyte production, overexpression of GATA-1 in an early mouse myeloid cell line induces megakaryocyte differentiation (Visvader et al. 1992). Moreover, genes that are expressed within the megakaryocyte lineage depend on GATA consensus sites for full transcriptional activity (Shivdasani et al. 1997). In mice, conditional inactivation of GATA-1 in megakaryocytes significantly reduces megakaryocyte proliferation and cytoplasmic maturation (Shivdasani et al. 1997). Moreover, patients with inherited mutations within *GATA-1* present with platelet dysfunction and thrombocytopenia (Daly 2017). The functional role of GATA-1 in megakaryocytes is to recruit transcriptional cofactors, such as friend of GATA-1 (FOG) to megakaryocyte-expressed genes. Genetic studies have demonstrated that the interaction between GATA-1 and FOG1 is essential of megakaryocyte differentiation (Wang et al. 2002; Tsang et al. 1997).

Runt-related transcription factor (RUNX1 or AML1) is essential for definitive hematopoiesis and plays an important role in megakaryocyte differentiation. Germline inactivation of *Runx1* in mice is embryonically lethal due to severe hematopoietic defects. Moreover, hematopoietic-specific inactivation of RUNX1 in adult mice results in abnormal megakaryopoiesis and thrombocytopenia (Ichikawa et al. 2004). Clinically, mutations or inactivation of RUNX1 observed in patients is associated with leukemia, myelodysplastic syndromes, and a familial platelet disorder with a predisposition to acute myeloid leukemia (Daly 2017). An important mechanism by which RUNX1 controls megakaryocyte differentiation is through the downregulation of non-muscle myosin IIB heavy chain (MYH10) that contributes to megakaryocyte polyploidization (Lordier et al. 2012). MYH10 expression in platelets is a biomarker for RUNX1 and FLI1 alterations in patients with platelet disorders and myeloid neoplasms (Antony-Debre et al. 2012).

The basic region leucine zipper transcription factor NF-E2 plays a critical role in platelet formation. NF-E2 is a heterodimer that is comprised of a hematopoietic restricted 45 kDa (p45) subunit and a widely expressed 18 kDa (p18) subunit. Deletion of the p45 subunit in mice leads to absolute thrombocytopenia and mortality from hemorrhage. While NF-E2 inactivation does not affect megakaryocyte proliferation in response to TPO, NF-E2-deficient megakaryocytes fail to form platelets in their cytoplasm (Shivdasani et al. 1995). Moreover, expression of p45 along with Mafg and Mafk is sufficient to convert mouse 3T3 and human dermal fibroblasts into megakaryocytes (Ono et al. 2012).

The ETS family transcription factor, Fli-1, is an important regulator of the late stages of megakaryocyte differentiation. Germline inactivation of Fli-1 in mice results in embryonic lethality associated with an early block in the differentiation of megakaryocytes (Hart et al. 2000). Moreover, germline mutations in FLI1 have been associated with platelet dysfunction, thrombocytopenia, and bleeding disorders in human patients underscoring the importance of FLI-1 in platelet formation (Daly 2017). Functionally, Fli-1 cooperates with GATA-1 for the activation of genes associated with the terminal differentiation of megakaryocytes. Another ETS family transcription factor, PU.1, is important in the development of platelets, whereby PU.1 repression is needed for the normal development of megakaryocyte-erythroid progenitors (DeKoter et al. 2007; Niswander et al. 2014).

1.4.2 Growth Factor Signaling

Megakaryopoiesis and platelet formation occur within the bone marrow microenvironment. Cytokines and other factors within the microenvironment play an important role in megakaryocyte differentiation and platelet formation. In vitro studies have demonstrated that human interleukin-3 (IL-3), interleukin-6 (IL-6), stem cell factor (SCF), and thrombopoietin (TPO) promote megakaryocyte differentiation and proliferation (Guo et al. 2015). Among these factors, TPO is the primary regulator of MK development and platelet formation (Kaushansky et al. 1995). TPO binds to the MPL receptor that is expressed on megakaryocyte progenitor cells to induce proliferation and differentiation (Gurney et al. 1994). TPO is primarily produced by the liver at constitutive levels and is cleared by MPL receptor in platelets (Emmons et al. 1996).

1.4.3 Microenvironment

Within the bone marrow microenvironment, an important role for the vascular niche in the regulation of megakaryocyte maturation and platelet formation has recently been described. MK association with the sinusoidal vasculature promotes proplatelet formation and platelet release into the circulation (Niswander et al. 2014; Junt et al. 2007; Pitchford et al. 2012). Future studies are needed to further explore the cellular and molecular mechanisms controlling platelet formation in the bone marrow microenvironment.

1.5 Monocyte

Monocytes are produced in the bone marrow and circulate in the blood stream and enter tissues where they differentiate into macrophages and dendritic cells. Both macrophages and dendritic cells contribute to host defense, tissue remodeling, and repair (Gordon and Taylor 2005).

1.5.1 Genetic and Epigenetic Regulation

The development of monocytes from pluripotent HSCs occurs through several myeloid progenitors including the common myeloid progenitor (CMP), granulocyte/macrophage precursor (GMP), and a macrophage/DC precursor (MDP). Recently, a DC-restricted progenitor (CDP) and a monocyte/macrophage-restricted progenitor (cMoP) downstream of the MDP have been described. Monopoiesis occurs in the bone marrow through the coordination of transcription factor expression. There are a number of transcription factors that coordinate this process.

The ETS transcription factor PU.1 plays an important role in monocyte differentiation. While PU.1 expression inhibits the differentiation of the granulocyte lineage, PU.1 is required for macrophage and dendritic cell development (Dahl et al. 2003). PU.1 is expressed in early myeloid lineage commitment and activates the expression of monocyte-specific factors including IRF8 and KLF4 to support monocyte differentiation (Schonheit et al. 2013; Feinberg et al. 2007).

The interferon-gamma (IFN-g)-regulated transcription factor, IRF8, plays a key role in monocyte differentiation. While IRF8-deficient mice are viable, these mice accumulate GMP, expand neutrophils, and are deficient in macrophages and dendritic cells (recently reviewed in (Terry and Miller 2014)).

The Kruppel-like factor KLF4 plays an important role in monocyte differentiation. KLF4 is expressed in monocyte-restricted progenitors (Feinberg et al. 2007). Overexpression of KLF4 in HSCs promotes monocyte differentiation, whereas KLF4 knockdown inhibits monocyte differentiation (Feinberg et al. 2007). Furthermore, introduction of KLF4 into PU.1 or IRF8-deficient cells is sufficient to rescue monocyte development (Terry and Miller 2014). In support of this notion, KLF4-deficient mice die within a few days after birth. Transplantation of KLF4-deficient fetal liver cells into lethally irradiated mice resulted in a complete loss of circulating monocytes (Alder et al. 2008). Together these studies suggest that KLF4 is an important downstream factor controlling monocyte development.

The nuclear receptor NR4A1 (Nur77) is a transcription factor that has recently been identified in the differentiation of Ly6C$^-$ monocytes. Ly6C$^-$ monocytes are surveillance monocytes present in the circulation that have recently been implicated in controlling metastasis, monitoring endothelial cells, inflammation, and tissue repair (Terry and Miller 2014). Germline inactivation of NR4A1 resulted in a specific depletion of Ly6C$^-$ monocytes. NR4A1 is important in promoting the survival and differentiation of Ly6C$^-$ monocytes (Hanna et al. 2011).

1.5.2 Growth Factor Signaling

There are a number of cytokines and growth factors that promote monocyte differentiation and regulate macrophage and dendritic cell development. The receptor tyrosine kinase CD115 (CSF-1R) is expressed by early myeloid progenitors and is required for monocyte survival, proliferation, and differentiation. Mice that are deficient for CSF-1R lack most monocyte and macrophage populations (Dai et al. 2002). There are two ligands for CSF-1R, CSF-1, and IL-34. Germline inactivation of these factors results in monocyte and macrophages deficiencies (for recent review (Terry and Miller 2014)). During inflammatory conditions, the cytokines interferon-gamma (IFN-gamma) and type I interferon (IFN-1) promote monocyte development. Flt3 ligand (Flt3L) is an important regulator of dendritic cell development. The Flt3 receptor is expressed by dendritic cells throughout development and is maintained on terminally differentiated macrophages (Satpathy et al. 2012). Loss of Flt3L, Flt3, or its key downstream signaling molecule STAT3 results in dendritic cell depletion in mice (McKenna et al. 2000; Waskow et al. 2008; Laouar et al. 2003).

1.6 Neutrophil

Neutrophils represent 50–75% of the total circulating leukocytes, play an important role in inflammation, and are early responders to pathogens including bacteria, fungi, and viruses. They mediate direct antimicrobial activities through the release of enzymes and toxic factors, the generation of reactive oxygen species, and the release of nuclear material into extracellular traps. In addition, neutrophils regulate adaptive and innate immune responses through the release of cytokines and pattern recognition receptors. Granulocyte differentiation occurs in the bone marrow through a series of developmental stages. The myeloblast is a neutrophil and monocyte progenitor that arises from the common myeloid progenitor. After the myeloblast stage, granulopoiesis promotes the differentiation of neutrophils through the formation of promyelocytes, myelocytes, metamyelocytes, and band cells ultimately leading to polymorphonuclear neutrophils. Neutrophils then exit the bone marrow and undergo terminal maturation in the bloodstream. Neutrophils have a half-life of 4–10 h in circulation and survive in tissues for up to 2 days. Therefore, these cells need to be continuously replenished through the coordinated regulation of growth factor receptor signaling and transcriptional regulation of neutrophil-specific gene programs (for a recent review, see (Ostuni et al. 2016; Barreda et al. 2004)).

1.6.1 Transcription Factors

There are a number of transcription factors that regulate neutrophil development. Early in monocyte/granulocyte lineage commitment, the balance between PU.1 and C/EBPα expression plays an important role in specifying monocyte and neutrophil production. High PU.1 levels favor the development of macrophages and dendritic cells, whereas high levels of C/EBPα promote neutrophil differentiation (for a recent review, see (Ostuni et al. 2016)). Later during terminal neutrophil commitment, the transcription factors C/EBPε, GFI-1, and LEF-1 play important roles in the terminal differentiation of neutrophils.

The CCAAT/enhancer-binding protein-E (C/EBPε) transcription factor promotes the terminal differentiation and maturation of neutrophils. C/EBPε is highly expressed in granulocytes where it is essential for their terminal differentiation. Mice with an inactivating mutation in C/EBPε are viable. However, C/EBPε-deficient mice fail to produce functional neutrophils and eosinophils and succumb to opportunistic infections by 3–5 months of age (Yamanaka et al. 1997). C/EBPε is essential for the expression neutrophil granule proteins including lactoferrin and defensins (Khanna-Gupta et al. 2003; Tsutsumi-Ishii et al. 2000). Interestingly, many of the features observed in in C/EBPε-deficient mice are observed in patients with SGD, a rare autosomal recessive primary immunodeficiency that develops from a neutrophil-specific granule deficiency. Recent studies have identified a variety of mutations within C/EBPε in patients with SGD supporting an important role for C/EBPε in the physiologic and pathophysiologic regulation of neutrophils (Lekstrom-Himes et al. 1999; Gombart et al. 2001; Wada et al. 2015).

The zinc finger transcriptional repressor Gfi-1 plays an essential role in neutrophil differentiation. Genetic inactivation of Gfi-1 in mice results in growth retardation, early lethality, and bacterial infection. Peripheral blood analysis in Gfi-1-deficient mice revealed a specific defect in neutrophils associated with a block in neutrophil differentiation at the myeloblast to promyelocyte transition (Hock et al. 2004). Mechanistically, Gfi-1 is required for the expression of neutrophil-specific genes including MPO, C/EBPε, and elastase (Hock et al. 2004; Person et al. 2003). Clinically, mutations within GFI1 have been found in patients with severe congenital neutropenia (SCN), a rare autosomal recessive disorder characterized by a defect in neutrophil maturation and a risk of life-threatening bacterial and fungal infections (Person et al. 2003).

Another important transcription factor in neutrophil differentiation is the lymphoid enhancer-binding factor (LEF-1). LEF-1 is a transcription factor that is normally expressed in lymphoid cells. However, promoter analysis of ELA2 (protease neutrophil elastase), a gene linked to severe congenital neutropenia, revealed a functional LEF-1 binding site within the ELA2 promoter that cooperates with core-binding factor (CBFalpha) in the activation of ELA2 expression (Li et al. 2004). Clinically, low LEF-1 levels are associated with congenital neutropenia where neutrophils arrest at the promyelocytic stage. Functional studies in early hematopoietic progenitor cells from patients with congenital neutropenia demonstrated that reconstitution of LEF-1 is sufficient to rescue defective myelopoiesis and granulocyte maturation (Skokowa et al. 2006).

1.6.2 Growth Factor Signaling

Neutrophil production is regulated by the expression of granulocyte colony-stimulating factor (G-CSF). G-CSF promotes neutrophil proliferation, differentiation, and survival through the activation of the G-CSF receptor expressed on neutrophilic progenitors and mature neutrophils. During neutrophil maturation, the expression of G-CSFR increases with mature neutrophils expressing 200–1000 receptors per cell. The G-CSF receptor is a member of the type I cytokine receptor superfamily that binds to G-CSF as a homodimer. The extracellular domain contains an immunoglobulin-like (Ig-like) domain, a cytokine receptor homology (CRH) module that is required for G-CSF binding, and three fibronectin type II domains. The cytoplasmic domain contains Box1 and Box2 domains that have homology to other cytokine receptors and a STAT3 binding site. Intracellular signaling downstream of the G-CSF receptor relies upon cytoplasmic enzymes because the G-CSFR does not have an intrinsic tyrosine kinase activity. G-CSF binding to G-CSFR results in homodimerization of the receptor and the formation of a tetrameric complex containing two ligand and two receptor complexes. G-CSFR activation results in the activation of JAK, STAT, Erk, and Src family kinase signaling that mediates the biologic activities associated with G-CSF signaling in neutrophils (for a recent review, see (Barreda et al. 2004)).

1.6.3 Microenvironment

A variety of cells within the microenvironment regulate neutrophil production under homeostatic and stress conditions. Among these cell types, macrophages play an important in the regulation of steady state and stress granulopoiesis. Under homeostatic conditions, apoptotic neutrophils in the periphery and bone marrow are ingested by resident tissue macrophages. This results in the suppression of proinflammatory cytokine production by macrophages and a reduction of G-CSF production by T cells (Stark et al. 2005). Under stress conditions, bacterial lipopolysaccharide (LPS) IL-1, M-CSF, and other factors stimulate macrophages and monocytes to produce G-CSF (for a review, see (Barreda et al. 2004)). In addition to macrophages, dendritic cells regulate neutrophil homeostasis by regulating the recruitment and survival of neutrophils in peripheral tissues. Conditional depletion of dendritic cells results in increased mobilization of neutrophils from the bone marrow to the liver. Increased neutrophils in the liver of dendritic cell depleted mice were associated with the increased expression of neutrophil-mobilizing cytokines and reduced neutrophil apoptosis in the liver (Jiao et al. 2014). Finally, recent studies have highlighted a role for the microbiota in the regulation of neutrophil aging through the activation of Toll-like receptor and myeloid differentiation factor 88-mediated signaling (Zhang et al. 2015).

1.7 Eosinophil

Eosinophils are granulocytic white blood cells that play an important role in innate and adaptive immunity. Eosinophils differentiate in the bone marrow and exit the bone marrow as terminally differentiated cells. Under homeostatic conditions, eosinophils are found at low levels in the blood (<5% of leukocytes) and primarily reside in tissues such as the gut mucosa; there they maintain homeostasis with resident microbiota (Davoine and Lacy 2014). Eosinophils are not capable of proliferating and have high rates of spontaneous apoptosis. It is estimated that their lifespan is 2–5 days within resident tissues. Therefore, the production of eosinophils is a tightly regulated process that is needed to maintain eosinophil levels within tissues while maintaining low levels of these sensitive cells within the blood. Eosinophils develop in the bone marrow over 3–4 days from pluripotent stem cells and granulocyte-monocyte progenitors to an eosinophil lineage-committed progenitor (EoP) (Doyle et al. 2013). There are number of genetic, epigenetic, and microenvironmental factors that control eosinophil differentiation and survival in the bone marrow that will be discussed below.

1.7.1 Genetic

Eosinophil development results from carefully coordinated activation of transcription factors. The transcription factors GATA-1, PU.1, C/

EBPa, C/EBPe, IRF8, and XBP-1 are expressed by eosinophils and are required for their specification and differentiation (Yu et al. 2002; McKercher et al. 1999; Zhang et al. 1997; Tamura et al. 2015; Bettigole et al. 2015). GATA-1 is particularly important in the specification of the eosinophil lineage. Targeted deletion of the high-affinity GATA-1 binding site in the GATA-1 promoter results in eosinophil lineage depletion in mice (Yu et al. 2002). Moreover, a high-affinity double-GATA site is present within the regulatory elements of eosinophil-specific genes including the eotaxin receptor CC chemokine receptor 3 (CCR3), MBP, and the IL-5 receptor alpha (IL-5Rα) genes (Du et al. 2002; Kim et al. 2010; Yamaguchi et al. 1998).

Recent studies have demonstrated a key role for the transcription factor XBP-1 in eosinophil differentiation. XBP-1 is a transcription factor that mediates the cellular response to endoplasmic reticulum (ER) stress by activating the expression of genes that encode proteins that regulate protein folding, maturation, and degradation within the ER (Lee et al. 2003). During differentiation, eosinophils activate the expression of XBP1 to enhance the posttranslational maturation of key granule proteins, which are thought to allow for the progression of the eosinophil transcriptional developmental program (Bettigole et al. 2015).

Eosinophils are unique among granulocytes in that they must safely store a variety of cytotoxic proteins including eosinophil major basic proteins (MBP-1, MBP-2), eosinophil-associated ribonucleases, and eosinophil peroxidase (EPX) (Lee et al. 2012). The survival of eosinophils during differentiation is also dependent upon granule formation. Gene-targeting studies in mice have demonstrated that granule protein expression, specifically MBP-1 and EPX, is required for eosinophilopoiesis suggesting that granule protein expression and/or formation is not a passive consequence of differentiation but also plays an important role in the differentiation process (Doyle et al. 2013).

Studies investigating gene expression and chromatin changes during eosinophil development have been limited, likely because of the rarity of the cell population under homeostatic conditions. A recent study utilized chromatin immunoprecipitation coupled with massively parallel sequencing (ChIP-seq) and RNA sequencing (RNA-seq) to identify transcription factors and genetic regulatory elements that are active during homeostatic eosinophil production in the bone marrow (Bouffi et al. 2015). This study found that genes that are induced eosinophil lineage-committed cells (EoPs) were poised with active chromatin marks in GMPs. In contrast genes that are highly and specifically expressed during eosinophil maturation were not marked with open chromatin at early stages, suggesting that a subset of genes associated with Eos effector functions may be poised for expression early in lineage commitment (Bouffi et al. 2015).

1.7.2 Growth Factor Signaling

There are three cytokines that are important in eosinophil development including IL-5, IL-3, and GM-CSF. IL-5 is particularly important both eosinophil differentiation and release from the bone marrow into the circulation. Overproduction of IL-5 in transgenic mice leads to eosinophilia, whereas IL-5 or the IL-5 receptor α chain (IL-5Rα)-deficient mice fail to develop parasite-induced eosinophilia (Kopf et al. 1996; Tominaga et al. 1991; Dent et al. 1990; Yoshida et al. 1996). Clinically, overproduction of IL-5 is associated with eosinophilia (Agache et al. 2016; Van Gool et al. 2014; Pavord et al. 2012).

Interleukin-5, IL-3, and GM-CSF signal through the common beta-receptor chain (βc) to provide proliferative and differentiation signals to eosinophil progenitors. Mice lacking the common beta-receptor have a reduced number of peripheral eosinophils under homeostatic conditions highlighting the importance of IL-5/IL-3/GM-CSF signaling in eosinophil production (Nishinakamura et al. 1996). The IL-5 receptor complex is comprised of an IL-5 homodimer, two IL-5Ralpha subunits, and one beta-receptor chain (Broughton et al. 2015). IL-5 receptor signaling activates Lyn, Syk, and JAK2 and signals through the Ras-MAPK, JAK-STAT, and PI3K/

AKT pathways to promote eosinophil proliferation, differentiation, and survival (Adachi and Alam 1998).

1.7.3 Microenvironment

The primary cellular source of serum IL-5 during homeostatic conditions is maintained by long-lived type II innate lymphoid cells resident in peripheral tissues (Nussbaum et al. 2013). Within the bone marrow niche, eosinophils are localized with plasma cells. While eosinophils are important in providing plasma cells with survival factors, the role of plasma cells on eosinophil function remains poorly understood (Chu et al. 2011).

1.8 Basophil and Mast Cells

Basophils and mast cells are granulocytes that play an important role in mediating allergy and parasite immune responses. Both cell types express high-affinity immunoglobulin E (IgE) receptors on their cell surface that leads to the release of cytokines and chemical mediators upon antigen stimulation. Basophils and mast cells develop in the bone marrow from common myeloid progenitors (CMP) and granulocyte-monocyte progenitors (CMP). Current models suggest that bipotential granulocyte progenitors differentiate into pre-basophil and mast cell progenitors (pre-BMPs) and then to basophil or mast cell progenitors. While basophil maturation occurs in the bone marrow, mast maturation occurs primarily within peripheral tissues. Basophil and mast cell differentiation utilizes cues from the microenvironment to coordinate transcription factor gene expression that is necessary for lineage differentiation (for a recent review, see (Sasaki et al. 2016)).

1.8.1 Transcription Factors

There are multiple transcription factors that coordinate basophil and mast cell differentiation in the bone marrow including IRF8, C/EBPa, GATA2, microphthalmia-associated transcription factor MITF, STAT5, and RUNX1.

The interferon regulatory factor-8 (IRF-8) is a transcription factor required for the development of several myeloid lineages described above. Recent studies have identified an important role for IRF-8 in the differentiation of basophil and mast cells. Irf8 inactivation in mice led to a severe defect in peripheral basophil counts that was associated with a block in GMP to pre-BMP differentiation in the bone marrow. While tissue resident mast cells were maintained in Irf8-deficient mice, GMP cells from these mice failed to differentiate into mast cells suggesting an important role for Irf8 in mast cell and basophil production in vivo (Sasaki et al. 2015). Future studies are needed to elucidate the mechanisms by which IRF8 controls mast and basophil differentiation.

Recent studies have demonstrated that the coordinate regulation of STAT5, C/EBPa, and MITF controls the differentiation and specification of basophil and mast cell progenitors in the bone marrow. The transcription factor C/EBPa plays an important role in promoting the differentiation of pre-BMPs into basophils. Cebpa mRNA is upregulated during the GMP to pre-BMP transition through STAT5, an essential signaling molecule for basophils and mast cells as conditional inactivation of Cebpa in adult mice resulted in a block in pre-BMP development in the bone marrow (Sasaki et al. 2016; Qi et al. 2013). At the molecular level, C/EBPa promotes basophil differentiation and identity by actively repressing genes that are highly expressed within the mast cell lineage. In particular, C/EBPa directly binds to and suppresses the activation of Mitf, a transcription factor that is required for mast cell differentiation in vivo (Sasaki et al. 2016; Qi et al. 2013).

As described above, GATA2 is an important factor in the early stages of hematopoiesis. Recent studies have revealed an important role for GATA2 in mast cell and basophil differentiation. Gene expression profiling of factors that are highly expressed in the GMP to pre-BMP transition identified GATA2 as a factor highly expressed in pre-BMPs. Conditional inactivation of GATA2 in pre-BMPs leads to a block in pre-BMP differentiation to mast and basophils demonstrating as essential for this factor in mast cell and basophil differentiation. At the molecular level, GATA2 is important in maintaining the expression of genes that control basophil and mast cell function and histamine synthesis. Interestingly, STAT5 which signals downstream of IL-3 and other growth factors activate GATA2 expression in pre-BMP cells (Li et al. 2015).

RUNX1 is a key transcription factor in the regulation of early hematopoiesis (see discussion above). Runx1 has two promoters, a distal (P1) and proximal (P2) promoter that can be differentially regulated during development. The functional role of Runx1 variants during hematopoiesis remains poorly understood. However, recent studies have shown that P1-Runx1-deficient mice have a severe reduction of bone marrow, blood, and spleen basophils, while other granulocyte lineages, including mast cells, were not affected. Future studies are needed to further elucidate the mechanisms by which P1-Runx1 controls basophil differentiation in the bone marrow.

1.8.2 Growth Factor Signaling

The cytokines IL-3, GM-CSF, SCF, and thymic stromal lymphopoietin (TSLP) activate STAT5 signaling to promote basophil and mast cell proliferation, activation, and cytokine secretion (Voehringer 2012). In vitro, SCF and IL-3 are sufficient to stimulate mouse bone marrow production of basophils and mast cells (Metcalf et al. 2013). SCF is required for the production of mature mast cells in vivo (Alexander et al. 1991).

Overproduction of IL-3 during parasite infection is associated with basophilia and mastocytosis (Voehringer 2012; Lantz et al. 1998). IL-3 signals through the IL-3 receptor that is comprised of an IL-3 receptor alpha chain and a common beta chain. IL-3R signaling promotes mast and basophil proliferation, survival, and activation through JAK2/STAT5 signaling.

Overproduction of TSLP results in IL-3 independent basophilia in response to allergy (Siracusa et al. 2011). TSLP signals through a heterodimeric receptor comprised of the IL-7 receptor alpha chain and the TSLP receptor. Downstream signaling from the TSLPR/IL-7Ralpha complex leads to the activation of pSTAT5 through mechanisms that remain unclear (Voehringer 2012).

1.9 B Cell

B cells are antibody-producing cells that mediate protection from pathogens. B lymphocytes are continuously produced throughout life although infection and age significantly influence the numbers produced. In the bone marrow, B cells develop through a series of stages based on the rearrangement status of the immunoglobulin heavy-chain locus, the expression of stage-specific surface markers, and growth factor dependence where HSCs and CLPs lead to the development of the pre-pro-B cell, pro-B cell, large pre-B cell, small pre-B cell, and immature B cell that exits the bone marrow to continue maturation in the blood and spleen (De Obaldia and Bhandoola 2015).

1.9.1 Genetic

Among these factors, five transcription factors play a well-established role in B-lineage differentiation including PU.1, Ikaros, E2A/E47, Ebf1, and Pax5. PU.1, Ikaros, and E2A/E47 are expressed in early progenitor cells and are involved in multilineage determination, whereas Ebf1 and Pax5 are important in B-lineage progenitors (Yokota et al. 2013).

As described above, PU.1 is important in the regulation of myeloid fate. PU.1 expression is also important in the regulation of T and B cell differentiation as PU.1-deficient mice die during fetal development and lack B, T, and myeloid progenitors. PU.1-deficient progenitors fail to proliferate and differentiate into pro-B cells in response to stromal cell contact and IL-7 (Scott et al. 1997). At the molecular level, PU.1 is essential for the expression of the IL-7 receptor alpha chain, an essential component of IL-7 signaling, that drives B cell progenitor proliferation and survival (DeKoter et al. 2002).

The Ik3f1 transcription factor, which encodes IKAROS, plays an important role in B cell differentiation. Conditional inactivation of Ik3f1 in pro-B cells lead to an arrest in B cell development (Heizmann et al. 2013; Schwickert et al. 2014). Ikaros regulates the expression of genes important in B cell survival, metabolism, cell signaling, and function (Schwickert et al. 2014).

The early B cell factor (EBF-1) is an atypical helix-loop-helix transcription factor that is exclusively expressed by cells within the B cell lineage (Hagman et al. 1993). Targeted inactivation of EBF-1 leads to a block in B cell development (Lin and Grosschedl 1995). EBF works together with E2A, another helix-loop-helix transcription factor required for early B cell development, to activate the transcription of early B-lineage genes (O'Riordan and Grosschedl 1999; Zhuang et al. 1994).

The pax family transcription factor Pax5 plays an essential role in early B-lymphoid development. Pax5 is exclusively expressed within the B cell lineage within the hematopoietic system where it is required for B-lymphopoiesis at the pro-B cell stage (Nutt et al. 1999).

1.9.2 Growth Factor Signaling

Interleukin-7 (IL-7) is a key factor for the proliferation and survival of B cells during B-lymphopoiesis. IL-7 signals through the IL-7 receptor (IL-7R) that is comprised of the IL-7Ralpha chain and the common gamma chain. Inactivation of IL-7 or IL-7Ra blocks B-lymphopoiesis in the adult bone marrow (Peschon et al. 1994; Clark et al. 2014). IL-7R signaling promotes B cell development through the activation of JAK3/STAT5 signaling. While the IL-7Ra and common gamma chain do not have intrinsic kinase activity, the common gamma chain is constitutively associated with JAK3. IL-7 binding to the receptor complex results in the phosphorylation of JAK3 and tyrosine residue Y449 on the IL-7Ra chain that leads to the recruitment of STAT5A and STAT5B (Clark et al. 2014). STAT5 is a critical effector of IL-7 signaling in B-lymphopoiesis as inactivation of Stat5a and Stat5b arrests B-lymphocyte development at the pre-pro-B cell stage, whereas constitutive STAT5 activation is sufficient to rescue B cell development in IL-7Ra-deficient mice (Yao et al. 2006; Goetz et al. 2004). The Tec family cytoplasmic protein tyrosine kinase, Bruton's tyrosine kinase (BTK), is an important regulator of B cell differentiation and controls IL-7 responsiveness in pro-B and pre-B cells (Middendorp et al. 2002; Christie et al. 2015).

1.9.3 Microenvironment

There are multiple niches in the bone marrow microenvironment that contribute to the proliferation and survival of B lymphocytes cells (Tokoyoda et al. 2004). First, the CXCR4 receptor expressed on B cell progenitors plays an important role in controlling B cell lineage motility and retention in the bone marrow (Beck et al. 2014). CXCL12, the ligand for CXCR4, is a potent chemoattractant and is expressed by stromal cells, osteoblasts, endothelial cells, and perivascular cells in the bone marrow (Ding and Morrison 2013). Osteoblastic CXCL12 is particularly important in the retention of lymphoid progenitors in the bone marrow (Ding and Morrison 2013).

Osteoblasts are also an important source of IL-7 during B-lymphopoiesis. Conditional inactivation of Gsa, a critical component of PTH/PPR signaling in osteoblasts, leads to severe osteoporosis and impaired B-lymphopoiesis in mice. IL-7 mRNA levels in osteoblasts of Gsa-deficient mice were significantly decreased, and exogenous treatment of IL-7 was sufficient to rescue to the B-lymphopoiesis defect in Gsa-deficient mice (Wu et al. 2008).

1.10 T Cell

T cells promote cell-mediated immune responses that are antigen specific. Among the hematopoietic lineages, T cells are unique in that uncommitted lymphoid progenitors migrate to the thymus where they undergo T cell maturation in response to ligands that activate the Notch signaling pathway (for a recent review on thymic T cell development, see (De Obaldia and Bhandoola 2015)). The early phases of lymphoid development in the bone marrow are similar for B and T cells. Similar to B cell precursors, T cell precursors arise from HSCs and CLPs. As described above, the generation and retention of CLPs in the bone marrow are dependent upon IL-7, kit ligand, Flt3 ligand, and CXCL12/CXCR4 signaling. Additionally, the transcription factors Ikaros, Bcl11a, E2A, Pu.1, Myb, Gfi1, STAT5, Hoxa9, and Miz-1 contribute to the production of lymphoid precursors in the bone marrow (for a recent review, see (Rothenberg 2014)).

Notch1 is particularly important for T cell fate specification. In the absence of Notch1, bone marrow progenitors enter the thymus and develop into B cells (Wilson et al. 2001). In contrast, Notch1-IC domain or DLL4 expression in bone marrow progenitors results in ectopic T cell development in the bone marrow that is associated with a block in B cell development. Together these studies demonstrate that Notch1 plays an important role in determining T-lymphoid versus B-lymphoid lineage decisions. Recent studies have revealed that osteocalcin (Ocn)-positive bone-producing cells produce the Notch ligand DLL4 to promote the production of thymus-seeding progenitors under homeostatic conditions (Yu et al. 2015). Moreover, conditional deletion of DLL4 in Ocn-positive cells within the bone marrow resulted in impaired T-lymphopoiesis, suggesting that Ocn-positive cells in the bone marrow may promote T cell production and thymus seeding through the production of DLL4 (Yu et al. 2015). These findings suggest that Notch1 is important in both bone marrow and thymic regulation of T cell development.

1.11 Natural Killer Cells and Innate Lymphoid Cells

Natural killer cells are innate lymphoid cells that are important in controlling virally infected as well as tumor cells. Recent studies have demonstrated that NK cells have features of adaptive immunity as well through their antigen specificity and ability to mount long-livered memory responses. They primarily function through the rapid release of inflammatory cytokines such as interferon-gamma and can directly kill infected cells through the secretion of lytic granules. Within the bone marrow, NK differentiate and mature through a series of stages. NK are derived from a common lymphoid progenitor cell that develops into an NK cell precursor (NKP) and immature NK cells (iNK). As they mature in the bone marrow (marked by the expression of CD11b, CD43, Ly49, CD49b), they gain functional competence in cytotoxicity and interferon-gamma expression and egress from the bone marrow (for a recent review, see (Geiger and Sun 2016)).

It has also recently been recognized that NK cells are the founding members of innate lymphoid cells (ILCs) that play an important role in mediating tissue repair, host defense, and metabolic homeostasis. ILCs are categorized into three groups based on the transcription factors that activate their functions and the cytokines they produce. Studies are ongoing to define the molecular basis for lineage restriction within the ILC groups. For a recent review on this rapidly expanding area of research, see (Zook and Kee 2016).

1.11.1 Transcription Factors

NK development and maturation requires the coordinated expression of multiple lineage-specific transcription factors. A complex network of transcription factors promotes the differentiation and maturation of NKs cells including Nfil3, PU.1, Id2, Tox, Eomes, and T-bet.

The basic leucine zipper transcription factor nuclear factor interleukin-3 regulated (Nfil3) is critical for NK cell lineage commitment at the CLP stage. Both NK cells and ILCs require Nfil3 for their development (Geiger and Sun 2016). While NFIL3 is highly expressed in CLP cells, germline inactivation of Nfil3 resulted in a specific loss of NK cells, whereas B cells and T cells were not affected (Gascoyne et al. 2009; Kamizono et al. 2009). To determine if Nfil3 is required throughout NK cell differentiation, Firth et al. specifically inactivated Nfil3 in immature

NK cells. NK-lineage maintenance or homeostasis was not affected in these mice indicating that Nfil3 is particularly important for in the early stages of NK cell commitment (Firth et al. 2013). Mechanistically, Nfil3 directly regulates the expression of downstream transcription factors Eomes and Id2 to promote the early stages of NK cell commitment (Male et al. 2014).

The inhibitor of DNA-binding protein-2 ID2 plays a critical role in the development of NK cells. Both NK and ILCs require Id2 for their development. Id2-deficient mice have a defect in peripheral NK cells that is associated with an arrest at the iNK stage (Yokota et al. 1999; Boos et al. 2007). Moreover, conditional inactivation of Id2 from HSCs or NK cells resulted in a rapid loss of NK cells from the periphery. The canonical role for Id2 is to dimerize with E-proteins and prevent E-protein transcription factors from binding to E-box sequences in target genes. In mature NK cells, Id2 is important to suppress the expression of E-box targets including Socs3, Cxcr5, and Il-10, which compromise interleukin-15 (IL-15) signaling (Delconte et al. 2016).

The Ets family transcription factors PU.1, Ets-1, and Mef are important in NK cell maturation. PU.1 is expressed early in the CLP cells and is important in the differentiation of NKP cells. Chimeric PU.1-deficient mice have reduced numbers of both NKP and immature NK cells. Ets-1 appears to be important at a later stage of NK cell development as peripheral NK cells are significantly decreased in Ets-1-deficient mice and are associated with an arrest at the NKP-cell stage. Ets-1 controls NK cell maturation at least in part through the regulation of other NK cell transcription factors Id2 and T-bet (Boos et al. 2007; Townsend et al. 2004). Finally, Mef controls both NK cell numbers and function. Mef-deficient mice have a significant reduction in NK cells as well as reduced cell cytotoxicity ability and IFN-gamma secretion (Lacorazza et al. 2002). Together these findings highlight the role of Ets family members in the regulation of NK cell differentiation and maturation.

The thymocyte selection-associated HMG-box factor Tox plays an important role in NK cell maturation. Mice that are deficient for Tox have a specific defect in mature NK cells as immature NK cells are not affected in these mice (Aliahmad et al. 2010).

The T-box transcription factors eomesodermin (Eomes) and T-box expressed in T cells (T-bet) are required for NK cell development and maturation. T-bet-deficient mice fail to develop mature NK cells and have decreased numbers in peripheral lymphoid organs (Townsend et al. 2004). At the molecular level, T-bet regulated the expression of cytolytic effector molecules including perforin and granzyme B (Townsend et al. 2004). Eomes is required to maintain a differentiated NK cell state as deletion of Eomes from mature NK cells caused a reversion to an immature state (Gordon et al. 2012).

1.11.2 Growth Factor Signaling

NK cells are dependent upon the interleukin-15 (IL-15) for their proliferation, survival, and activation (Geiger and Sun 2016). IL-15 signals through the common gamma chain and IL-2RB receptor complex to activate JAK3/STAT5 signaling (Mishra et al. 2014). Inactivation of IL-15, JAK3, or STAT5 in mice leads to defective lymphoid development highlighting the importance of this pathway in the homeostatic regulation of NK cell specification (Eckelhart et al. 2011; Imada et al. 1998; Kennedy et al. 2000; Nosaka et al. 1995). IL-15 signaling promotes NK survival through the regulation of antiapoptotic genes such as MCL1 and the repression of pro-apoptotic BIM and NOXA gene expression (Huntington et al. 2007).

References

Adachi T, Alam R (1998) The mechanism of IL-5 signal transduction. Am J Physiol 275(3 Pt 1): C623–C633

Agache I, Strasser DS, Klenk A, Agache C, Farine H, Ciobanu C et al (2016) Serum IL-5 and IL-13 consistently serve as the best predictors for the blood eosinophilia phenotype in adult asthmatics. Allergy 71(8):1192–1202

Alder JK, Georgantas RW III, Hildreth RL, Kaplan IM, Morisot S, Yu X et al (2008) Kruppel-like factor 4 is essential for inflammatory monocyte differentiation in vivo. J Immunol 180(8):5645–5652

Alexander WS, Lyman SD, Wagner EF (1991) Expression of functional c-kit receptors rescues the genetic defect of W mutant mast cells. EMBO J 10(12): 3683–3691

Aliahmad P, de la Torre B, Kaye J (2010) Shared dependence on the DNA-binding factor TOX for the development of lymphoid tissue-inducer cell and NK cell lineages. Nat Immunol 11(10):945–952

Antony-Debre I, Bluteau D, Itzykson R, Baccini V, Renneville A, Boehlen F et al (2012) MYH10 protein expression in platelets as a biomarker of RUNX1 and FLI1 alterations. Blood 120(13):2719–2722

Barreda DR, Hanington PC, Belosevic M (2004) Regulation of myeloid development and function by colony stimulating factors. Dev Comp Immunol 28(5):509–554

Beck TC, Gomes AC, Cyster JG, Pereira JP (2014) CXCR4 and a cell-extrinsic mechanism control immature B lymphocyte egress from bone marrow. J Exp Med 211(13):2567–2581

Bettigole SE, Lis R, Adoro S, Lee AH, Spencer LA, Weller PF et al (2015) The transcription factor XBP1 is selectively required for eosinophil differentiation. Nat Immunol 16(8):829–837

Boos MD, Yokota Y, Eberl G, Kee BL (2007) Mature natural killer cell and lymphoid tissue-inducing cell development requires Id2-mediated suppression of E protein activity. J Exp Med 204(5):1119–1130

Bouffi C, Kartashov AV, Schollaert KL, Chen X, Bacon WC, Weirauch MT et al (2015) Transcription Factor Repertoire of Homeostatic Eosinophilopoiesis. J Immunol 195(6):2683–2695

Broughton SE, Nero TL, Dhagat U, Kan WL, Hercus TR, Tvorogov D et al (2015) The betac receptor family - structural insights and their functional implications. Cytokine 74(2):247–258

Calvi LM, Adams GB, Weibrecht KW, Weber JM, Olson DP, Knight MC et al (2003) Osteoblastic cells regulate the haematopoietic stem cell niche. Nature 425(6960):841–846

Chow A, Huggins M, Ahmed J, Hashimoto D, Lucas D, Kunisaki Y et al (2013) CD169(+) macrophages provide a niche promoting erythropoiesis under homeostasis and stress. Nat Med 19(4):429–436

Christie DA, Xu LS, Turkistany SA, Solomon LA, Li SK, Yim E et al (2015) PU.1 opposes IL-7-dependent proliferation of developing B cells with involvement of the direct target gene bruton tyrosine kinase. J Immunol 194(2):595–605

Chu VT, Frohlich A, Steinhauser G, Scheel T, Roch T, Fillatreau S et al (2011) Eosinophils are required for the maintenance of plasma cells in the bone marrow. Nat Immunol 12(2):151–159

Clark MR, Mandal M, Ochiai K, Singh H (2014) Orchestrating B cell lymphopoiesis through interplay of IL-7 receptor and pre-B cell receptor signalling. Nat Rev Immunol 14(2):69–80

Cullen SM, Mayle A, Rossi L, Goodell MA (2014) Hematopoietic stem cell development: an epigenetic journey. Curr Top Dev Biol 107:39–75

Dahl R, Walsh JC, Lancki D, Laslo P, Iyer SR, Singh H et al (2003) Regulation of macrophage and neutrophil cell fates by the PU.1:C/EBPalpha ratio and granulocyte colony-stimulating factor. Nat Immunol 4(10):1029–1036

Dai XM, Ryan GR, Hapel AJ, Dominguez MG, Russell RG, Kapp S et al (2002) Targeted disruption of the mouse colony-stimulating factor 1 receptor gene results in osteopetrosis, mononuclear phagocyte deficiency, increased primitive progenitor cell frequencies, and reproductive defects. Blood 99(1):111–120

Daly ME (2017) Transcription factor defects causing platelet disorders. Blood Rev 31:1

Davoine F, Lacy P (2014) Eosinophil cytokines, chemokines, and growth factors: emerging roles in immunity. Front Immunol 5:570

De Obaldia ME, Bhandoola A (2015) Transcriptional regulation of innate and adaptive lymphocyte lineages. Annu Rev Immunol 33:607–642

DeKoter RP, Lee HJ, Singh H (2002) PU.1 regulates expression of the interleukin-7 receptor in lymphoid progenitors. Immunity 16(2):297–309

DeKoter RP, Kamath MB, Houston IB (2007) Analysis of concentration-dependent functions of PU.1 in hematopoiesis using mouse models. Blood Cells Mol Dis 39(3):316–320

Delconte RB, Shi W, Sathe P, Ushiki T, Seillet C, Minnich M et al (2016) The helix-loop-helix protein ID2 governs NK cell fate by tuning their sensitivity to interleukin-15. Immunity 44(1):103–115

Dent LA, Strath M, Mellor AL, Sanderson CJ (1990) Eosinophilia in transgenic mice expressing interleukin 5. J Exp Med 172(5):1425–1431

Ding L, Morrison SJ (2013) Haematopoietic stem cells and early lymphoid progenitors occupy distinct bone marrow niches. Nature 495(7440):231–235

Doulatov S, Notta F, Laurenti E, Dick JE (2012) Hematopoiesis: a human perspective. Cell Stem Cell 10(2):120–136

Doyle AD, Jacobsen EA, Ochkur SI, McGarry MP, Shim KG, Nguyen DT et al (2013) Expression of the secondary granule proteins major basic protein 1 (MBP-1) and eosinophil peroxidase (EPX) is required for eosinophilopoiesis in mice. Blood 122(5):781–790

Du J, Stankiewicz MJ, Liu Y, Xi Q, Schmitz JE, Lekstrom-Himes JA et al (2002) Novel combinatorial interactions of GATA-1, PU.1, and C/EBPepsilon isoforms regulate transcription of the gene encoding eosinophil granule major basic protein. J Biol Chem 277(45):43481–43494

Ebert BL, Bunn HF (1999) Regulation of the erythropoietin gene. Blood 94(6):1864–1877

Eckelhart E, Warsch W, Zebedin E, Simma O, Stoiber D, Kolbe T et al (2011) A novel Ncr1-Cre mouse reveals the essential role of STAT5 for NK-cell survival and development. Blood 117(5):1565–1573

Emmons RV, Reid DM, Cohen RL, Meng G, Young NS, Dunbar CE et al (1996) Human thrombopoietin levels are high when thrombocytopenia is due to megakaryocyte deficiency and low when due to increased platelet destruction. Blood 87(10):4068–4071

Feinberg MW, Wara AK, Cao Z, Lebedeva MA, Rosenbauer F, Iwasaki H et al (2007) The Kruppel-like factor KLF4 is a critical regulator of monocyte differentiation. EMBO J 26(18):4138–4148

Firth MA, Madera S, Beaulieu AM, Gasteiger G, Castillo EF, Schluns KS et al (2013) Nfil3-independent lineage maintenance and antiviral response of natural killer cells. J Exp Med 210(13):2981–2990

Fujimaki S, Harigae H, Sugawara T, Takasawa N, Sasaki T, Kaku M (2001) Decreased expression of transcription factor GATA-2 in haematopoietic stem cells in patients with aplastic anaemia. Br J Haematol 113(1):52–57

Gascoyne DM, Long E, Veiga-Fernandes H, de Boer J, Williams O, Seddon B et al (2009) The basic leucine zipper transcription factor E4BP4 is essential for natural killer cell development. Nat Immunol 10(10):1118–1124

Geiger TL, Sun JC (2016) Development and maturation of natural killer cells. Curr Opin Immunol 39:82–89

Giger KM, Kalfa TA (2015) Phylogenetic and ontogenetic view of erythroblastic islands. Biomed Res Int 2015:873628

Goetz CA, Harmon IR, O'Neil JJ, Burchill MA, Farrar MA (2004) STAT5 activation underlies IL7 receptor-dependent B cell development. J Immunol 172(8):4770–4778

Gombart AF, Shiohara M, Kwok SH, Agematsu K, Komiyama A, Koeffler HP (2001) Neutrophil-specific granule deficiency: homozygous recessive inheritance of a frameshift mutation in the gene encoding transcription factor CCAAT/enhancer binding protein--epsilon. Blood 97(9):2561–2567

Gordon S, Taylor PR (2005) Monocyte and macrophage heterogeneity. Nat Rev Immunol 5(12):953–964

Gordon SM, Chaix J, Rupp LJ, Wu J, Madera S, Sun JC et al (2012) The transcription factors T-bet and Eomes control key checkpoints of natural killer cell maturation. Immunity 36(1):55–67

Guo T, Wang X, Qu Y, Yin Y, Jing T, Zhang Q (2015) Megakaryopoiesis and platelet production: insight into hematopoietic stem cell proliferation and differentiation. Stem Cell Investig 2:3

Gurney AL, Carver-Moore K, de Sauvage FJ, Moore MW (1994) Thrombocytopenia in c-mpl-deficient mice. Science 265(5177):1445–1447

Hadland BK, Huppert SS, Kanungo J, Xue Y, Jiang R, Gridley T et al (2004) A requirement for Notch1 distinguishes 2 phases of definitive hematopoiesis during development. Blood 104(10):3097–3105

Hagman J, Belanger C, Travis A, Turck CW, Grosschedl R (1993) Cloning and functional characterization of early B-cell factor, a regulator of lymphocyte-specific gene expression. Genes Dev 7(5):760–773

Hanna RN, Carlin LM, Hubbeling HG, Nackiewicz D, Green AM, Punt JA et al (2011) The transcription factor NR4A1 (Nur77) controls bone marrow differentiation and the survival of Ly6C- monocytes. Nat Immunol 12(8):778–785

Hart A, Melet F, Grossfeld P, Chien K, Jones C, Tunnacliffe A et al (2000) Fli-1 is required for murine vascular and megakaryocytic development and is hemizygously deleted in patients with thrombocytopenia. Immunity 13(2):167–177

Heizmann B, Kastner P, Chan S (2013) Ikaros is absolutely required for pre-B cell differentiation by attenuating IL-7 signals. J Exp Med 210(13):2823–2832

Hock H, Hamblen MJ, Rooke HM, Schindler JW, Saleque S, Fujiwara Y et al (2004) Gfi-1 restricts proliferation and preserves functional integrity of haematopoietic stem cells. Nature 431(7011):1002–1007

Huang HT, Kathrein KL, Barton A, Gitlin Z, Huang YH, Ward TP et al (2013) A network of epigenetic regulators guides developmental haematopoiesis in vivo. Nat Cell Biol 15(12):1516–1525

Huntington ND, Puthalakath H, Gunn P, Naik E, Michalak EM, Smyth MJ et al (2007) Interleukin 15-mediated survival of natural killer cells is determined by interactions among Bim, Noxa and Mcl-1. Nat Immunol 8(8):856–863

Ichikawa M, Asai T, Saito T, Seo S, Yamazaki I, Yamagata T et al (2004) AML-1 is required for megakaryocytic maturation and lymphocytic differentiation, but not for maintenance of hematopoietic stem cells in adult hematopoiesis. Nat Med 10(3):299–304

Imada K, Bloom ET, Nakajima H, Horvath-Arcidiacono JA, Udy GB, Davey HW et al (1998) Stat5b is essential for natural killer cell-mediated proliferation and cytolytic activity. J Exp Med 188(11): 2067–2074

Jiao J, Dragomir AC, Kocabayoglu P, Rahman AH, Chow A, Hashimoto D et al (2014) Central role of conventional dendritic cells in regulation of bone marrow release and survival of neutrophils. J Immunol 192(7):3374–3382

Junt T, Schulze H, Chen Z, Massberg S, Goerge T, Krueger A et al (2007) Dynamic visualization of thrombopoiesis within bone marrow. Science 317(5845):1767–1770

Kamizono S, Duncan GS, Seidel MG, Morimoto A, Hamada K, Grosveld G et al (2009) Nfil3/E4bp4 is required for the development and maturation of NK cells in vivo. J Exp Med 206(13):2977–2986

Kaushansky K (2008) Historical review: megakaryopoiesis and thrombopoiesis. Blood 111(3):981–986

Kaushansky K, Broudy VC, Lin N, Jorgensen MJ, McCarty J, Fox N et al (1995) Thrombopoietin, the Mpl ligand, is essential for full megakaryocyte development. Proc Natl Acad Sci U S A 92(8):3234–3238

Kennedy MK, Glaccum M, Brown SN, Butz EA, Viney JL, Embers M et al (2000) Reversible defects in natural killer and memory CD8 T cell lineages in interleukin 15-deficient mice. J Exp Med 191(5):771–780

Khanna-Gupta A, Zibello T, Sun H, Gaines P, Berliner N (2003) Chromatin immunoprecipitation (ChIP) studies indicate a role for CCAAT enhancer binding proteins alpha and epsilon (C/EBP alpha and C/EBP epsilon) and CDP/cut in myeloid maturation-induced lactoferrin gene expression. Blood 101(9):3460–3468

Kim BS, Uhm TG, Lee SK, Lee SH, Kang JH, Park CS et al (2010) The crucial role of GATA-1 in CCR3 gene transcription: modulated balance by multiple GATA elements in the CCR3 regulatory region. J Immunol 185(11):6866–6875

Knudsen KJ, Rehn M, Hasemann MS, Rapin N, Bagger FO, Ohlsson E et al (2015) ERG promotes the maintenance of hematopoietic stem cells by restricting their differentiation. Genes Dev 29(18):1915–1929

Kopf M, Brombacher F, Hodgkin PD, Ramsay AJ, Milbourne EA, Dai WJ et al (1996) IL-5-deficient mice have a developmental defect in CD5+ B-1 cells and lack eosinophilia but have normal antibody and cytotoxic T cell responses. Immunity 4(1):15–24

Korolnek T, Hamza I (2015) Macrophages and iron trafficking at the birth and death of red cells. Blood 125(19):2893–2897

Kosan C, Godmann M (2016) Genetic and epigenetic mechanisms that maintain hematopoietic stem cell function. Stem Cells Int 2016:5178965

Lacorazza HD, Miyazaki Y, Di Cristofano A, Deblasio A, Hedvat C, Zhang J et al (2002) The ETS protein MEF plays a critical role in perforin gene expression and the development of natural killer and NK-T cells. Immunity 17(4):437–449

Lantz CS, Boesiger J, Song CH, Mach N, Kobayashi T, Mulligan RC et al (1998) Role for interleukin-3 in mast-cell and basophil development and in immunity to parasites. Nature 392(6671):90–93

Laouar Y, Welte T, Fu XY, Flavell RA (2003) STAT3 is required for Flt3L-dependent dendritic cell differentiation. Immunity 19(6):903–912

Laurenti E, Varnum-Finney B, Wilson A, Ferrero I, Blanco-Bose WE, Ehninger A et al (2008) Hematopoietic stem cell function and survival depend on c-Myc and N-Myc activity. Cell Stem Cell 3(6):611–624

Lee AH, Iwakoshi NN, Glimcher LH (2003) XBP-1 regulates a subset of endoplasmic reticulum resident chaperone genes in the unfolded protein response. Mol Cell Biol 23(21):7448–7459

Lee JJ, Jacobsen EA, Ochkur SI, McGarry MP, Condjella RM, Doyle AD et al (2012) Human versus mouse eosinophils: "that which we call an eosinophil, by any other name would stain as red". J Allergy Clin Immunol 130(3):572–584

Lekstrom-Himes JA, Dorman SE, Kopar P, Holland SM, Gallin JI (1999) Neutrophil-specific granule deficiency results from a novel mutation with loss of function of the transcription factor CCAAT/enhancer binding protein epsilon. J Exp Med 189(11):1847–1852

Levine RL, Wadleigh M, Cools J, Ebert BL, Wernig G, Huntly BJ et al (2005) Activating mutation in the tyrosine kinase JAK2 in polycythemia vera, essential thrombocythemia, and myeloid metaplasia with myelofibrosis. Cancer Cell 7(4):387–397

Li FQ, Person RE, Takemaru K, Williams K, Meade-White K, Ozsahin AH et al (2004) Lymphoid enhancer factor-1 links two hereditary leukemia syndromes through core-binding factor alpha regulation of ELA2. J Biol Chem 279(4):2873–2884

Li Y, Qi X, Liu B, Huang H (2015) The STAT5-GATA2 pathway is critical in basophil and mast cell differentiation and maintenance. J Immunol 194(9):4328–4338

Lin H, Grosschedl R (1995) Failure of B-cell differentiation in mice lacking the transcription factor EBF. Nature 376(6537):263–267

Lordier L, Bluteau D, Jalil A, Legrand C, Pan J, Rameau P et al (2012) RUNX1-induced silencing of non-muscle myosin heavy chain IIB contributes to megakaryocyte polyploidization. Nat Commun 3:717

Male V, Nisoli I, Kostrzewski T, Allan DS, Carlyle JR, Lord GM et al (2014) The transcription factor E4bp4/Nfil3 controls commitment to the NK lineage and directly regulates Eomes and Id2 expression. J Exp Med 211(4):635–642

McKenna HJ, Stocking KL, Miller RE, Brasel K, De Smedt T, Maraskovsky E et al (2000) Mice lacking flt3 ligand have deficient hematopoiesis affecting hematopoietic progenitor cells, dendritic cells, and natural killer cells. Blood 95(11):3489–3497

McKercher SR, Henkel GW, Maki RA (1999) The transcription factor PU.1 does not regulate lineage commitment but has lineage-specific effects. J Leukoc Biol 66(5):727–732

Metcalf D, Ng AP, Baldwin TM, Di Rago L, Mifsud S (2013) Concordant mast cell and basophil production by individual hematopoietic blast colony-forming cells. Proc Natl Acad Sci U S A 110(22):9031–9035

Middendorp S, Dingjan GM, Hendriks RW (2002) Impaired precursor B cell differentiation in Bruton's tyrosine kinase-deficient mice. J Immunol 168(6):2695–2703

Mishra A, Sullivan L, Caligiuri MA (2014) Molecular pathways: interleukin-15 signaling in health and in cancer. Clin Cancer Res 20(8):2044–2050

Morrison SJ, Scadden DT (2014) The bone marrow niche for haematopoietic stem cells. Nature 505(7483):327–334

Neubauer H, Cumano A, Muller M, Wu H, Huffstadt U, Pfeffer K (1998) Jak2 deficiency defines an essential developmental checkpoint in definitive hematopoiesis. Cell 93(3):397–409

Nishinakamura R, Miyajima A, Mee PJ, Tybulewicz VL, Murray R (1996) Hematopoiesis in mice lacking the entire granulocyte-macrophage colony-stimulating factor/interleukin-3/interleukin-5 functions. Blood 88(7):2458–2464

Niswander LM, Fegan KH, Kingsley PD, McGrath KE, Palis J (2014) SDF-1 dynamically mediates megakaryocyte niche occupancy and thrombopoiesis at steady state and following radiation injury. Blood 124(2):277–286

Nosaka T, van Deursen JM, Tripp RA, Thierfelder WE, Witthuhn BA, McMickle AP et al (1995) Defective lymphoid development in mice lacking Jak3. Science 270(5237):800–802

Nussbaum JC, Van Dyken SJ, von Moltke J, Cheng LE, Mohapatra A, Molofsky AB et al (2013) Type 2 innate lymphoid cells control eosinophil homeostasis. Nature 502(7470):245–248

Nutt SL, Heavey B, Rolink AG, Busslinger M (1999) Commitment to the B-lymphoid lineage depends on the transcription factor Pax5. Nature 401(6753):556–562

O'Riordan M, Grosschedl R (1999) Coordinate regulation of B cell differentiation by the transcription factors EBF and E2A. Immunity 11(1):21–31

Oguro H, Iwama A, Morita Y, Kamijo T, van Lohuizen M, Nakauchi H (2006) Differential impact of Ink4a and Arf on hematopoietic stem cells and their bone marrow microenvironment in Bmi1-deficient mice. J Exp Med 203(10):2247–2253

Oguro H, Yuan J, Ichikawa H, Ikawa T, Yamazaki S, Kawamoto H et al (2010) Poised lineage specification in multipotential hematopoietic stem and progenitor cells by the polycomb protein Bmi1. Cell Stem Cell 6(3):279–286

Ono Y, Wang Y, Suzuki H, Okamoto S, Ikeda Y, Murata M et al (2012) Induction of functional platelets from mouse and human fibroblasts by p45NF-E2/Maf. Blood 120(18):3812–3821

Ostuni R, Natoli G, Cassatella MA, Tamassia N (2016) Epigenetic regulation of neutrophil development and function. Semin Immunol 28(2):83–93

Palis J (2014) Primitive and definitive erythropoiesis in mammals. Front Physiol 5:3

Paul F, Arkin Y, Giladi A, Jaitin DA, Kenigsberg E, Keren-Shaul H et al (2015) Transcriptional heterogeneity and lineage commitment in myeloid progenitors. Cell 163(7):1663–1677

Pavord ID, Korn S, Howarth P, Bleecker ER, Buhl R, Keene ON et al (2012) Mepolizumab for severe eosinophilic asthma (DREAM): a multicentre, double-blind, placebo-controlled trial. Lancet 380(9842):651–659

Perie L, Duffy KR, Kok L, de Boer RJ, Schumacher TN (2015) The branching point in erythro-myeloid differentiation. Cell 163(7):1655–1662

Perkins AC, Sharpe AH, Orkin SH (1995) Lethal beta-thalassaemia in mice lacking the erythroid CACCC-transcription factor EKLF. Nature 375(6529):318–322

Perkins A, Xu X, Higgs DR, Patrinos GP, Arnaud L, Bieker JJ et al (2016) Kruppeling erythropoiesis: an unexpected broad spectrum of human red blood cell disorders due to KLF1 variants. Blood 127(15):1856–1862

Person RE, Li FQ, Duan Z, Benson KF, Wechsler J, Papadaki HA et al (2003) Mutations in proto-oncogene GFI1 cause human neutropenia and target ELA2. Nat Genet 34(3):308–312

Peschon JJ, Morrissey PJ, Grabstein KH, Ramsdell FJ, Maraskovsky E, Gliniak BC et al (1994) Early lymphocyte expansion is severely impaired in interleukin 7 receptor-deficient mice. J Exp Med 180(5):1955–1960

Pevny L, Simon MC, Robertson E, Klein WH, Tsai SF, D'Agati V et al (1991) Erythroid differentiation in chimaeric mice blocked by a targeted mutation in the gene for transcription factor GATA-1. Nature 349(6306):257–260

Pevny L, Lin CS, D'Agati V, Simon MC, Orkin SH, Costantini F (1995) Development of hematopoietic cells lacking transcription factor GATA-1. Development 121(1):163–172

Pitchford SC, Lodie T, Rankin SM (2012) VEGFR1 stimulates a CXCR4-dependent translocation of megakaryocytes to the vascular niche, enhancing platelet production in mice. Blood 120(14):2787–2795

Qi X, Hong J, Chaves L, Zhuang Y, Chen Y, Wang D et al (2013) Antagonistic regulation by the transcription factors C/EBPalpha and MITF specifies basophil and mast cell fates. Immunity 39(1):97–110

Rothenberg EV (2014) Transcriptional control of early T and B cell developmental choices. Annu Rev Immunol 32:283–321

Sasaki H, Kurotaki D, Osato N, Sato H, Sasaki I, Koizumi S et al (2015) Transcription factor IRF8 plays a critical role in the development of murine basophils and mast cells. Blood 125(2):358–369

Sasaki H, Kurotaki D, Tamura T (2016) Regulation of basophil and mast cell development by transcription factors. Allergol Int 65(2):127–134

Satpathy AT, Wu X, Albring JC, Murphy KM (2012) Re(de)fining the dendritic cell lineage. Nat Immunol 13(12):1145–1154

Schonheit J, Kuhl C, Gebhardt ML, Klett FF, Riemke P, Scheller M et al (2013) PU.1 level-directed chromatin structure remodeling at the Irf8 gene drives dendritic cell commitment. Cell Rep 3(5):1617–1628

Schwickert TA, Tagoh H, Gultekin S, Dakic A, Axelsson E, Minnich M et al (2014) Stage-specific control of early B cell development by the transcription factor Ikaros. Nat Immunol 15(3):283–293

Scott EW, Fisher RC, Olson MC, Kehrli EW, Simon MC, Singh H (1997) PU.1 functions in a cell-autonomous manner to control the differentiation of multipotential lymphoid-myeloid progenitors. Immunity 6(4):437–447

Seita J, Weissman IL (2010) Hematopoietic stem cell: self-renewal versus differentiation. Wiley Interdiscip Rev Syst Biol Med 2(6):640–653

Shivdasani RA, Rosenblatt MF, Zucker-Franklin D, Jackson CW, Hunt P, Saris CJ et al (1995) Transcription factor NF-E2 is required for platelet formation independent of the actions of thrombopoietin/MGDF in megakaryocyte development. Cell 81(5):695–704

Shivdasani RA, Fujiwara Y, McDevitt MA, Orkin SH (1997) A lineage-selective knockout establishes the critical role of transcription factor GATA-1 in megakaryocyte growth and platelet development. EMBO J 16(13):3965–3973

Silberstein L, Goncalves KA, Kharchenko PV, Turcotte R, Kfoury Y, Mercier F et al (2016) Proximity-based differential single-cell analysis of the niche to identify stem/progenitor cell regulators. Cell Stem Cell 19:530

Siracusa MC, Saenz SA, Hill DA, Kim BS, Headley MB, Doering TA et al (2011) TSLP promotes interleukin-3-independent basophil haematopoiesis and type 2 inflammation. Nature 477(7363):229–233

Skokowa J, Cario G, Uenalan M, Schambach A, Germeshausen M, Battmer K et al (2006) LEF-1 is crucial for neutrophil granulocytopoiesis and its expression is severely reduced in congenital neutropenia. Nat Med 12(10):1191–1197

Socolovsky M, Nam H, Fleming MD, Haase VH, Brugnara C, Lodish HF (2001) Ineffective erythropoiesis in Stat5a(-/-)5b(-/-) mice due to decreased survival of early erythroblasts. Blood 98(12):3261–3273

Stark MA, Huo Y, Burcin TL, Morris MA, Olson TS, Ley K (2005) Phagocytosis of apoptotic neutrophils regulates granulopoiesis via IL-23 and IL-17. Immunity 22(3):285–294

Tamura T, Kurotaki D, Koizumi S (2015) Regulation of myelopoiesis by the transcription factor IRF8. Int J Hematol 101(4):342–351

Taoudi S, Bee T, Hilton A, Knezevic K, Scott J, Willson TA et al (2011) ERG dependence distinguishes developmental control of hematopoietic stem cell maintenance from hematopoietic specification. Genes Dev 25(3):251–262

Terry RL, Miller SD (2014) Molecular control of monocyte development. Cell Immunol 291(1-2):16–21

Tokoyoda K, Egawa T, Sugiyama T, Choi BI, Nagasawa T (2004) Cellular niches controlling B lymphocyte behavior within bone marrow during development. Immunity 20(6):707–718

Tominaga A, Takaki S, Koyama N, Katoh S, Matsumoto R, Migita M et al (1991) Transgenic mice expressing a B cell growth and differentiation factor gene (interleukin 5) develop eosinophilia and autoantibody production. J Exp Med 173(2):429–437

Townsend MJ, Weinmann AS, Matsuda JL, Salomon R, Farnham PJ, Biron CA et al (2004) T-bet regulates the terminal maturation and homeostasis of NK and Valpha14i NKT cells. Immunity 20(4):477–494

Tsai FY, Keller G, Kuo FC, Weiss M, Chen J, Rosenblatt M et al (1994) An early haematopoietic defect in mice lacking the transcription factor GATA-2. Nature 371(6494):221–226

Tsang AP, Visvader JE, Turner CA, Fujiwara Y, Yu C, Weiss MJ et al (1997) FOG, a multitype zinc finger protein, acts as a cofactor for transcription factor GATA-1 in erythroid and megakaryocytic differentiation. Cell 90(1):109–119

Tsutsumi-Ishii Y, Hasebe T, Nagaoka I (2000) Role of CCAAT/enhancer-binding protein site in transcription of human neutrophil peptide-1 and -3 defensin genes. J Immunol 164(6):3264–3273

Van Gool F, Molofsky AB, Morar MM, Rosenzwajg M, Liang HE, Klatzmann D et al (2014) Interleukin-5-producing group 2 innate lymphoid cells control eosinophilia induced by interleukin-2 therapy. Blood 124(24):3572–3576

Visvader JE, Elefanty AG, Strasser A, Adams JM (1992) GATA-1 but not SCL induces megakaryocytic differentiation in an early myeloid line. EMBO J 11(12):4557–4564

Voehringer D (2012) Basophil modulation by cytokine instruction. Eur J Immunol 42(10):2544–2550

Wada T, Akagi T, Muraoka M, Toma T, Kaji K, Agematsu K et al (2015) A novel in-frame deletion in the leucine zipper domain of C/EBPepsilon leads to neutrophil-specific granule deficiency. J Immunol 195(1):80–86

Wang X, Crispino JD, Letting DL, Nakazawa M, Poncz M, Blobel GA (2002) Control of megakaryocyte-specific gene expression by GATA-1 and FOG-1: role of Ets transcription factors. EMBO J 21(19):5225–5234

Wang H, Diao D, Shi Z, Zhu X, Gao Y, Gao S et al (2016) SIRT6 controls hematopoietic stem cell homeostasis through epigenetic regulation of wnt signaling. Cell Stem Cell 18(4):495–507

Waskow C, Liu K, Darrasse-Jeze G, Guermonprez P, Ginhoux F, Merad M et al (2008) The receptor tyrosine kinase Flt3 is required for dendritic cell development in peripheral lymphoid tissues. Nat Immunol 9(6):676–683

Wilkinson AC, Gottgens B (2013) Transcriptional regulation of haematopoietic stem cells. Adv Exp Med Biol 786:187–212

Wilson A, MacDonald HR, Radtke F (2001) Notch 1-deficient common lymphoid precursors adopt a B cell fate in the thymus. J Exp Med 194(7):1003–1012

Wilson A, Murphy MJ, Oskarsson T, Kaloulis K, Bettess MD, Oser GM et al (2004) c-Myc controls the balance between hematopoietic stem cell self-renewal and differentiation. Genes Dev 18(22):2747–2763

Wu H, Liu X, Jaenisch R, Lodish HF (1995) Generation of committed erythroid BFU-E and CFU-E progenitors does not require erythropoietin or the erythropoietin receptor. Cell 83(1):59–67

Wu H, Lee SH, Gao J, Liu X, Iruela-Arispe ML (1999) Inactivation of erythropoietin leads to defects in cardiac morphogenesis. Development 126(16):3597–3605

Wu JY, Purton LE, Rodda SJ, Chen M, Weinstein LS, McMahon AP et al (2008) Osteoblastic regulation of B lymphopoiesis is mediated by Gs{alpha}-dependent signaling pathways. Proc Natl Acad Sci U S A 105(44):16976–16981

Yamaguchi Y, Ackerman SJ, Minegishi N, Takiguchi M, Yamamoto M, Suda T (1998) Mechanisms of transcription in eosinophils: GATA-1, but not GATA-2, transactivates the promoter of the eosinophil granule major basic protein gene. Blood 91(9):3447–3458

Yamanaka R, Barlow C, Lekstrom-Himes J, Castilla LH, Liu PP, Eckhaus M et al (1997) Impaired granulopoiesis, myelodysplasia, and early lethality in CCAAT/enhancer binding protein epsilon-deficient mice. Proc Natl Acad Sci U S A 94(24):13187–13192

Yao Z, Cui Y, Watford WT, Bream JH, Yamaoka K, Hissong BD et al (2006) Stat5a/b are essential for normal lymphoid development and differentiation. Proc Natl Acad Sci U S A 103(4):1000–1005

Yokota Y, Mansouri A, Mori S, Sugawara S, Adachi S, Nishikawa S et al (1999) Development of peripheral lymphoid organs and natural killer cells depends on the helix-loop-helix inhibitor Id2. Nature 397(6721):702–706

Yokota T, Sudo T, Ishibashi T, Doi Y, Ichii M, Orirani K et al (2013) Complementary regulation of early B-lymphoid differentiation by genetic and epigenetic mechanisms. Int J Hematol 98(4):382–389

Yoshida T, Ikuta K, Sugaya H, Maki K, Takagi M, Kanazawa H et al (1996) Defective B-1 cell development and impaired immunity against Angiostrongylus cantonensis in IL-5R alpha-deficient mice. Immunity 4(5):483–494

Yu C, Cantor AB, Yang H, Browne C, Wells RA, Fujiwara Y et al (2002) Targeted deletion of a high-affinity GATA-binding site in the GATA-1 promoter leads to selective loss of the eosinophil lineage in vivo. J Exp Med 195(11):1387–1395

Yu VW, Saez B, Cook C, Lotinun S, Pardo-Saganta A, Wang YH et al (2015) Specific bone cells produce DLL4 to generate thymus-seeding progenitors from bone marrow. J Exp Med 212(5):759–774

Zanjani ED, Ascensao JL, McGlave PB, Banisadre M, Ash RC (1981) Studies on the liver to kidney switch of erythropoietin production. J Clin Invest 67(4):1183–1188

Zeng H, Yucel R, Kosan C, Klein-Hitpass L, Moroy T (2004) Transcription factor Gfi1 regulates self-renewal and engraftment of hematopoietic stem cells. EMBO J 23(20):4116–4125

Zhang DE, Zhang P, Wang ND, Hetherington CJ, Darlington GJ, Tenen DG (1997) Absence of granulocyte colony-stimulating factor signaling and neutrophil development in CCAAT enhancer binding protein alpha-deficient mice. Proc Natl Acad Sci U S A 94(2):569–574

Zhang J, Niu C, Ye L, Huang H, He X, Tong WG et al (2003) Identification of the haematopoietic stem cell niche and control of the niche size. Nature 425(6960):836–841

Zhang D, Chen G, Manwani D, Mortha A, Xu C, Faith JJ et al (2015) Neutrophil ageing is regulated by the microbiome. Nature 525(7570):528–532

Zhang X, Su J, Jeong M, Ko M, Huang Y, Park HJ et al (2016) DNMT3A and TET2 compete and cooperate to repress lineage-specific transcription factors in hematopoietic stem cells. Nat Genet 48: 1014

Zhuang Y, Soriano P, Weintraub H (1994) The helix-loop-helix gene E2A is required for B cell formation. Cell 79(5):875–884

Zook EC, Kee BL (2016) Development of innate lymphoid cells. Nat Immunol 17(7):775–782

2 Acquired Aplastic Anemia

Yigal Dror and Michaela Cada

Contents

Y. Dror (✉)
Marrow Failure and Myelodysplasia Program, Haematology Section, Division of Haematology Oncology, Paediatrics, The Hospital for Sick Children, The University of Toronto, Toronto, ON, Canada

Genetics and Genome Biology Program, Research Institute, Institute of Medical Sciences, The Hospital for Sick Children, The University of Toronto, Toronto, ON, Canada
e-mail: yigal.dror@sickkids.ca

M. Cada
Marrow Failure and Myelodysplasia Program, Division of Haematology Oncology, Paediatrics, The Hospital for Sick Children, University of Toronto, Toronto, ON, Canada

Haematology Oncology Education Program, The Hospital for Sick Children, University of Toronto, Toronto, ON, Canada
e-mail: michaela.cada@sickkids.ca

G. M. Kupfer et al. (eds.), *Bone Marrow Failure*, Pediatric Oncology,
https://doi.org/10.1007/978-3-319-61421-2_2

Abbreviations

AA	Aplastic anemia
AML	Acute myeloid leukemia
ATG	Antithymocyte globulin
G-CSF	Granulocyte colony-stimulating factor
GM-CSF	Granulocyte-monocyte colony-stimulating factor
HSCT	Hematopoietic stem cell transplantation
IST	Immunosuppressive therapy
MDS	Myelodysplastic syndrome
PNH	Paroxysmal nocturnal hemoglobinuria
SAA	Severe aplastic anemia
TBI	Total body irradiation

2.1 Introduction

Aplastic anemia (AA) is characterized by reduced peripheral blood cell counts with a hypocellular bone marrow and no evidence of evolution into myelodysplastic syndrome (MDS) or leukemia. Despite its historic name, anemia is neither the only feature of this disease nor the most life-threatening; bi-lineage cytopenia or pancytopenia is seen in the majority of patients. Although severe hypocellular bone marrow (aplasia) is seen in most cases, mildly to moderately hypocellular bone marrow (hypoplasia) is also common.

Little population-based data are available about the proportion of children with AA who are ultimately diagnosed with acquired versus inherited disease in the era of advanced genetics and genomics. An inherited etiology can be identified in about 25% of cases. These cases are referred to as inherited bone marrow failure syndromes (IBMFSs). In a small proportion of children (probably <10%), a definitive environmental cause can be identified (e.g., infections, drugs, toxins, cancer, and autoimmune disorders), and the AA resolves after treatment that targets the causal factor. In such cases the AA can confidently be determined as acquired. About 70% of cases are labeled as idiopathic. The efficacy of immunosuppressive therapy in about 70–75% of these idiopathic cases strongly suggests an acquired cause in those with a prominent response and potentially another etiology in those without a response. Therefore, the overall proportion of acquired AA among all cases of AA is estimated to be about 60%. The current chapter is about definitive acquired and idiopathic AA. For simplicity, we will herein refer to both as acquired AA.

2.2 Epidemiology

In developed countries, the incidence of AA in childhood in those <15 years of age was reported as 1–3 per million children per year (Linet et al. 1986; *Blood* 1987; Mary et al. 1990; Clausen et al. 1996). Most reports from Asia cite a two to threefold higher incidence of AA than that of the West, possibly due to environmental or genetic differences (Young et al. 1986; Issaragrisil 1999). There is a strong inverse association between incidence of disease and socioeconomic status (Issaragrisil 1999).

AA can occur at any age. However, there are two age groups during which the incidence of presentation with AA peaks, at 15–25 years and older than 60 years (*Blood* 1987; Mary et al. 1990). There is a slight male predominance. Over 70% of children with AA have severe disease at the time of presentation (Mary et al. 1990; Howard et al. 2004; Locasciulli et al. 2007).

2.3 Etiology

Acquired AA can sometimes be attributed to a definable cause including drugs and toxins, viral infections, autoimmune disorders, and cancer (Gupta et al. 2013). About 70% of AA cases are idiopathic (Mary et al. 1990; Howard et al. 2004; Gupta et al. 2013; Camitta et al. 1979). In a large prospective study by the French Cooperative Group (Mary et al. 1990), the suspected etiology was recorded for 243 cases of AA in children and adults: 79% were idiopathic (including 5% with hepatitis-associated AA), 13% were associated with drugs and 5% with toxins, and the rest were categorized as miscellaneous including two cases that were pregnancy related.

Many case reports, case series, and large epidemiological studies have implicated a multitude of drugs in the etiology of AA, but these associations might be circumstantial rather than causative (Mary et al. 1990; Issaragrisil 1999; Imashuku et al. 2003; Baumelou et al. 1993; *JAMA* 1986). Some studies have implicated certain medications convincingly. In a meta-analysis of three large-scale studies by Kaufman and colleagues (1996), the evidence for implication of drugs in the etiology of AA was studied. Comparisons were made between 454 patients and AA, and 6458 controls. The strongest associations between AA and drugs were for penicillamine, gold, and carbamazepine. The other associated drugs included butazones, indomethacin, diclofenac, sulfonamides, and furosemide. These studies, however, lacked accurate data about the drug exposure period and dose.

The French Cooperative Group studied 147 cases of AA compared to 287 hospitalized controls and 108 neighbors (Baumelou et al. 1993). The results implicated gold salts, D-penicillamine, salicylates, and colchicine as risk factors for AA. However, the association between rheumatoid arthritis and AA confounded the ability to clearly link anti-inflammatory agents with AA. Similarly, the use of non-phenicol antibiotics appeared to be linked to AA, but the history of a recent infectious episode confounded the interpretation of this result. The use of chloramphenicol and thiamphenicol was too limited to allow any conclusions.

In a study from Latin America, exposure to azithromycin, chloramphenicol, benzene, and pesticides was statistically higher in patients with AA compared to controls; however, in multivariant analysis only azithromycin and benzene remained significant (Maluf et al. 2009).

Most of the patients in the abovementioned studies were adults. The incidence of drug-related AA in children was generally low, as the commonly implicated drugs are less frequently used in childhood, with the exception of anticonvulsants (e.g., valproate and carbamazepine) and some nonsteroidal anti-inflammatories (e.g., indomethacin).

Chloramphenicol exposure has been reported in several cases of young children with AA, but a causal relationship is controversial. Since the first publications, chloramphenicol exposures in this age population became very rare (Mary et al. 1990; Kaufman et al. 1996), and the estimated risk is difficult to predict. In studies from Thailand, there was no evidence of an association between chloramphenicol and AA (Issaragrisil 1999; Issaragrisil et al. 1997). As mentioned above, in multivariant analysis, also in a study from Latin America, exposure to chloramphenicol was not significant (Maluf et al. 2009). Global reductions in the use of chloramphenicol have not been accompanied by a parallel reduction in the incidence of AA (Mizuno et al. 1982; Bottiger et al. 1979).

Exposure to environmental toxins, such as pesticides (e.g., DDT, chlordane, lindane) (Issaragrisil 1999; Maluf et al. 2009; Roberts 1990; Rugman and Cosstick 1990), paints (Guiguet et al. 1995), and solvents (Issaragrisil 1999), has often been implicated as a cause of AA, but not in all studies (Issaragrisil 1999). Prolonged exposure to benzene and its derivatives carries a particularly high risk of hematological toxicities. Its metabolites have been implicated as a cause of aplasia (Maluf et al. 2009; Yardley-Jones et al. 1991), DNA damage (Pellack-Walker and Blumer 1986), and apoptosis of hematopoietic cells (Moran et al. 1996). A recent report demonstrated that chronic low-level exposure to benzene, at air levels considered to be safe by occupational guidelines, was also toxic to hematopoietic cells, particularly in susceptible individuals (Lan et al. 2004).

A number of viruses have been implicated in the development of AA in a small proportion of patients. However, attributing causality to some viral agents may be difficult due to their ubiquitous nature. Implicated viruses include Epstein-Barr virus (Baranski et al. 1988), cytomegalovirus (Sing and Ruscetti 1995), human herpesvirus 6 (Carrigan and Knox 1994), human immunodeficiency virus (Shah and Murthy 2005), parvovirus B19 (Goto et al. 2004; Qian et al. 2002; Mishra et al. 2005), hepatitis A (Shah and Murthy 2005; Domenech et al. 1986) and B (Goto et al. 2004; McSweeney et al. 1988), measles, mumps, rubella (Qian et al. 2002; Kook et al. 2000), varicella, and flaviviruses (Nakao et al. 1989), as well as varicella-zoster virus, hepatitis C virus, and dengue (Klco et al. 2010; Morinet et al. 2011). Viruses may trigger expansion of oligoclonal CD8+ T cells, which secrete IFNγ and TNFα, and cause hematopoietic cell death (de Bruin et al. 2014). Persistent secretion of these pro-inflammatory cytokines may lead to HSC exhaustion (de Bruin et al. 2014; Libregts and Nolte 2014).

Hepatitis-associated AA occurs several weeks to several months after the onset of acute hepatitis of variable severity (Linet et al. 1986; Clausen et al. 1996; Baumelou et al. 1993; *JAMA* 1986; Brown et al. 1997). Most commonly, the hepatitis is seronegative for any known hepatitis viruses (Brown et al. 1997; Pol et al. 1993; Hibbs et al. 1992). It appears to be more common in young males (Brown et al. 1997). The hepatitis may follow a relatively benign course; however, the aplasia is associated with high mortality if untreated (Klco et al. 2010) or if refractory to therapy. Preceding hepatitis is seen in about 2–34% of patients with AA in studies (Mary et al. 1990; Young et al. 1986; Hibbs et al. 1992; Li et al. 2016; Babushok et al. 2016). A recent study of ten patients with hepatitis-associated aplastic anemia found significantly shorter telomeres and lower lymphocyte counts in patients with hepatitis-associated AA than in other types of idiopathic AA (Babushok et al. 2016). Four of the patients had telomere lengths below the first percentile. Detailed outcome of the patients who received IST were not provided. In three cases, whole-exome sequencing revealed variants in telomere-related genes that were deemed nonpathogenic by the group. In one case, familial occurrence of hepatitis-associated aplastic anemia and acute lymphoblastic leukemia was reported (Breakey et al. 2009).

Hematological and non-hematological tumors have been reported in patients with preceding aplastic anemia. A systemic autoimmune process, such as in the case of thymoma, is one possible mechanism. A paraneoplastic process involving inhibitory cytokines is possible although not proven. In the case of acute myeloid leukemia, an inhibitory effect of mouse cells on mouse hematopoietic differentiation has been shown; however, the mechanism and the relevance to aplastic anemia are unknown. All cases of cancer with preceding or concomitant aplastic anemia should be carefully evaluated for the possibility of underlying IBMFSs, which are known to carry a predisposition for various types of cancer.

Systemic autoimmune disorders are occasionally associated with acquired AA, albeit they are rare. AA has been reported in patients with eosinophilic fasciitis (Kim et al. 1997; Ritchie et al. 2002), thymoma (Ritchie et al. 2002), Graves' disease (Das et al. 2007), systemic lupus erythematosus (Chute et al. 1996; Quiquandon et al. 1997), rheumatoid arthritis (Baumelou et al. 1993), Sjogren's syndrome (Quiquandon et al. 1997), and transfusion-related graft-versus-host disease (GVHD) (Anderson and Weinstein 1990).

Hemophagocytic lymphohistiocytosis is a rare hyper-inflammatory syndrome that can be caused by either inherited mutations in genes that regulate granule-dependent cytotoxicity of cytotoxic T cells and NK cells (e.g., PRF1, UNC13D, STX11, or STXBP2) or secondary to autoimmune and infectious processes. Frequently, bone marrow specimens are normocellular, and hemophagocytic cells are absent. However, a mild to severe hypocellular bone marrow may present along with bone marrow hemophagocytosis and/or systemic evidence of macrophage activation. Although old studies recommended excluding the diagnosis of AA in cases of evidence of hemophagocytosis, cases that fit the diagnostic criteria of both severe AA and hemophagocytic lymphohistiocytosis have been described (Celkan 2010; Chandar et al. 2017) and also observed by the authors (unpublished). Further mutations in PRF1 genes have been identified in a small percentage of patients with classical severe AA (Solomou et al. 2007).

In severe cases of hepatitis-associated AA, the liver disease progresses to fulminant liver failure.

It appears to be more common in younger individuals with a mean age of 10 years (Itterbeek et al. 2002). Aplastic anemia was reported in 28–33% of children and 5% of adults who underwent orthotopic liver transplantation for fulminant seronegative hepatitis (Cattral et al. 1994; Tzakis et al. 1988). In contrast, AA was reported in <1% of liver transplant patients for other reasons (Itterbeek et al. 2002; Tzakis et al. 1988). Although the cause of hepatitis and the associated AA is not known, there is evidence to support a T-cell, immune-mediated mechanism against both systems (Brown et al. 1997; Lu et al. 2004).

Clinical paroxysmal nocturnal hemoglobinuria (PNH) is very uncommon in childhood, particularly before adolescence; however, with modern sensitive flow cytometry testing for this condition, laboratory evidence of PNH clones occurs in about 40% of children with AA (Narita et al. 2015). Clinical PNH is characterized by episodic hemolysis, thrombosis, AA, and increased risk for MDS. It is an acquired clonal disorder of hematopoietic stem cells due to an X-linked somatic mutation of the PIGA gene (Nishimura et al. 1999). This results in abnormal biosynthesis of the cell membrane-anchoring protein, glycosylphosphatidylinositol, and an absence of glycosylphosphatidylinositol-linked proteins, including the complement regulatory proteins, CD55 and CD59. Approximately 25% of adult patients with PNH present with or develop AA, and about 15% of adult patients with AA develop PNH in the recovery phase after IST (de Planque et al. 1989; Doney et al. 1997; Tichelli et al. 1992; Locasciulli 2002). A small percentage of patients with PNH progress to leukemia.

An important differential diagnosis of acquired AA is an IBMFS. IBMFSs have been estimated to represent approximately one-third of childhood AA. Some patients may present with AA without characteristic physical anomalies, even in their fifth and sixth decades (Yamaguchi et al. 2005; Keel et al. 2016). Pathogenic mutations in IBMFS genes (e.g., *TERC*, *TERT*, and *TIN2*) have been identified in some patients with apparent clinical presentation of acquired AA (Yamaguchi et al. 2005; Vulliamy et al. 2005; Ghemlas et al. 2015), indicating that some of these patients may indeed have an inherited disorder. Advances in genetic and genomic diagnostic techniques allow the diagnosis of these cases of seemingly "acquired" aplastic anemia. Differentiating IBMFSs from acquired AA is crucial since their therapy and prognoses differ. As well, genetic and family counselling is warranted. There is a debate between adult bone marrow failure experts who encounter AA of mainly acquired nature and pediatric hematologists who commonly diagnose AA in patients with IBMFSs, whether patients with mutations in IBMFS genes should be diagnosed as having an IBMFS or as having acquired AA with an underlying genetic risk factor. Even if patients are considered to have acquired AA with a genetic predisposition, the management of these patients and their families should resemble that of patients with IBMFSs, including careful consideration of treatment options.

Low-risk variants in certain genes may occur in AA and increase its risk. For example, variants in HLA-DR2 are more common in patients with AA compared to healthy subjects (Nimer et al. 1994). Monoallelic mutations in genes that are associated with autosomal recessive IBMFSs are reported in patients with idiopathic AA, for example, *SBDS* (Calado et al. 2007). The occurrence of these variants may represent a predisposition for developing AA and/or poor response to immunosuppressive therapy.

2.4 Pathophysiology

Three main mechanisms have been implicated in the pathophysiology of acquired AA: (1) autoimmune damage to hematopoietic progenitor cells, (2) inherent stem cell defects, and (3) defects of the bone marrow stroma or microenvironment. Most of the studies that aimed to decipher the pathophysiology of AA have been done on adult patients or a mixed population of adults and children with AA.

Cellular-mediated autoimmunity was proposed as a major mechanism in the pathophysiology of acquired AA. The strongest evidence comes from the observed clinical response to IST. Also, there is an overrepresentation of

HLA-DR2 among patients with AA as in autoimmune diseases (Nimer et al. 1994). In vitro hematopoietic colony formation was inhibited by patients' lymphocytes from both the circulation and bone marrow (Nakao et al. 1997).

Predominance of CD8+ phenotype (Viale et al. 1991) or CD4+ cytotoxic cells (Nakao et al. 1997) has been reported in patients with AA. Many investigators also demonstrated oligoclonal expansion of specific T cells and a skewed T-cell receptor Vβ repertoire (Nakao et al. 1997; Zeng et al. 2001; Risitano et al. 2004; Piao et al. 2005; Krell et al. 2013). The restricted T-cell clones can be cytotoxic to both autologous and allogeneic hematopoietic progenitor cells (Nakao et al. 1997). The size of the expanded T-cell clones correlates with disease activity, but clones persist at low levels even after remission is achieved with IST (Zeng et al. 2001; Risitano et al. 2004). Interestingly, there is molecular homology of these clones between patients, suggesting a limited number of antigens driving the immune response (Zeng et al. 2001). In one study, the TCR/CD3 complex regulator, CD3ζ, the co-stimulatory factor, and CD28 were found to be overexpressed in peripheral blood mononuclear cells of AA patients, and the T-cell attenuating molecules, CTLA-4 and Cbl-b, were decreased (Li et al. 2016). In other studies of AA patients, where specifically CD4+/CD25+ T-cell regulatory cells were studied, CTLA-4 expression levels were reduced (Yan et al. 2015; Shi et al. 2012). Total peripheral blood Tregs in AA were also found to have impaired migratory ability due to reduced CXCR4 expression and had reduced potential to inhibit interferon-γ production by effector T cells (Shi et al. 2012). Total T-regulatory cells were also found to be reduced in AA patients, possibly due to apoptosis (Yan et al. 2015). All of the above suggest that increased activity of cytotoxic T cells and decreased activity of T-regulatory cells may lead to hyperactivation of the adaptive immune response and suppression of self-tolerance mechanisms.

Interestingly, patients with AA also show imbalanced levels of dendritic cell subsets (elevated DC1), enhancement of dendritic cell DC function, and imbalance of Th1/Th2 subsets (enhanced Th1) (Zonghong et al. 2011). This is consistent with an increase in *in vitro* and *in vivo* type I lymphoid factors, including interferon-γ, interleukin-2, and tumor necrosis factor-α (Viale et al. 1991; Zeng et al. 2001, 2004; Hara et al. 2004; Sloand et al. 2002). These suppressive factors interfere with the mitotic cycle of hematopoietic precursors (Zeng et al. 2001), upregulate Fas receptors on CD34+ hematopoietic stem cells, and cause apoptosis (Liu et al. 2014; Philpott et al. 1995; Maciejewski et al. 1995). The hematopoietic progenitor cells in patients who develop AA may have an enhanced sensitivity to lymphokines such as tumor necrosis factor-α (Kasahara et al. 2002).

The detection of autoantibodies against hematopoietic antigens such as kinectin in some patients with AA (Hirano et al. 2003) also suggests an immune mechanism.

Primary hematopoietic stem cell and progenitor abnormalities have been demonstrated in acquired AA, including reduced numbers of CD34+ cells (Scopes et al. 1996), reduced multipotent and committed colony-forming cells, reduced long-term culture-initiating cells (Maciejewski et al. 1996; Marsh et al. 1990), and decreased cobblestone area-forming cells (Schrezenmeier et al. 1996). In a recent study where multiparametric flow cytometry was performed, markedly reduced levels of hematopoietic stem cells, multipotent stem cells, common myeloid progenitors, and megakaryocyte-erythroid progenitors were observed (Notta et al. 2016). The cure of AA following an infusion of hematopoietic stem cells implicates this deficiency. This is further supported by crossover experiments in which patients' marrow cells, which have been depleted of adherent cells, grew poorly on normal stroma (Marsh et al. 1990; Novitzky and Jacobs 1995). In addition, the observations of clonal evolution and persistence of stem cell deficiency and macrocytosis in some patients after recovery following IST further supports an underlying stem cell abnormality. It is important to note that bone marrow stroma has been shown to be of host origin, rather than donor, after HSCT (Sagmeister et al. 1999).

Patients with acquired AA may have normal or slightly short telomere length in peripheral blood leukocytes (Fig. 2.1a, b). The average telomere length in peripheral blood leukocytes from children with AA is shorter than normal age-matched controls, and the length improves after successful treatment with IST (Narita et al. 2015; Ball et al. 1998; Sakaguchi et al. 2014). Like hemoglobin F, this might reflect "stress" hematopoiesis (Ball et al. 1998). Very short telomere lengths (<1% of normal telomere distribution for age) have also been reported in cases of patients with apparently acquired AA; however, detailed clinical and genetic testing is required in such cases to rule out an underlying diagnosis of dyskeratosis congenita. As discussed above in the section about Etiology, mutations in telomere homeostasis genes have been reported in patients with apparently acquired AA, and these patients are considered by most pediatric hematologists to have IBMFSs.

A recent study of patients with AA and short telomeres demonstrated improvement in telomere length after treatment with danazol (Townsley et al. 2016). However, many of these patients either had mutations in telomere-related disorders or did not respond to immunosuppressive therapy, raising the possibility that a substantial proportion of these patients had IBMFSs rather than acquired AA.

The fact that a proportion of patients do not respond to IST and that there is a relative increased risk of graft failure in patients with AA despite marked depletion of hematopoietic cells

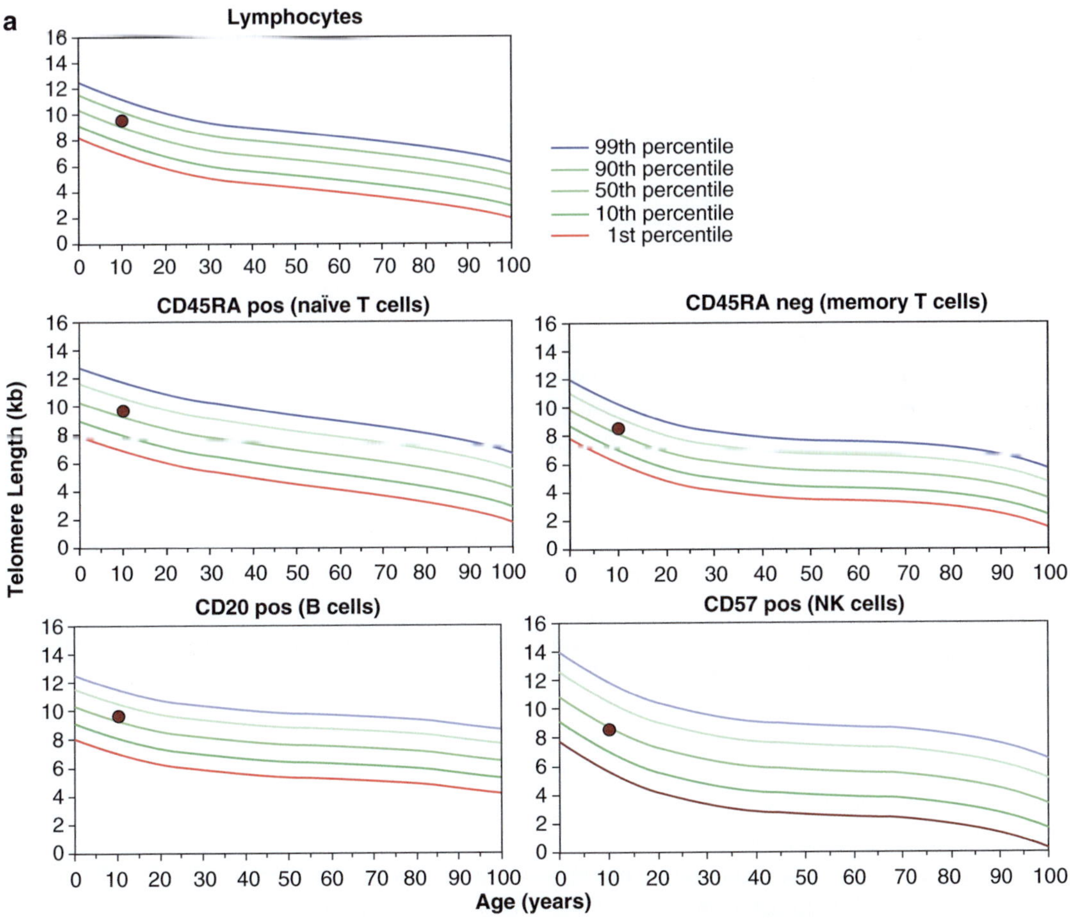

Fig. 2.1 Telomere lengths in patients with aplastic anemia. (**a**) Patient with normal telomere lengths who responded to immunosuppressive therapy. (**b**) Patient with very short telomere lengths (<1% for age), who did not respond to immunosuppressive therapy

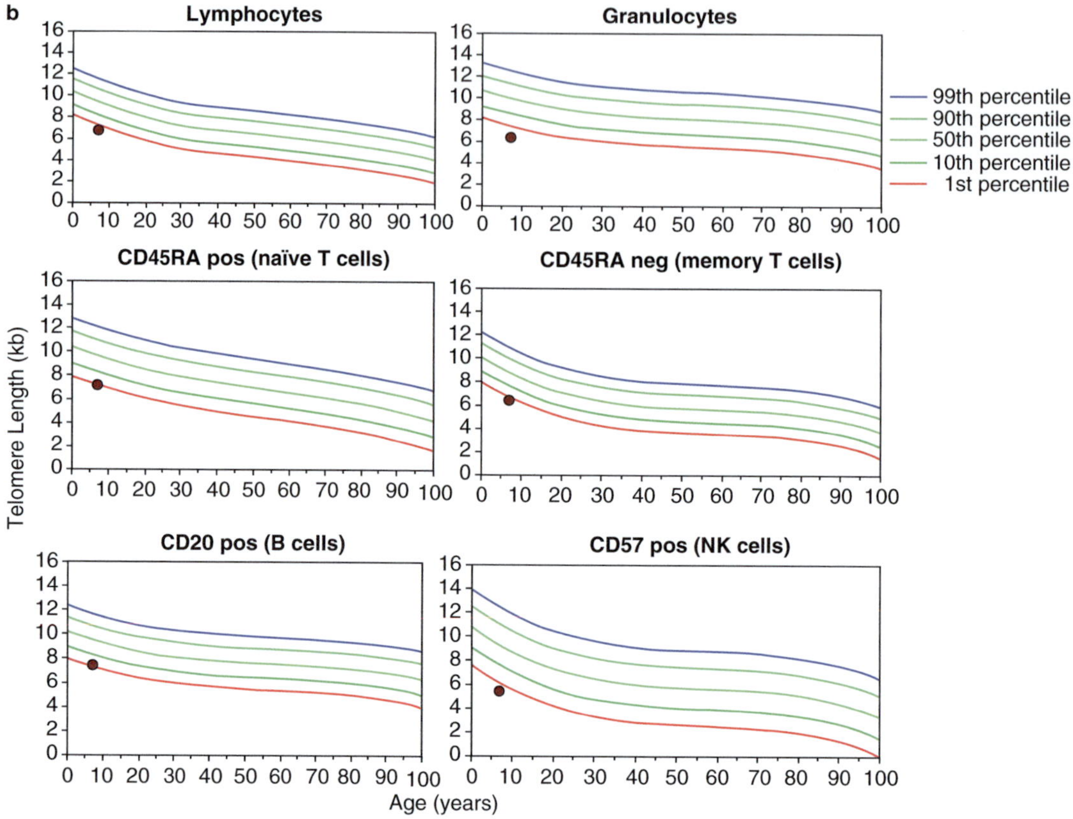

Fig. 2.1 (continued)

and frequently also of peripheral blood lymphocytes, is intriguing. Although these observations could be explained by additional impairment of the bone marrow stroma, the contribution of AA stroma to the pathogenesis of the disease is controversial. Abnormalities of the marrow stroma have been reported in a proportion of patients with AA. Approximately 50% of patients have abnormal stromal cell proliferation (Yan et al. 2015; Holmberg et al. 1994), do not form a confluent stromal layer in long-term cultures, or have morphologic differences from normal stroma (Marsh et al. 1990). Patients with no stromal cell growth have a longer duration of aplasia (Holmberg et al. 1994). Abnormal stromal secretion of hematopoietic growth factors has been found in patients with AA, including higher levels of macrophage inflammatory protein-1α and leukemia-inhibitory factor, a decrease in interleukin-1 receptor antagonist, and decreased inteleukin-6 production in response to interleukin-1, tumor necrosis factor-α, and cytomegalovirus (Holmberg et al. 1994; Dilloo et al. 1995). Some studies have also reported that AA-derived mesenchymal stromal cells display aberrant morphology and transcriptome profile, as well as impaired proliferation, clonogenic potential, and adipogenic and osteogenic differentiation (Xu et al. 2009; Chao et al. 2010; Li et al. 2012; Hamzic et al. 2015). Other studies, however, reported that AA-derived mesenchymal stromal cells display normal morphology and differentiation properties (Bueno et al. 2014). In some studies, the capacity of AA-derived mesenchymal stromal cells to sustain hematopoiesis in an *in vitro* co-culture was reduced (Hamzic et al. 2015), while others reported a normal ability of AA-derived mesenchymal stromal cells to support normal hematopoiesis (Bueno et al. 2014; Michelozzi et al. 2017). Finally, since patients with AA can be cured by HSCT despite preservation of their marrow stroma, the role of marrow stroma in the pathogenesis of acquired AA is likely minor.

Toxins, drugs, or their metabolites may be directly injurious to the bone marrow or may trigger an immune response against stem or stromal cells. Due to the rarity of identified antibodies in patients with AA, drugs may not serve as simple haptens that trigger an immune response. Viruses can directly infect stem cells, progenitor cells, or stromal cells leading to cytokine-mediated cell death by cytotoxic lymphocytes (Zonghong et al. 2011; Frickhofen et al. 1990). These mechanisms can lead either to stem cell loss through direct toxicity, microenvironmental failure, or immune suppression of marrow elements by an activated immune system (Hara et al. 2004; Torok-Storb 1990). Some individuals might also be genetically more susceptible to toxins or viruses.

2.5 Grading of Severity

Severe aplastic anemia (SAA) is diagnosed when the bone marrow cellularity is <25% (*Blood* 1987) or the cellularity is <30% (Barone et al. 2015) of normal bone marrow cellularity for age, determined by bone marrow biopsy, and when at least two of the following peripheral blood findings are present: granulocytes $<0.5 \times 10^9$/L, platelets $<20 \times 10^9$/L, or absolute reticulocyte $\leq 20 \times 10^9$/L (Barone et al. 2015) or $\leq 40 \times 10^9$/L (*Blood* 1987). Mild and moderate AA are diagnosed when criteria for severe disease are not met.

Very severe AA is defined when the above criteria for SAA are met and the granulocyte count is $<0.2 \times 10^9$/L. Recently, the term fulminant aplastic anemia was introduced by Yagasaki and colleague (Yagasaki et al. 2014) and was referred to in cases with neutrophil counts of 0×10^9/L for a duration of at least 2 weeks.

In one study of 70% of patients who presented with apparently acquired AA, 70% had severe disease, 27.5% had moderated disease and 2.5% had very severe disease (Jain et al. 2012). The category of disease severity is vital in dictating the urgency and choice of therapy, and is valuable in assessing prognosis.

2.6 Clinical Presentation

Children with AA usually present with symptoms related to cytopenias. Increased bruising with or without mucosal bleeding due to thrombocytopenia is the most common initial presentation (Clausen et al. 1996). Pallor and fatigue due to anemia are also common at presentation (Clausen et al. 1996). However, severe anemia of gradual onset is usually well compensated for by young children. Serious infections due to neutropenia are uncommon presenting symptoms. Apart from these signs and symptoms, patients generally appear well, have normal physical examinations, and have no dysmorphic features. Lymphadenopathy and hepatosplenomegaly are atypical and should raise the possibility of other diagnoses such as leukemia. Most children have symptoms for <1 month and >80% for <3 months (Mary et al. 1990; Clausen et al. 1996).

Family history is typically unremarkable, and history of bone marrow hypoplasia and hematologic malignancies in first-degree relatives should raise the possibility of an IBMFS.

2.7 Natural History

In a series of 112 children with idiopathic AA, 71% met the criteria for SAA, 21% for moderate AA, and <5% for mild AA (Howard et al. 2004). Two-thirds of patients with moderate disease progressed to SAA at a median of 9.5 months (range of 2–290 months) after diagnosis. The remaining patients persisted with moderate disease (21%), with a median of 32 months of follow-up, or underwent spontaneous complete resolution (12%), at a median of 7 months.

Untreated SAA has a high mortality due to either infections or hemorrhagic events. Improved supportive care modalities, including transfusions for severe thrombocytopenia and anemia, and broad-spectrum antibiotics for febrile episodes, have substantially improved survival. Specific therapies (i.e., IST or HSCT) have dramatically changed the outlook for children diagnosed with AA. In this era of supportive and specific therapies, survival closely depends on the neutrophil count and duration of severe neutropenia. Causes of death include infections, internal bleeding, and treatment-related complications. About one-third of the documented infections in AA are due to fungi (Clausen et al. 1996). The actuarial survival of children treated between 1989 and 1996 was improved to 84% at 8 years (Pitcher et al. 1999). The 10-year overall survival of patients treated with IST or HSCT after 2000 has frequently been reported as >90% (Nishikawa et al. 2017; Deyell et al. 2011).

2.8 Diagnosis and Laboratory Evaluation

Evaluation of a child with AA should include a detailed medical history. Symptoms related to the present illness, time when the symptoms started, and recent jaundice should be determined. A history of any previous hematological derangements, drug and viral exposure, and history which may suggest non-hematological manifestations, development milestones, surgeries, and hospitalization should be elucidated. Family history should include information about the medical health of the core and extended family, as well as consanguinity, ethnic background, and previous pregnancy outcomes. Careful physical examination should be performed to evaluate degree of bleeding, organ function, and infections, as well as to exclude other diagnoses such as IBMFSs and leukemia.

Complete blood count demonstrates pancytopenia and absolute reticulocytopenia. The peripheral blood smear commonly shows red blood cell macrocytosis and hemoglobin F is high, although less frequently and to a lesser degree compared to that observed in IBMFSs with pancytopenia, such as Fanconi anemia and dyskeratosis congenita. These levels may remain elevated in patients who have clinically recovered. A direct antiglobulin test is useful to rule out an autoimmune hemolytic process and as preparation for a potential prolonged period of transfusion need.

Bone marrow examination by an aspirate and a trephine biopsy is essential for confirmation of hypoplasia and its severity, and to rule out other causes of pancytopenia. Bone marrow aspirates usually show empty particles and increased fat, reticulum, plasma, and mast cells but are inadequate for accurate assessment of cellularity. Cellular morphology is usually normal. Bone marrow biopsy is essential for the work-up of AA and allows the determination of architecture and percentage of residual cellularity (Fig. 2.2). Prominent fibrosis is usually absent. Bone marrow cytogenetics should be performed to rule out a clonal disorder suggesting hypoplastic MDS. Rarely, an acute leukemia presents ini-

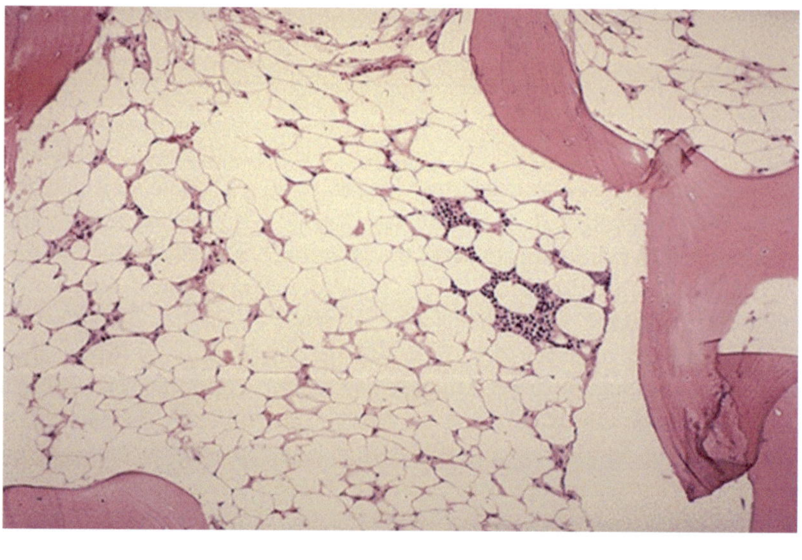

Fig. 2.2 Bone marrow biopsy specimen from a patient with severe aplastic anemia showing active hematopoiesis in <25% of the bone marrow space

tially with a period of bone marrow failure (Liang et al. 1993; Sharathkumar et al. 2003). Clonogenic assays of marrow CD34+ cells can provide additional evidence for reduced production by showing abnormally low colony-forming potential.

AA in children should be differentiated from true refractory cytopenia (RC), which is an early stage of MDS (Niemeyer and Baumann 2011). Criteria for diagnosis of RC have been published, but there is no consensus. Objective discriminatory features include (1) clonal marrow cytogenetic abnormalities, particularly complex cytogenetic abnormalities or −7/−7q, and (2) prominent dysplasia in at least two cell lineages and in at least 10% of the cells in each lineage. Unfortunately, even these criteria are not entirely predictive of no response to IST (Hama et al. 2015). Some other features that have been used to define RC are difficult to reproduce and may sometimes reflect evolving stages of the aplastic process. Also, if mainly morphological criteria are used to define RC, the overall response to treatment with IST and risk of malignant progression is similar between RC and AA (Hama et al. 2015; Yoshimi et al. 2014).

The tests above are mainly aimed to determine whether the child's cytopenia is due to AA. After establishing this diagnosis, a second set of tests are performed to discover a potential cause or associated disorders.

Careful attention should be paid to a possible diagnosis of underlying IBMFS. These patients do not achieve remission if treated with standard medical treatment for acquired AA and may suffer substantial toxicity if treated with nonmodified regimens for HSCT. The patient past medical history, family medical history, and careful physical examination likely allow most cases of IBMFSs to be ruled out. However, a yet undetermined proportion of patients with AA that do not have a family history suggestive of an IBMFS or physical malformations, may still have an underlying IBMFS (Ghemlas et al. 2015). Therefore, whenever possible, screening tests for an underlying IBMFS should be urgently initiated before treatment decisions are made. An ultrasonographic examination of the patient's abdomen is useful in the setting of AA as it may reveal physical malformations. X-rays of the large bones and joints may reveal osteopenia (as seen in many IBMFSs), radial anomalies (as seen in Fanconi anemia), metaphyseal dysplasia (as seen in dyskeratosis congenita), and radioulnar synostosis (as seen in thrombocytopenia associated with radioulnar synostosis). However, unless necessary for ruling out acute complications such as infections or bleeding, the authors do not recommend performing these tests before a diagnosis of an IBMFSs has been attempted by other methods. The reason is the high risk of cancer in several IBMFSs, which may be augmented by radiation from certain imaging modalities. Other screening testing for IBMFSs may vary and is based on clinical suspicion, time, and cost/effectiveness of testing. As of 2016, the most widely performed tests to rule out specific common IBMFSs are chromosome fragility testing, telomere length assessment, and exocrine pancreatic enzyme-level measurement (Williams et al. 2014). Chromosome fragility testing with mitomycin C and/or diepoxybutane to rule out Fanconi anemia and telomere length measurement to identify cases with very short telomeres and to rule out telomere-related disorders are critically important and have a relatively rapid turnaround time. Measurement of exocrine pancreatic enzyme levels (particularly serum pancreatic isoamylase and trypsinogen), together with ultrasonographic examination of the abdomen, are useful screening tests for Shwachman-Diamond syndrome (Dror et al. 2011). Improvement in performing and interpreting results of next-generation sequencing panels of genes that are mutated in IBMFSs might prove to be cost-effective and may replace some or all other screening tests for IBMFSs.

A work-up for PNH is recommended, although this is a very uncommon finding in childhood AA. Deficiency of CD55 and CD59 on erythrocytes, granulocytes, and monocytes can be demonstrated by flow cytometry, which is a reliable test for detecting PNH clones with a sensitivity of 1% (Philpott et al. 1995). Fluorescein-labeled proaerolysin (FLAER) is a modified compound of aerolysin that is conjugated to fluorochrome and binds to cell surface GPI-linked structures without causing cell lysis. Aerolysin is a virulent factor of the bacterium *Aeromonas hydrophila*. This test increases the sensitivity of detecting GPI-negative clones to 0.01–0.5% but cannot be used for red blood cells. These tests have largely replaced the Ham's acid serum test, in which lowering the pH of fresh plasma from 7.0 to 6.5 resulted in the lysis of PNH red blood cells, as they are deficient in the complement inhibitors, CD55 and CD59.

Measurement of serum vitamin B12 and red blood cell folate should also be made to exclude dietary deficiency as a cause of pancytopenia and red blood cell macrocytosis or factors that may aggravate cytopenia related to AA. A limited immune work-up may implicate other etiologies and direct therapy differently. This might include quantitative immunoglobulin levels. Testing for a systemic autoimmune disorder may include antinuclear antibody, rheumatic factor, and C3/C4 complement factors.

Testing for a possible viral etiology may include cytomegalovirus; Epstein-Barr virus; parvovirus B19; hepatitis A, B, and C; human immunodeficiency virus; and herpes simplex virus type 6. These tests are also useful as a baseline before transfusion and before IST that may increase the risk of viral activation. Bone marrow may also be tested for viruses by culture or polymerase chain reaction if aplasia is suspected to be due to a viral infection. If leukoreduced products are not available, a patient's cytomegalovirus status may have an impact on the choice of blood products used in supportive measures; under such circumstances, the authors recommend that a cytomegalovirus-negative patient should ideally be offered cytomegalovirus-safe blood products wherever possible and cytomegalovirus-negative products within 4 weeks of HSCT.

A third set of tests is required to evaluate the general health of the child and to rule out associated illnesses. Liver function tests, plasma electrolytes, urea, creatinine, glucose, and urinalysis are useful before specific therapy is administered. Extended red blood cell antigen phenotyping is recommended, in addition to routine blood group and antibody screen. Provision of phenotypically matched red blood cells for transfusion would reduce sensitization, particularly in patients requiring long-term transfusion support. This is not always feasible or practical.

HLA typing of the patient and first-degree relatives is advisable at diagnosis, even when HSCT is not conducted as the first-line treatment, to facilitate the search for a suitable bone marrow donor in case treatment with IST is unsuccessful.

2.9 Treatment

2.9.1 Supportive Care

The mainstay of therapy is supportive care, while investigations into etiology of AA are ongoing, and specific treatment options are being considered and arranged. Chronic platelet and red blood cell transfusions treat and prevent major bleeding episodes and maintain hemoglobin, and antibiotics treat infections. Blood products should be matched, irradiated, and leukoreduced to prevent the risk of transfusion reactions, transfusion-associated GVHD, and to provide CMV-safe blood, respectively. CMV-negative blood products are not necessary if products are properly leukoreduced and processed to be CMV safe. Single-donor platelet units may be considered if readily available to reduce the risk of alloimmunization. Although transfusion of leukoreduced platelets has been shown to reduce refractoriness to repeated platelet transfusions, there is no data that this practice reduces the risk of graft failure post-HSCT. Donation of blood products from family members is not advisable, as HSCT using related donors might be warranted in the future. Using family members may increase the recipient risk of developing major and minor HLA alloantibodies to family donor products that can then persist into transplant and increase the risk of graft rejection.

Maintaining hemoglobin with transfusion of red blood cells allows for normal activities. Children can generally handle transfusion thresholds between 60 and 70 g/L. Platelet transfusion support to treat and prevent life-threatening bleeding has probably resulted in the largest impact on the survival of patients with SAA. It has changed the leading cause of death from bleeding to infections. Reducing the transfusion threshold to 10 × 10^9/L in a stable patient has been found to be safe (Sagmeister et al. 1999). Other measures to prevent bleeding include avoidance of antiplatelet agents (e.g., nonsteroidal anti-inflammatory drugs) and activities that increase risk of falls, head injury, and trauma.

The risk of serious bacterial and fungal infections correlates with the neutrophil count and duration of severe neutropenia. This risk is exacerbated during IST or HSCT. Prophylaxis for *Pneumocystis jiroveci* and fungal infections should be considered during IST. Neutropenic patients with fever should be treated aggressively with broad-spectrum antibiotics. Antifungal agents at treatment dosages should be added when a fungus is identified or suspected, when patients are prescribed broad-spectrum antibiotics for longer than 4–5 days and/or when fever persists despite adequate antibiotic coverage for more than 4–5 days.

2.9.2 Hematopoietic Stem Cell Transplantation: Matched Sibling Donor Hematopoietic Stem Cell Transplant

The first successful HSCT in a patient with SAA was reported in 1970 (Mathe et al. 1970). HSCT from an HLA-matched first-degree-related donor was established as the best therapy for children and young adults with SAA during the 1970s (Camitta et al. 1976), and early HSCT with such donors is widely considered as standard of care first-line therapy for children and young adults afflicted with SAA. Several trials report overall survivals of 79–100% following matched sibling donor HSCT (Locasciulli 2002; Sanders et al. 1994; Ades et al. 2004; Storb et al. 2001; Kojima et al. 2000a; Bacigalupo et al. 2015; Dufour et al. 2015a, b). In a large report, 16 of 23 patients given syngeneic marrow without preparation failed to engraft (Hinterberger et al. 1997). Thus, the need for conditioning therapy was established as essential. Cyclophosphamide (200 mg/kg over 4 days) is the most commonly used conditioning agent in HSCT for SAA. Following the publication of excellent results from the Seattle group, there has been increasing enthusiasm for the use of cyclophosphamide with ATG without irradiation (Ades et al. 2004; Storb et al. 2001), showing superior survival outcomes, in the order of 80–90% (Locasciulli 2002; Storb et al. 2001), in contrast to 55–67% when irradiation-based conditioning is used (Passweg et al. 1997).

Failed engraftment in up to 32% of patients was a significant problem in matched sibling HSCT for SAA in the 1970s (McCann et al. 1994). Early transplantation with minimal pretransplant transfusions, the addition of irradiation and a marrow nucleated cell dose of >3 × 10^8 cells/kg all decreased the incidence of graft rejection (Sanders et al. 1994; McCann et al. 1994; Gluckman et al. 1992). The use of cyclosporine in the GVHD prophylactic regimens was also associated with lower rates of graft failure (McCann et al. 1994; Gluckman et al. 1992). Thus, recent favored conditioning regimens incorporate cyclophosphamide and ATG without irradiation, followed by cyclosporine and a short course of methotrexate as GVHD prophylaxis. These reduce the engraftment failure rate to <5%, even in heavily pretreated patients (Storb et al. 2001).

Acute GVHD of grades II–IV (Ades et al. 2004; Gluckman et al. 1992), with a cumulative incidence of over 40%, was seen in a French study when regimens incorporating thoracoabdominal irradiation were used (Ades et al. 2004). The use of cyclosporine with methotrexate, in particular when ATG is in the conditioning regimen, reduces the incidence of acute GVHD to ~11% (Storb et al. 1991). The incidence of chronic GVHD has not been influenced by cyclosporine and occurs in about 30% of patients (Sanders et al. 1994; Storb et al. 2001), one-fifth of whom die of associated complications (Sanders et al. 1994).

Recently, there have been single- and multicenter reports on the successful use of the fludarabine/cyclophosphamide/campath H (FCC) regimen in adults and a smaller number of children. This regimen consists of fludarabine (30 mg/m^2 over 4 days), low-dose cyclophosphamide

(300 mg/m^2 over 4 days), and alemtuzumab (40–100 mg). Overall survival and event-free survival are between 95% and 100% and similar to those observed with the current ATG and cyclophosphamide regimens (Marsh et al. 2011, 2014; Deeg 2011; Siegal et al. 2008). Acute and chronic GVHD are seen in decreased numbers compared to ATG-based regimens, and in only ~11–13% of patients, with the majority of GVHD being mild (acute I–II and chronic mild) (Marsh et al. 2014; Grimaldi et al. 2017). Stable mixed T-cell chimerism is seen alongside full donor myeloid engraftment with the FCC regimen even after cessation of post-graft immunosuppression, suggesting a state of mutual immunological tolerance, without an increase in incidence of viral disease.

2.9.3 Immunosuppressive Therapy

There is a one in four chance that each fully biological sibling of an individual with SAA will be an HLA match for HSCT. In fact, only ~15% of patients with SAA have a sibling-matched donor. Less than 1% of patients have a fully HLA-matched parent donor. Clearly, alternative therapy to related HLA-matched HSCT is the reality for the large majority of patients with SAA. Until recently, IST was widely accepted as the next best therapeutic option. Currently, some are advocating for well-matched unrelated donor HSCT instead of IST as the second treatment of choice due to the risks of no response, relapse, and leukemic transformation seen with IST therapy.

Autologous bone marrow reconstitution was noted in the late 1960s and early 1970s, in a number of patients who received mismatched marrows (Mathe et al. 1970; Jeannet et al. 1976). This was also observed in some patients who were conditioned with cyclophosphamide and ATG but did not proceed to HSCT. These clinical observations, combined with the extensive laboratory data discussed in the Pathogenesis and Etiology sections above, strongly suggested immune mechanisms in the pathogenesis of AA and led to the development of IST regimens in the treatment of SAA (Speck et al. 1977).

Antilymphocyte globulin even without other agents or modalities has been shown to be more effective than supportive care alone (Champlin et al. 1983). Survival ranged from 30% to 70%, with responses typically occurring within the first 3–6 months following therapy. Two ATG products are widely available for the treatment of SAA: equine ATG (e.g., Atgam; Pharmacia & Upjohn, Milton Keynes, UK) usually administered at 100–160 mg/kg, in divided doses over 4–10 days and rabbit ATG (e.g., Thymoglobulin; Imtix-Sangstat, Lyon, France) given in doses of 2.5–3.5 mg/kg/day for 4–5 days (Di Bona et al. 1999). Cyclosporine was also shown to be effective in the treatment of AA (Frickhofen et al. 1991, 2003; Rosenfeld et al. 2003). The German group compared ATG and methylprednisolone versus ATG, methylprednisolone, and cyclosporine (Frickhofen et al. 1991, 2003). The response rate at 3 months was significantly higher in the group receiving cyclosporine (65% versus 39%; $p < 0.03$), primarily because of an increased response rate in patients with severe disease. Response was achieved sooner in the group receiving cyclosporine and plateaued by 6 months (Frickhofen et al. 2003). Recent smaller studies are showing similar response rates when tacrolimus is used instead of cyclosporine, with fewer side effects such as hirsutism and gingival hyperplasia (Macartney et al. 2009; Alsultan et al. 2009; Zhu et al. 2014).

A landmark randomized trial done in children and adults showed clear superiority of equine over rabbit ATG when used with cyclosporine with respect to response rates at 6 months (68% versus 37%; $p < 0.001$) and 3-year overall survival (96% versus 76%; $p = 0.04$) when events were censored at time of transplant (Scheinberg et al. 2011). Similar results were seen in a single-center retrospective trial of adults and children in Brazil (Atta et al. 2010) and a multicenter prospective trial of adults (Marsh et al. 2012). A multicenter prospective trial of children also showed superiority of equine ATG when compared to rabbit ATG with respect to response at 6 months (65% versus 34%; $p = 0.003$) and transplantation-free survival at 3 years (73% versus 30%; $p < 0.001$). Overall survival at 3 years was 92% in both groups, due to early successful salvage with HSCT (Yoshimi et al. 2013). A larger, retrospective study showed no difference in response at 6 months but demonstrated a significant improvement in survival at 2 and 10 years in the equine ATG group versus rabbit ATG (2-year overall survival, 96% versus 87%; 10-year overall survival, 92% versus 84%; $p = 0.004$). On the basis of multivariate analysis, use of rabbit ATG was a significant adverse factor for overall survival (hazard ratio = 3.56, 95% confidence interval, 1.53–8.28, $p = 0.003$) (Jeong et al. 2014). Thus, unless equine ATG is not available, children with SAA who require IST should receive this formulation of ATG. Acute allergic reactions are common. Immune complex-mediated serum sickness typically manifests 10–14 days after initiation of therapy. These adverse effects have largely been ameliorated by the concurrent administration of prednisone, usually at 1–2 mg/kg/day, and premedication with antihistamines and acetaminophen.

The EBMT compared ATG and methylprednisolone with or without oxymetholone (Bacigalupo et al. 1993). Responses were significantly higher in the oxymetholone arm at 120 days (68% versus 48%; $p = 0.02$). Unfortunately, the overall survival at 3 years did not reach statistical difference (71% with versus 65% without). Similarly, the addition of G-CSF to the combination of ATG and cyclosporine has shown no significant benefit either in terms of morbidity or survival (Tichelli et al. 2011; Gluckman et al. 2002; Teramura et al. 2007), although it may reduce infectious complications and duration of hospital admissions (Tichelli et al. 2011).

Children treated with IST generally have better survival outcomes compared to adults (Rosenfeld et al. 2003; Locasciulli et al. 2004). The reported response and survival rates over the last two decades are variable and range from 54% to 100%, averaging about 70–80% for response rate and about 90% for overall survival rate (Locasciulli 2002; Dufour et al. 2015a; Yoshimi et al. 2013; Jeong et al. 2014; Gillio et al. 1997; Fouladi et al. 2000; Fuhrer et al. 1998; Kojima et al. 2000b; Samarasinghe et al. 2014; Narita and Kojima 2016). This variability in outcomes may reflect the heterogeneity of treatment response definitions and treatment regimes, including administration of hematopoietic growth factors, length and dose of immunosuppression with cyclosporine, the inclusion of patients with clonal marrow cytogenetic abnormalities, and the inclusion of patients with IBMFSs. Combination of IST commonly used in most centers treating children with acquired AA consists of equine ATG, cyclosporine, and low- or intermediate-dose corticosteroids. The authors use Atgam 40 mg/kg/day for 4 days, prednisone 1 mg/kg/dose twice daily for 7 days followed by a slow wean over 3 weeks, and cyclosporine 6 mg/kg/dose twice daily to maintain blood levels of 150–200 μg/L.

There are a many studies in adults and children that have assessed predictive factors for response to IST. Some of these factors should be studied prospectively (Narita and Kojima 2016; Scheinberg et al. 2009). Very severe disease and having a minor PNH clone seem to be associated with an increased chance at response and better overall survival in children (Narita et al. 2015; Narita and Kojima 2016). Telomere lengths are generally viewed as markers of aging because they shorten with each cell division (Mather et al. 2011). In patients with AA, short telomeres are thought to be secondary to hematopoietic stress (Brummendorf et al. 2001). Mutations in telomerase complex genes resulting in extremely short telomeres have been described in some patients clinically diagnosed with acquired SAA (Yamaguchi et al. 2005; Ball et al. 1998; Brummendorf et al. 2001; Calado and Young 2008). A large study including mostly adult patients reported that shorter baseline leukocyte telomere lengths were associated with increased risk of relapse and clonal transformation, and decreased overall survival, but not hematologic response. A small study of children with SAA showed that very short telomeres in granulocytes, but not other leukocyte subsets, were associated with worse response to IST (Tutelman et al. 2014). Other studies limited to children showed that short lymphocyte telomere lengths were associated with significantly poorer response to IST, but not to relapse rate, clonal evolution, or overall survival (Narita et al. 2015; Sakaguchi et al. 2014). In a study from Japan, children with AA who had very short telomere lengths (typically considered as <1st percentile for age) had only a 12% chance of responding to IST (Narita et al. 2015). The magnitude and duration of response was not mentioned in this study. Thus, it seems that both in adults and children, having shorter telomere lengths is associated with poorer response to IST. This, in combination with the degree of severity of AA and the presence of minor PNH clones, should be considered when weighing options of IST versus other treatment modalities for SAA.

Patients who fail to respond to the initial course of IST still have a chance of response to a repeat course using ATG from the same or an alternative animal source (Camitta et al. 1976; Di Bona et al. 1999; Schrezenmeier et al. 1995; Tichelli et al. 1998; Scheinberg et al. 2006; Kosaka et al. 2008). There does not appear to be value in repeating more than two courses of IST in non-responders (Gupta et al. 2005). The EBMT SAA studied a group of children and adults and reported a 43% chance of response to a second treatment with the same equine ATG source after initial failure. In this study, actuarial survival at 13 years of those who responded after two courses was 68.5% versus 24.4% in those who did not receive a second course. There was no significant increase in adverse effects following repeated ATG (Schrezenmeier et al. 1995). A few years later, a study looking at patients under 40 years of age showed a 64% response rate to a second course of ATG in those who failed the first course. The cumulative survival at 10 years was 55%, and there was an increased risk of allergic reactions, namely, type I hypersensitivity reactions, with the second course of the same equine ATG source (Tichelli et al. 1998). Both studies noted a longer time to response with the second course of IST compared to the first, requiring 6 months or longer. A more recent prospective multicenter study looking only at children reported a mere 33% chance of response at 12 months with the same equine ATG source (Kosaka et al. 2008). A few studies have looked at using rabbit ATG for a second course of treatment in non-responders who received equine ATG as first-line therapy, as a way to potentially decrease allergic reactions and theoretically increase response rate by using a different ATG source. Response rates have varied between 33% and 77%, and short-term survival at 2–3 years has varied between 70% and 100% (Di Bona et al. 1999; Scheinberg et al. 2006), not showing clear superiority of using rabbit ATG over equine ATG in non-responders. There are no reported increases in side effects using this regimen, and there does not seem to be a significant difference in the risk of clonal disorders between patients receiving a single or multiple courses of ATG, irrespective of ATG source (Tichelli et al. 1992; Marsh et al. 2011; Siegal et al. 2008).

Relapse of disease occurs in a significant proportion of patients with SAA who are treated with IST. An older study on pediatric SAA showed a 33% relapse rate at 10 years (Marsh et al. 2014); however, more recent data in pediatric SAA show much lower relapse rates of about 15% at 10 years post diagnosis and treatment (Pitcher et al. 1999; Ades et al. 2004; Frickhofen et al. 2003; Kamio et al. 2011).

Finally, patients treated with IST continue to manifest defects in the number and function of hematopoietic progenitors (Maciejewski et al. 1996; Marsh et al. 1990; Schrezenmeier et al. 1996; Novitzky and Jacobs 1995). IST reduces, but does not eradicate, pathogenic T-cell clones even in patients who respond, paving the way for clonal diseases such a MDS and AML later on (Zeng et al. 2001; Risitano et al. 2004). In fact, the risk of pediatric patients developing MDS or AML when treated with IST is about 10% at 5–10 years from diagnosis with SAA (Ades et al. 2004; Frickhofen et al. 2003; Jeong et al. 2014; Kamio et al. 2011; Jiang et al. 2013; Kulasekararaj et al. 2014; Scheinberg et al. 2008), one of the major driving forces behind improving HSCT outcomes and thus decreasing this risk to ~1%.

There were promising results from an early pilot study of high-dose cyclophosphamide without HSCT in SAA (Brodsky et al. 1996). However, a prospective randomized study comparing ATG and cyclosporine with or without cyclophosphamide had to be terminated prematurely due to unacceptable incidence of invasive fungal infections and early deaths in the later arm (Tisdale et al. 2000). Follow-up of the survivors showed responses in 46% compared to 75% in the ATG group, with no difference in relapse rate or clonal evolution (Tisdale et al. 2002). A recent pediatric study showed good response to cyclophosphamide monotherapy, but cumulative incidences of bacterial and fungal infections remained high with this regimen (86% and 62%, respectively) (Gamper et al. 2016). Overall, this treatment has not received wide acceptance (Williams et al. 2014); however, selected patients may benefit from cyclophosphamide. The authors have successfully treated a patient with severe aplastic anemia and symptomatic central nervous system vasculitis with cyclophosphamide 500 mg/m^2 per dose for 7 monthly doses, followed by maintenance therapy with mycophenolate mofetil for 18 months (unpublished data from the Canadian Aplastic Anemia and Myelodysplasia Study, Approved by The Hospital for Sick Children's Research Ethics Board—REB#1000048159).

2.9.4 Hematopoietic Stem Cell Transplantation: Alternative Donor Hematopoietic Stem Cell Transplant

Matched sibling donors for HSCT are available in only ~15% of cases. Less than 1% of patients have a fully HLA-matched parent donor. Thus, much attention has been given in recent years to unrelated matched donor HSCT for patients with SAA. This is because when compared to IST, transplantation offers a more complete restoration of hematopoiesis, lower relapse rates, and better protection against secondary cancers. However, unrelated donor HSCT generally requires more intensive conditioning therapy to prevent graft failure and greater post-infusion immunosuppression to prevent GVHD than transplant from a related donor. Thus, unrelated donor HSCT introduces higher treatment-related mortality than IST and raises the concern for significant morbidity secondary to organ toxicity from conditioning chemotherapy and GVHD. Finally, since earlier treatment is associated with better outcome, availability of donors and length of time from diagnosis to HSCT plays an important role in decision-making.

The outcomes of HSCT from a fully matched unrelated donor for SAA are improving dramatically, due to availability of high-resolution HLA typing allowing for better donor selection, improvement in supportive care, and use of less toxic conditioning regimens. In a multicentered North American report of 141 pretreated patients (median age 17.7 years) who received HSCT from unrelated donors for SAA, favorable outcomes were associated with age <20 years (overall survival of 63%), HSCT within 3 years of diagnosis, and HLA-DRB1 matching (56% vs. 15% at 3 years) (Deeg et al. 1999). Investigators in Japan reported overall survival of 69% at 5 years for those under the age of 20 years. In addition to older age, other unfavorable factors for outcome were transplantation after 3 years from diagnosis, molecularly determined HLA-A or B mismatch, and conditioning without ATG (Kojima et al. 2002a). More recent retrospective reports in pediatric patients pretreated with immunosuppressive therapy, who failed this treatment, show failure-free survivals at 5 years approaching 95% (Samarasinghe et al. 2012).

Outcomes with HSCT have improved over the last decade, such that some support proceeding directly to unrelated donor HSCT if there is no matched sibling donor available and if it can be done in a timely fashion, rather than the standard procedure of using IST (Samarasinghe et al. 2014). A collaborative study in nine UK pediatric centers between 2005 and 2014 included 29 children who proceeded to upfront unrelated HSCT, and compared them to matched historical controls, who had undergone first-line therapy with a matched sibling/family donor HSCT, or IST with equine ATG and cyclosporine, or second-line therapy with unrelated donor HSCT post-failed IST. The 2-year overall survival in the upfront cohort was ~96% compared to 91% in the matched sibling donor controls, 94% in the IST controls, and 74% in the unrelated donor HSCT post-IST failure controls. The 2-year event-free survival in the upfront cohort was 92%, compared to 87% in the matched sibling donor controls, 40% in IST controls, and 74% in the unrelated donor HSCT post-IST failure controls. In fact, upfront unrelated donor HSCT was significantly superior in overall survival and event-free survival to unrelated donor HSCT after failed IST and significantly superior to event-free survival with IST (Dufour et al. 2015b). Similar results have been reported in other smaller studies (Choi et al. 2017; Mortensen et al. 2016). The cumulative incidence of acute and chronic GVHD was higher in the unrelated donor HSCT group compared to the matched sibling group, but similar when compared to the unrelated donor HSCT group after failed IST (Bacigalupo et al. 2015; Dufour et al. 2015b). For children, a benefit of unrelated donor HSCT over a second course of IST was reported from Japan and others. The 5-year overall survival in the Japanese cohort was similar between the two groups, but failure-free survival was significantly lower (84%) for transplanted patients compared to those who received further IST (9%) (Yagasaki et al. 2014). A recent multicenter trial showed success with a conditioning regimen that includes equine/rabbit ATG 30 mg/kg/day or 3 mg/kg/day, respectively, cyclophosphamide 50 mg/kg, fludarabine 30 mg/m^2/day, and low-dose total body irradiation (Anderlini et al. 2015). Cyclophosphamide toxicity was reduced, and engraftment and long-term survival were improved with this regimen combination. In addition, excellent results with conditioning regimens using alemtuzumab have been reported, showing excellent overall survival and decreased incidence of GVHD (Dufour et al. 2015b; Marsh et al. 2011; Vassiliou et al. 2001).

HSCT with hematopoietic stem cells from an HLA-haploidentical family member donor (usually a parent) has gradually improved and has also been successfully applied in the setting of SAA (Bacigalupo et al. 1988; Wagner et al. 1996; Esteves et al. 2015; Liu et al. 2016), although the reported cases are small. Haploidentical transplant has a role in patients with SAA who fail conventional treatment with IST or develop clonal disease and have no other curative options.

The use of umbilical cord blood (UCB) as a source of stem cells for HSCT has been expanding. Although unrelated UCB was shown to be a promising source of hematopoietic stem cells for transplantation in general, the results of its use specifically in the setting of AA have been inferior to several other transplant cell sources. In adult and pediatric patients with SAA, using UCB as the stem cell source resulted in a 3-year overall survival of ~40% (Peffault de Latour et al. 2011; Kuwatsuka et al. 2016), which is substantially inferior to results of transplantation from live-unrelated donors. In one study, the only factor associated with improved survival was a total nucleated cell dose of >3.7 × 10^7/kg (Peffault de Latour et al. 2011). The main challenge with using UCB in transplanting patients with AA has been lower engraftment rates. The relatively longer time to engraftment when UCB is used might be another factor that increases the risk of infections in patients who have had a long time of severe neutropenia before transplant. A smaller study with Japanese adult patients reported a 3-year overall survival of 83% with UCB transplant with no grade III or IV acute GVHD or extensive chronic GVHD (Yamamoto et al. 2011). Thus, modifications of the transplant preparatory regimens and/or usage of multiple UCB samples might improve outcome. Currently, the use of UCB should probably be reserved to patients with AA who do not have other curative options (including haploidentical donors) or to participation in clinical trials.

2.9.5 Late Effects

Long-term sequelae post-HSCT for SAA are not well studied. A recent large multicenter retrospective study looked at 1718 patients from 186 centers. One thousand, one hundred, and seventy-six patients received a matched sibling HSCT at a median age of 20 years, while 542 patients received an unrelated HSCT at a median age of 20 years, between 1995 and 2006. Median follow-up for both groups was ~5.5 years (Buchbinder et al. 2012). The prevalence of at least one late effect at 5 years was 11% in the matched sibling group and 25% in the unrelated donor group. Multiple late effects at this time point were seen in 2% of patients in the matched sibling group versus 14% in the unrelated donor group. Among the matched sibling donor group, the cumulative incidence of late effects was ≤3% and was not significantly different in those transplanted during pediatric age versus adult age. Gonadal dysfunction represented the most common late effect in both matched sibling and unrelated donor groups. The cumulative incidence of developing gonadal dysfunction over the next 5 years in the matched sibling group was 3% versus 10.5% in the unrelated donor group. Cumulative growth disturbance in the next 5 years in the matched sibling versus unrelated donor groups was 0.5% versus 7.2%, respectively. Pediatric patients were more likely to experience growth disturbance (14% of patients) compared to adult patients (0% of patients). Inclusion of irradiation in preparatory regimens has been shown to be a risk factor for reduced ultimate height in pediatric patients (Cohen et al. 1999). Sixty-eight percent of patients who received an unrelated donor HSCT received irradiation in this large retrospective study.

A retrospective study of 137 pediatric patients transplanted for idiopathic SAA between 1971 and 2009, at a median age of 11 years and followed for a median of 21.8 years assessed the development of late effect over four decades (Sanders et al. 2011). Height growth was not significantly affected by HSCT, the majority of pediatric patients progress normally through puberty, and pregnancies were successful in this group, even after high-dose cyclophosphamide. Twenty-three percent of patients who had TBI in their conditioning regimen and 8.4% of patients who did not receive TBI developed thyroid function abnormalities.

Secondary malignant tumors are of concern after successful HSCT. Although MDS and leukemia of donor origin can develop in up to 1% of patients after HSCT for AA (Townsley et al. 2016; Holmberg et al. 1994; Dilloo et al. 1995), the more common concern is solid tumors. Older studies reported an incidence of 3.5% of secondary malignancies among patients with AA at 10 years (Kolb et al. 1999), ~12% at 15 years (Ades et al. 2004; Kolb et al. 1999), and 13% at 20 years post-HSCT (Deeg et al. 1996), respectively. Risk factors include treatment of GVHD with azathioprine and cyclosporine, use of irradiation, chronic GVHD, and male sex (Ades et al. 2004; Sanders et al. 2011; Kolb et al. 1999; Deeg et al. 1996). In the more recent multicentered study, the cumulative incidence of developing a solid tumor at 5 years post-transplant was 0.3% in the matched sibling group versus 1.6% in the unrelated donor group (Buchbinder et al. 2012). Sites of disease included thyroid, esophagus, lung, colon, and soft tissue, among others. The risk of lymphoma was low in both groups: 0.1% and 0.6% for matched sibling donor and unrelated donor, respectively, at 5 years of follow-up. In a smaller pediatric study, 13% of patients developed a secondary malignancy at 1–31 years post-transplant (Fouladi et al. 2000). The most common malignancy was squamous cell carcinoma, occurring mostly in patients with significant skin chronic GVHD, followed by breast cancer and thyroid malignancy. Others included hepatocarcinoma secondary to hepatitis C, melanoma, and myelodysplastic syndrome. The outcome of patients who develop secondary malignancy is poor.

2.9.6 Androgens and Growth Factors

Androgens have no role as a single-treatment agent for acquired SAA (Camitta et al. 1979) and have not proven to improve response or survival when given in combination with other therapy. One study demonstrated an increased rate of response in females with severe aplasia, who received oxymetholone with IST, but this did not translate into improved survival (Bacigalupo et al. 1993). Responses have been described in a small proportion of patients with acquired disease (Marwaha et al. 2004). Since most patients with an IBMFS respond to androgens, it is possible that the reported responses are in patients with an undiagnosed inherited disorder, rather than acquired AA.

Growth factors such as G-CSF, GM-CSF, and IL-3 have been used as single agents in AA (Gluckman et al. 2002; Kojima et al. 2000b;

Guinan et al. 1990; Hord et al. 1995; Kojima and Matsuyama 1994; Ganser et al. 1990), but responses are rare and transient, and very high doses are sometimes necessary to achieve response. Several studies have examined the impact of adding G-CSF to IST on response and long-term survival (Gluckman et al. 2002; Kojima et al. 2000b). Although the use of G-CSF improved neutrophil counts in many patients, there did not seem to be significant differences in the rates of infectious episodes, overall hematological response, or survival (Gluckman et al. 2002; Kojima et al. 2000b). In the presences of documented or suspected bacterial or fungal infection and very severe neutropenia, it is reasonable to administer G-CSF in an attempt to raise neutrophil production and assist in resolving the infection.

Old studies that evaluated the effect of thrombopoietics in patients with thrombocytopenia demonstrated a high incidence of developing life-threatening refractory thrombocytopenia due to autoantibody formation. Two thrombomimetic small molecules, eltrombopag and romiplostim, have been developed for refractory immune thrombocytopenia and have recently entered clinical trials of SAA. These molecules bind and activate the thrombopoietin receptor with high efficiency and specificity. Eltrombopag is a small molecule agonist of the thrombopoietin receptor (c-mpl), which is expressed on hematopoietic stem cells and on cells throughout megakaryocytic development. There are recent reports of its successful use in mostly adult patients with relapsed or refractory to therapy SAA. Some adults achieved trilineage response and improvement in blood counts, and in some, response was maintained even upon discontinuation of the growth factor (Desmond et al. 2014; Olnes et al. 2012). As with G-CSF, there is concern that eltrombopag may promote growth or survival of leukemic clones. Since the thrombopoietin receptor is expressed on hematopoietic stem cells, there is also concern that eltrombopag may increase the risk of clonal evolution. This needs to be further clarified with prospective, long-term follow-up studies. There are no published studies of eltrombopag use in children with SAA. Currently, clinical trials are under way to assess the benefit of adding eltrombopag upfront to standard IST in terms of response and overall and event-free survival. There are no published reports on the use of romiplostim in AA. One adult patient in a case series of refractory SAA patients received eltrombopag and romiplostim without effect (Gill et al. 2017).

2.9.7 Myelodysplastic Syndrome and Acute Myeloid Leukemia

Several large studies have demonstrated an increased risk of MDS and/or AML in survivors of SAA who have been treated with supportive care, androgens, or IST (Hibbs et al. 1992; Kim et al. 1997; Rosenfeld et al. 2003). Clonal marrow cytogenetic abnormalities can appear without morphological signs of MDS/AML. In one study, in 50% of cases with marrow cytogenetic abnormalities after IST, the aberrant clone was present at diagnosis but detected retrospectively (Fuhrer et al. 1998). Those with somatic mutations also have an increased risk of progressing to MDS/AML. The actuarial risk of MDS/AML in pediatric patients with AA is ~10% at 5–10 years post-IST (Doney et al. 1997; Jeong et al. 2014; Jiang et al. 2013; Kulasekararaj et al. 2014; Scheinberg et al. 2008; Maciejewski et al. 2002; Kojima et al. 2002b; Garanito et al. 2014). A recent pediatric study described clonal evolution in over 30% of their patients with SAA. All patients with clonal evolution had very severe disease, all but one developed monosomy 7, and all received G-CSF for more than 40 days. The cumulative incidence of clonal evolution at 10 years in this study was ~10% (Hama et al. 2015). The most common chromosomal abnormalities are monosomy 7 (40–50%) and trisomy 8 (Linet et al. 1986; Kulasekararaj et al. 2014; Maciejewski et al. 2002; Ohara et al. 1997; Maciejewski and Selleri 2004), and patients with monosomy 7 and complex cytogenetics have higher rates of transformation to AML (Maciejewski et al. 2002). As MDS/AML have also been reported in patients who received androgens or were treated with supportive care without IST (Najean and Haguenauer 1990; Mir and Geary 1980), it is likely that patients with AA have an inherent predisposition to malignant myeloid transformation, although the mechanism is unclear. MDS/AML secondary to AA are associated with poor survival.

Acquired AA is an immune-mediated bone marrow failure disorder with clonal hematopoiesis. The majority of adult (Kulasekararaj et al. 2014; Afable II et al. 2011; Marsh and Mufti 2016; Ogawa 2016; Lane et al. 2013; Yoshizato et al. 2015) and pediatric (Babushok et al. 2015) patients with AA have somatic mutations and/or structural chromosomal abnormalities detected as early as at diagnosis. In recent years, there has been a strong focus on understanding these mutations using single-nucleotide polymorphism array karyotyping, targeted next-generation deep sequencing, and whole-exome sequencing. The goal of these efforts is to better understand the etiology and pathophysiology of AA, to help tailor appropriate therapy, and to predict response to treatment and evolution to MDS/AML. In adults, the most common somatic alterations are nonmalignant clonal expansions of cells lacking glycophosphotidylinositol-anchored proteins and loss of human leukocyte antigen alleles, as well as leukemia-related mutations in *BCOR*/*BCORL1*, *ASXL1*, and *DNMT3A* (Afable II et al. 2011; Stanley et al. 2017; Shimamura 2016). In adult patients, mutations in *PIGA*, *BCOR*, and *BCORL1* have been shown to disappear or show stable clone size over time. This has correlated with a positive response to IST, and a significantly better outcome than that seen in patients with mutations is *ASXL1* and *DNMT3A*. Mutations in these genes have been shown likely to increase their clone size over time, and this has been associated with a lower response to IST, lower survival particularly in younger patients, and faster progression to MDS/AML. Despite these general findings, significant patient variability exists and makes it difficult to incorporate this information into clinical practice at this time. In addition, more comprehensive studies are needed in pediatric patients before this information can be extrapolated to this population. Testing for mutations that are proven to be associated with progression and can impact clinical decisions should be incorporated into the regular work-up and follow-up of patients with AA whenever possible.

In the past, genetic predisposition to AA, which comes with a significantly increased risk for MDS and AML compared to the acquired form of the disease, was thought to be rare. Diagnosis of a genetic predisposition relied on family history and physical examination. It is now well established that a significant number of patients with a genetic predisposition to AA, MDS or AML lack abnormal physical findings and have a negative family history for these disorders (Ghemlas et al. 2015; Zhang et al. 2015). Recent genomic screening of patients with idiopathic bone marrow failure or MDS identified germ line disorders in 5–10% of cases (Keel et al. 2016). Clearly, reliance solely on physical findings or family history when genetic tools are available is no longer appropriate. Therefore, easily accessible and timely genetic testing to help differentiate between germ line predisposition to AA and acquired disease is of utmost importance to have in the clinic and is crucial to choosing the correct treatment modality.

The relationship between G-CSF and MDS/AML in acquired AA is controversial (Kojima et al. 2002b; Bessho et al. 2003; Kaito et al. 1998). In a prospective randomized study of IST with and without G-CSF in children with acquired AA, the risk of clonal evolution was proportional to the duration of G-CSF administration, particularly if it was longer than 180 days. Failure to respond to IST at 6 months was another risk factor in multivariate analysis (Kojima et al. 2002b). An earlier report also identified the duration and cumulative dose of G-CSF therapy as risk factors in the development of MDS/AML in children with acquired AA (Ohara et al. 1997). Similar results have been reported in a randomized trial of adults and other retrospective studies (Hama et al. 2015; Teramura et al. 2007; Socie et al. 2007; Li et al. 2011). A more recent, non-randomized long-term follow-up study identified clonal evolution in over 30% of the children with AA. All patients had very severe disease and had been treated with G-CSF for more than 40 days (median 139 days; range 43–393 days) (Hama et al. 2015). Other studies, including a recent meta-analysis, have not confirmed these findings (Imashuku et al. 2003; Gluckman et al. 2002; Schrezenmeier et al. 1995; Locasciulli et al. 2001; Gurion et al. 2009). It is possible that G-CSF merely hastens the appearance of existing clones rather than triggering their evolution, since monosomy 7 is a common finding in AA and since G-CSF has been shown to promote the growth of monosomy 7 cells that express the class IV isoform of the G-CSF receptor (Sloand et al. 2006). No study has found a clear benefit of adding G-CSF to IST on overall mortality and survival. Therefore, unless clinically indicated for severe or frequent infections, G-CSF should not be routinely added to the IST regimen, and if added, the length and cumulative dose of treatment should be minimized.

2.9.8 Paroxysmal Nocturnal Hemoglobinuria

PNH is characterized by nonmalignant clonal expansion of hematopoietic cells due to acquired somatic mutations in the PIGA gene resulting in the absence of glycosyl phosphatidylinositol-anchored cell surface proteins. This disorder is associated with episodic intravascular hemolysis of red blood cells, and individuals with PNH are at increased risk of developing AA (Brodsky 2014). Clinical PNH rarely presents in childhood, but when it does, it presents as AA in the majority of children (Ware et al. 1991). Small numbers of PNH clones (<10%) are frequently observed in patients presenting with AA. Flow cytometry analysis indicates that 20–70% of pediatric AA patients possess minor PNH populations at the time of diagnosis but have no actual PNH disease (Tutelman et al. 2014; Kulagin et al. 2014; Yoshida et al. 2008). The cause of the high incidence of minor PNH populations in AA patients is unclear, but it is hypothesized that the absence of cell surface proteins allows cells to escape immune attack (Karadimitris et al. 2000). The absence of PNH in patients with hypocellular bone marrow due to chemotherapy, irradiation, and IBMFSs suggests that PNH clonal expansion is not merely the result of hematopoietic failure (Dunn et al. 1999; DeZern et al. 2014). Furthermore, the detection of PNH clones in treatment-naïve children and the absence of PNH in patients who received ATG for other reasons suggest that ATG-based therapy is not the cause (Dunn et al. 1999). Finally, the hypothesis that PNH is a late complication of AA is unlikely, given that PNH clones are present at the time of diagnosis with AA, and no patient with normal glycosylphosphatidylinositol-linked proteins at the time of diagnosis developed PNH clones after therapy (Dunn et al. 1999). Information is emerging that having minor PNH clones is associated with an increased chance of response to IST and better overall survival in children with SAA, but the mechanism of this remains to be elucidated (Narita and Kojima 2016).

Disclosure Informed written consent for participation in research studies was obtained from the patients whose figure was included in the present chapter, and the study was approved by The Hospital for Sick Children's Research Ethics Board.

References

Ades L, Mary JY, Robin M, Ferry C, Porcher R, Esperou H et al (2004) Long-term outcome after bone marrow transplantation for severe aplastic anemia. Blood 103(7):2490–2497

Afable MG II, Wlodarski M, Makishima H, Shaik M, Sekeres MA, Tiu RV et al (2011) SNP array-based karyotyping: differences and similarities between aplastic anemia and hypocellular myelodysplastic syndromes. Blood 117(25):6876–6884

Alsultan A, Goldenberg NA, Kaiser N, Graham DK, Hays T (2009) Tacrolimus as an alternative to cyclosporine in the maintenance phase of immunosuppressive therapy for severe aplastic anemia in children. Pediatr Blood Cancer 52(5):626–630

Anderlini P, Wu J, Gersten I, Ewell M, Tolar J, Antin JH et al (2015) Cyclophosphamide conditioning in patients with severe aplastic anaemia given unrelated marrow transplantation: a phase 1-2 dose de-escalation study. Lancet Haematol 2(9):e367–e375

Anderson KC, Weinstein HJ (1990) Transfusion-associated graft-versus-host disease. N Engl J Med 323(5):315–321

Atta EH, Dias DS, Marra VL, de Azevedo AM (2010) Comparison between horse and rabbit antithymocyte globulin as first-line treatment for patients with severe aplastic anemia: a single-center retrospective study. Ann Hematol 89(9):851–859

Babushok DV, Perdigones N, Perin JC, Olson TS, Ye W, Roth JJ et al (2015) Emergence of clonal hematopoiesis in the majority of patients with acquired aplastic anemia. Cancer Genet 208(4):115–128

Babushok DV, Grignon AL, Li Y, Atienza J, Xie HM, Lam HS et al (2016) Disrupted lymphocyte homeostasis in hepatitis-associated acquired aplastic anemia is associated with short telomeres. Am J Hematol 91(2):243–247

Bacigalupo A, Hows J, Gordon-Smith EC, Gluckman E, Van Lint MT, Congiu M et al (1988) Bone marrow transplantation for severe aplastic anemia from donors other than HLA identical siblings: a report of the BMT Working Party. Bone Marrow Transplant 3(6):531–535

Bacigalupo A, Chaple M, Hows J, Van Lint MT, McCann S, Milligan D et al (1993) Treatment of aplastic anaemia (AA) with antilymphocyte globulin (ALG) and methylprednisolone (MPred) with or without androgens: a randomized trial from the EBMT SAA working party. Br J Haematol 83(1):145–151

Bacigalupo A, Socie G, Hamladji RM, Aljurf M, Maschan A, Kyrcz-Krzemien S et al (2015) Current outcome of HLA identical sibling versus unrelated donor transplants in severe aplastic anemia: an EBMT analysis. Haematologica 100(5):696–702

Ball SE, Gibson FM, Rizzo S, Tooze JA, Marsh JC, Gordon-Smith EC (1998) Progressive telomere shortening in aplastic anemia. Blood 91(10):3582–3592

Baranski B, Armstrong G, Truman JT, Quinnan GV Jr, Straus SE, Young NS (1988) Epstein-Barr virus in the bone marrow of patients with aplastic anemia. Ann Intern Med 109(9):695–704

Barone A, Lucarelli A, Onofrillo D, Verzegnassi F, Bonanomi S, Cesaro S et al (2015) Diagnosis and management of acquired aplastic anemia in childhood. Guidelines from the Marrow Failure Study Group of the Pediatric Haemato-Oncology Italian Association (AIEOP). Blood Cells Mol Dis 55(1):40–47

Baumelou E, Guiguet M, Mary JY (1993) Epidemiology of aplastic anemia in France: a case-control study. I. Medical history and medication use. The French Cooperative Group for Epidemiological Study of Aplastic Anemia. Blood 81(6):1471–1478

Bessho M, Hotta T, Ohyashiki K, Takahashi T, Mizoguchi H, Asano S et al (2003) Multicenter prospective study of clonal complications in adult aplastic anemia patients following recombinant human granulocyte colony-stimulating factor (lenograstim) administration. Int J Hematol 77(2):152–158

(1987) Incidence of aplastic anemia: the relevance of diagnostic criteria. By the International Agranulocytosis and Aplastic Anemia Study. Blood 70(6):1718–1721

Bottiger LE, Furhoff AK, Holmberg L (1979) Drug-induced blood dyscrasias. A ten-year material from the Swedish Adverse Drug Reaction Committee. Acta Med Scand 205(6):457–461

Breakey VR, Meyn S, Ng V, Allen C, Dokal I, Lansdorp PM et al (2009) Hepatitis-associated aplastic anemia presenting as a familial bone marrow failure syndrome. J Pediatr Hematol Oncol 31(11):884–887

Brodsky RA (2014) Paroxysmal nocturnal hemoglobinuria. Blood 124(18):2804–2811

Brodsky RA, Sensenbrenner LL, Jones RJ (1996) Complete remission in severe aplastic anemia after high-dose cyclophosphamide without bone marrow transplantation. Blood 87(2):491–494

Brown KE, Tisdale J, Barrett AJ, Dunbar CE, Young NS (1997) Hepatitis-associated aplastic anemia. N Engl J Med 336(15):1059–1064

de Bruin AM, Voermans C, Nolte MA (2014) Impact of interferon-gamma on hematopoiesis. Blood 124(16):2479–2486

Brummendorf TH, Rufer N, Holyoake TL, Maciejewski J, Barnett MJ, Eaves CJ et al (2001) Telomere length dynamics in normal individuals and in patients with hematopoietic stem cell-associated disorders. Ann N Y Acad Sci 938:293–303. discussion 4.

Buchbinder D, Nugent DJ, Brazauskas R, Wang Z, Aljurf MD, Cairo MS et al (2012) Late effects in hematopoietic cell transplant recipients with acquired severe aplastic anemia: a report from the late effects working committee of the center for international blood and marrow transplant research. Biol Blood Marrow Transplant 18(12):1776–1784

Bueno C, Roldan M, Anguita E, Romero-Moya D, Martin-Antonio B, Rosu-Myles M et al (2014) Bone marrow mesenchymal stem cells from patients with aplastic anemia maintain functional and immune properties and do not contribute to the pathogenesis of the disease. Haematologica 99(7):1168–1175

Calado RT, Young NS (2008) Telomere maintenance and human bone marrow failure. Blood 111(9):4446–4455

Calado RT, Graf SA, Wilkerson KL, Kajigaya S, Ancliff PJ, Dror Y et al (2007) Mutations in the SBDS gene in acquired aplastic anemia. Blood 110(4):1141–1146

Camitta BM, Thomas ED, Nathan DG, Santos G, Gordon-Smith EC, Gale RP et al (1976) Severe aplastic anemia: a prospective study of the effect of early marrow transplantation on acute mortality. Blood 48(1):63–70

Camitta BM, Thomas ED, Nathan DG, Gale RP, Kopecky KJ, Rappeport JM et al (1979) A prospective study of androgens and bone marrow transplantation for treatment of severe aplastic anemia. Blood 53(3):504–514

Carrigan DR, Knox KK (1994) Human herpesvirus 6 (HHV-6) isolation from bone marrow: HHV-6-associated bone marrow suppression in bone marrow transplant patients. Blood 84(10):3307–3310

Cattral MS, Langnas AN, Markin RS, Antonson DL, Heffron TG, Fox IJ et al (1994) Aplastic anemia after liver transplantation for fulminant liver failure. Hepatology 20(4 Pt 1):813–818

Celkan T (2010) Aplastic anemia presenting as hemophagocytic lymphohistiocytosis. Turkish J Haematol 27(1):38–42

Champlin R, Ho W, Gale RP (1983) Antithymocyte globulin treatment in patients with aplastic anemia: a prospective randomized trial. N Engl J Med 308(3):113–118

Chandar R, Chandrasekaran V, Jagadisan B, Kumar D, Biswal N (2017) Hemophagocytic lymphohistiocytosis in a child with very severe aplastic anemia: double jeopardy resulting in fatality. J Pediatr Hematol Oncol 39:e43

Chao YH, Peng CT, Harn HJ, Chan CK, Wu KH (2010) Poor potential of proliferation and differentiation in bone marrow mesenchymal stem cells derived from children with severe aplastic anemia. Ann Hematol 89(7):715–723

Choi YB, Yi ES, Lee JW, Sung KW, Koo HH, Yoo KH (2017) Immunosuppressive therapy versus alternative donor hematopoietic stem cell transplantation for children with severe aplastic anemia who lack an HLA-matched familial donor. Bone Marrow Transplant 52:47

Chute JP, Hoffmeister K, Cotelingam J, Davis TA, Frame JN, Jamieson T (1996) Aplastic anemia as the sole presentation of systemic lupus erythematosus. Am J Hematol 51(3):237–239

Clausen N, Kreuger A, Salmi T, Storm-Mathisen I, Johannesson G (1996) Severe aplastic anaemia in the Nordic countries: a population based study of incidence, presentation, course, and outcome. Arch Dis Child 74(4):319–322

Cohen A, Duell T, Socie G, van Lint MT, Weiss M, Tichelli A et al (1999) Nutritional status and growth after bone marrow transplantation (BMT) during childhood: EBMT late-effects working party retrospective data. European Group for Blood and Marrow Transplantation. Bone Marrow Transplant 23(10):1043–1047

Das PK, Wherrett D, Dror Y (2007) Remission of aplastic anemia induced by treatment for Graves disease in a pediatric patient. Pediatr Blood Cancer 49(2):210–212

Deeg HJ (2011) GVHD-free with Campath? Blood 118(8):2033–2034

Deeg HJ, Socie G, Schoch G, Henry-Amar M, Witherspoon RP, Devergie A et al (1996) Malignancies after marrow transplantation for aplastic anemia and fanconi anemia: a joint Seattle and Paris analysis of results in 700 patients. Blood 87(1):386–392

Deeg HJ, Seidel K, Casper J, Anasetti C, Davies S, Gajeweski JL et al (1999) Marrow transplantation from unrelated donors for patients with severe aplastic anemia who have failed immunosuppressive therapy. Biol Blood Marrow Transplant 5(4):243–252

Desmond R, Townsley DM, Dumitriu B, Olnes MJ, Scheinberg P, Bevans M et al (2014) Eltrombopag restores trilineage hematopoiesis in refractory severe aplastic anemia that can be sustained on discontinuation of drug. Blood 123(12):1818–1825

Deyell RJ, Shereck EB, Milner RA, Schultz KR (2011) Immunosuppressive therapy without hematopoietic growth factor exposure in pediatric acquired aplastic anemia. Pediatr Hematol Oncol 28(6):469–478

DeZern AE, Symons HJ, Resar LS, Borowitz MJ, Armanios MY, Brodsky RA (2014) Detection of paroxysmal nocturnal hemoglobinuria clones to exclude inherited bone marrow failure syndromes. Eur J Haematol 92(6):467–470

Di Bona E, Rodeghiero F, Bruno B, Gabbas A, Foa P, Locasciulli A et al (1999) Rabbit antithymocyte globulin (r-ATG) plus cyclosporine and granulocyte colony stimulating factor is an effective treatment for aplastic anaemia patients unresponsive to a first course of intensive immunosuppressive therapy. Gruppo Italiano Trapianto di Midollo Osseo (GITMO). Br J Haematol 107(2):330–334

Dilloo D, Vohringer R, Josting A, Habersang K, Scheidt A, Burdach S (1995) Bone marrow fibroblasts from children with aplastic anemia exhibit reduced interleukin-6 production in response to cytokines and viral challenge. Pediatr Res 38(5):716–721

Domenech P, Palomeque A, Martinez-Gutierrez A, Vinolas N, Vela E, Jimenez R (1986) Severe aplastic anaemia following hepatitis A. Acta Haematol 76(4):227–229

Doney K, Leisenring W, Storb R, Appelbaum FR (1997) Primary treatment of acquired aplastic anemia: outcomes with bone marrow transplantation and immunosuppressive therapy. Seattle Bone Marrow Transplant Team. Ann Intern Med 126(2):107–115

Dror Y, Donadieu J, Koglmeier J, Dodge J, Toiviainen-Salo S, Makitie O et al (2011) Draft consensus guidelines for diagnosis and treatment of Shwachman-Diamond syndrome. Ann N Y Acad Sci 1242:40–55

Dufour C, Pillon M, Socie G, Rovo A, Carraro E, Bacigalupo A et al (2015a) Outcome of aplastic anaemia in children. A study by the severe aplastic anaemia and paediatric disease working parties of the European group blood and bone marrow transplant. Br J Haematol 169(4):565–573

Dufour C, Veys P, Carraro E, Bhatnagar N, Pillon M, Wynn R et al (2015b) Similar outcome of upfront-unrelated and matched sibling stem cell transplantation in idiopathic paediatric aplastic anaemia. A study on behalf of the UK Paediatric BMT Working Party, Paediatric Diseases Working Party and Severe Aplastic Anaemia Working Party of EBMT. Br J Haematol 171(4):585–594

Dunn DE, Tanawattanacharoen P, Boccuni P, Nagakura S, Green SW, Kirby MR et al (1999) Paroxysmal nocturnal hemoglobinuria cells in patients with bone marrow failure syndromes. Ann Intern Med 131(6):401–408

Esteves I, Bonfim C, Pasquini R, Funke V, Pereira NF, Rocha V et al (2015) Haploidentical BMT and post-transplant Cy for severe aplastic anemia: a multicenter retrospective study. Bone Marrow Transplant 50(5):685–689

Fouladi M, Herman R, Rolland-Grinton M, Jones-Wallace D, Blanchette V, Calderwood S et al (2000) Improved survival in severe acquired aplastic anemia of childhood. Bone Marrow Transplant 26(11):1149–1156

Frickhofen N, Liu JM, Young NS (1990 Winter) Etiologic mechanisms of hematopoietic failure. Am J Pediatr Hematol Oncol 12(4):385–395

Frickhofen N, Kaltwasser JP, Schrezenmeier H, Raghavachar A, Vogt HG, Herrmann F et al (1991) Treatment of aplastic anemia with antilymphocyte globulin and methylprednisolone with or without cyclosporine. The German Aplastic Anemia Study Group. N Engl J Med 324(19):1297–1304

Frickhofen N, Heimpel H, Kaltwasser JP, Schrezenmeier H (2003) German Aplastic Anemia Study G. Antithymocyte globulin with or without cyclosporin A: 11-year follow-up of a randomized trial comparing treatments of aplastic anemia. Blood 101(4):1236–1242

Fuhrer M, Burdach S, Ebell W, Gadner H, Haas R, Harbott J et al (1998) Relapse and clonal disease in children with aplastic anemia (AA) after immunosuppressive therapy (IST): the SAA 94 experience. German/Austrian Pediatric Aplastic Anemia Working Group. Klin Padiatr 210(4):173–179

Gamper CJ, Takemoto CM, Chen AR, Symons HJ, Loeb DM, Casella JF et al (2016) High-dose cyclophosphamide is effective therapy for pediatric severe aplastic anemia. J Pediatr Hematol Oncol 38(8):627–635

Ganser A, Lindemann A, Seipelt G, Ottmann OG, Eder M, Falk S et al (1990) Effects of recombinant human interleukin-3 in aplastic anemia. Blood 76(7):1287–1292

Garanito MP, Carneiro JD, Odone Filho V, Scheinberg P (2014) Outcome of children with severe acquired aplastic anemia treated with rabbit antithymocyte globulin and cyclosporine A. J Pediatr (Rio J) 90(5):523–527

Ghemlas I, Li H, Zlateska B, Klaassen R, Fernandez CV, Yanofsky RA et al (2015) Improving diagnostic precision, care and syndrome definitions using comprehensive next-generation sequencing for the inherited bone marrow failure syndromes. J Med Genet 52(9):575–584

Gill H, Leung GM, Lopes D, Kwong YL (2017) The thrombopoietin mimetics eltrombopag and romiplostim in the treatment of refractory aplastic anaemia. Br J Haematol 176:991

Gillio AP, Boulad F, Small TN, Kernan NA, Reyes B, Childs BH et al (1997) Comparison of long-term outcome of children with severe aplastic anemia treated with immunosuppression versus bone marrow transplantation. Biol Blood Marrow Transplant 3(1):18–24

Gluckman E, Horowitz MM, Champlin RE, Hows JM, Bacigalupo A, Biggs JC et al (1992) Bone marrow transplantation for severe aplastic anemia: influence of conditioning and graft-versus-host disease prophylaxis regimens on outcome. Blood 79(1):269–275

Gluckman E, Rokicka-Milewska R, Hann I, Nikiforakis E, Tavakoli F, Cohen-Scali S et al (2002) Results and follow-up of a phase III randomized study of recombinant human-granulocyte stimulating factor as support for immunosuppressive therapy in patients with severe aplastic anaemia. Br J Haematol 119(4):1075–1082

Goto H, Ishida A, Fujii H, Kuroki F, Takahashi H, Ikuta K et al (2004) Successful bone marrow transplantation for severe aplastic anemia in a patient with persistent human parvovirus B19 infection. Int J Hematol 79(4):384–386

Grimaldi F, Potter V, Perez-Abellan P, Veluchamy JP, Atif M, Grain R et al (2017) Mixed T cell chimerism after allogeneic hematopoietic stem cell transplantation for severe aplastic anemia using an alemtuzumab-containing regimen is shaped by persistence of recipient CD8 T cells. Biol Blood Marrow Transplant 23:293

Guiguet M, Baumelou E, Mary JY (1995) A case-control study of aplastic anaemia: occupational exposures. The French Cooperative Group for Epidemiological Study of Aplastic Anaemia. Int J Epidemiol 24(5):993–999

Guinan EC, Sieff CA, Oette DH, Nathan DG (1990) A phase I/II trial of recombinant granulocyte-macrophage colony-stimulating factor for children with aplastic anemia. Blood 76(6):1077–1082

Gupta V, Gordon-Smith EC, Cook G, Parker A, Duguid JK, Wilson KM et al (2005) A third course of anti-thymocyte globulin in aplastic anaemia is only beneficial in previous responders. Br J Haematol 129(1):110–117

Gupta V, Pratap R, Kumar A, Saini I, Shukla J (2013) Epidemiological features of aplastic anemia in Indian children. Indian J Pediatr

Gurion R, Gafter-Gvili A, Paul M, Vidal L, Ben-Bassat I, Yeshurun M et al (2009) Hematopoietic growth factors in aplastic anemia patients treated with immunosuppressive therapy-systematic review and meta-analysis. Haematologica 94(5):712–719

Hama A, Takahashi Y, Muramatsu H, Ito M, Narita A, Kosaka Y et al (2015) Comparison of long-term outcomes between children with aplastic anemia and refractory cytopenia of childhood who received immunosuppressive therapy with antithymocyte globulin and cyclosporine. Haematologica 100(11):1426–1433

Hamzic E, Whiting K, Gordon Smith E, Pettengell R (2015) Characterization of bone marrow mesenchymal stromal cells in aplastic anaemia. Br J Haematol 169(6):804–813

Hara T, Ando K, Tsurumi H, Moriwaki H (2004) Excessive production of tumor necrosis factor-alpha by bone marrow T lymphocytes is essential in causing bone marrow failure in patients with aplastic anemia. Eur J Haematol 73(1):10–16

Hibbs JR, Frickhofen N, Rosenfeld SJ, Feinstone SM, Kojima S, Bacigalupo A et al (1992) Aplastic anemia and viral hepatitis. Non-A, Non-B, Non-C? JAMA 267(15):2051–2054

Hinterberger W, Rowlings PA, Hinterberger-Fischer M, Gibson J, Jacobsen N, Klein JP et al (1997) Results of transplanting bone marrow from genetically identical twins into patients with aplastic anemia. Ann Intern Med 126(2):116–122

Hirano N, Butler MO, Von Bergwelt-Baildon MS, Maecker B, Schultze JL, O'Connor KC et al (2003)

Autoantibodies frequently detected in patients with aplastic anemia. Blood 102(13):4567–4575
Holmberg LA, Seidel K, Leisenring W, Torok-Storb B (1994) Aplastic anemia: analysis of stromal cell function in long-term marrow cultures. Blood 84(11):3685–3690
Hord JD, Gay JC, Whitlock JA, Janco RL, Edwards JR, Greer JP et al (1995) Long-term granulocyte-macrophage colony-stimulating factor and immunosuppression in the treatment of acquired severe aplastic anemia. J Pediatr Hematol Oncol 17(2):140–144
Howard SC, Naidu PE, Hu XJ, Jeng MR, Rodriguez-Galindo C, Rieman MD et al (2004) Natural history of moderate aplastic anemia in children. Pediatr Blood Cancer 43(5):545–551
Imashuku S, Hibi S, Bessho F, Tsuchida M, Nakahata T, Miyazaki S et al (2003) Detection of myelodysplastic syndrome/ acute myeloid leukemia evolving from aplastic anemia in children, treated with recombinant human G-CSF. Haematologica 88(11):ECR31
Issaragrisil S (1999) Epidemiology of aplastic anemia in Thailand. Thai Aplastic Anemia Study Group. Int J Hematol 70(3):137–140
Issaragrisil S, Kaufman DW, Anderson T, Chansung K, Thamprasit T, Sirijirachai J et al (1997) Low drug attributability of aplastic anemia in Thailand. The Aplastic Anemia Study Group. Blood 89(11):4034–4039
Itterbeek P, Vandenberghe P, Nevens F, Fevery J, Aerts R, Yap SH et al (2002) Aplastic anemia after transplantation for non-A, non-B, non-C fulminant hepatic failure: case report and review of the literature. Transpl Int 15(2-3):117–123
Jain D, Kumar R, Tyagi N, Negi A, Pande A, Mahajan A et al (2012) Etiology and survival of aplastic anemia: a study based on clinical investigation. J Clin Lab Anal 26(6):452–458
(1986) Risks of agranulocytosis and aplastic anemia. A first report of their relation to drug use with special reference to analgesics. The International Agranulocytosis and Aplastic Anemia Study. JAMA 256(13):1749–1757
Jeannet M, Speck B, Rubinstein A, Pelet B, Wyss M, Kummer H (1976) Autologous marrow reconstitutions in severe aplastic anaemia after ALG pretreatment and HL-A semi-incompatible bone marrow cell transfusion. Acta Haematol 55(3):129–139
Jeong DC, Chung NG, Cho B, Zou Y, Ruan M, Takahashi Y et al (2014) Long-term outcome after immunosuppressive therapy with horse or rabbit antithymocyte globulin and cyclosporine for severe aplastic anemia in children. Haematologica 99(4):664–671
Jiang J, Kulasekararaj AG, Smith AE, Mohamedali AM, Gandhi SA, Czepulkowski B et al (2013) Somatic mutations implicated in myeloid malignancies are frequent in idiopathic aplastic anaemia and its relevance to disease classification and treatment - a comprehensive analysis of 150 patients. Blood 122(21):803
Kaito K, Kobayashi M, Katayama T, Masuoka H, Shimada T, Nishiwaki K et al (1998) Long-term administration of G-CSF for aplastic anaemia is closely related to the early evolution of monosomy 7 MDS in adults. Br J Haematol 103(2):297–303
Kamio T, Ito E, Ohara A, Kosaka Y, Tsuchida M, Yagasaki H et al (2011) Relapse of aplastic anemia in children after immunosuppressive therapy: a report from the Japan Childhood Aplastic Anemia Study Group. Haematologica 96(6):814–819
Karadimitris A, Notaro R, Koehne G, Roberts IA, Luzzatto L (2000) PNH cells are as sensitive to T-cell-mediated lysis as their normal counterparts: implications for the pathogenesis of paroxysmal nocturnal haemoglobinuria. Br J Haematol 111(4):1158–1163
Kasahara S, Hara T, Itoh H, Ando K, Tsurumi H, Sawada M et al (2002) Hypoplastic myelodysplastic syndromes can be distinguished from acquired aplastic anaemia by bone marrow stem cell expression of the tumour necrosis factor receptor. Br J Haematol 118(1):181–188
Kaufman DW, Kelly JP, Jurgelon JM, Anderson T, Issaragrisil S, Wiholm BE et al (1996) Drugs in the aetiology of agranulocytosis and aplastic anaemia. Eur J Haematol Suppl 60:23–30
Keel SB, Scott A, Sanchez-Bonilla M, Ho PA, Gulsuner S, Pritchard CC et al (2016) Genetic features of myelodysplastic syndrome and aplastic anemia in pediatric and young adult patients. Haematologica 101(11):1343–1350
Kim SW, Rice L, Champlin R, Udden MM (1997) Aplastic anemia in eosinophilic fasciitis: responses to immunosuppression and marrow transplantation. Haematologia 28(3):131–137
Klco JM, Geng B, Brunt EM, Hassan A, Nguyen TD, Kreisel FH et al (2010) Bone marrow biopsy in patients with hepatitis C virus infection: spectrum of findings and diagnostic utility. Am J Hematol 85(2):106–110
Kojima S, Matsuyama T (1994) Stimulation of granulopoiesis by high-dose recombinant human granulocyte colony-stimulating factor in children with aplastic anemia and very severe neutropenia. Blood 83(6):1474–1478
Kojima S, Horibe K, Inaba J, Yoshimi A, Takahashi Y, Kudo K et al (2000a) Long-term outcome of acquired aplastic anaemia in children: comparison between immunosuppressive therapy and bone marrow transplantation. Br J Haematol 111(1):321–328
Kojima S, Hibi S, Kosaka Y, Yamamoto M, Tsuchida M, Mugishima H et al (2000b) Immunosuppressive therapy using antithymocyte globulin, cyclosporine, and danazol with or without human granulocyte colony-stimulating factor in children with acquired aplastic anemia. Blood 96(6):2049–2054
Kojima S, Matsuyama T, Kato S, Kigasawa H, Kobayashi R, Kikuta A et al (2002a) Outcome of 154 patients with severe aplastic anemia who received transplants from unrelated donors: the Japan Marrow Donor Program. Blood 100(3):799–803
Kojima S, Ohara A, Tsuchida M, Kudoh T, Hanada R, Okimoto Y et al (2002b) Risk factors for evolution of acquired aplastic anemia into myelodysplastic syn-

drome and acute myeloid leukemia after immunosuppressive therapy in children. Blood 100(3):786–790

Kolb HJ, Socie G, Duell T, Van Lint MT, Tichelli A, Apperley JF et al (1999) Malignant neoplasms in long-term survivors of bone marrow transplantation. Late Effects Working Party of the European Cooperative Group for Blood and Marrow Transplantation and the European Late Effect Project Group. Ann Intern Med 131(10):738–744

Kook H, Kim GM, Kim HJ, Kim CJ, Yoon WS, Hwang TJ (2000) Rubella-associated aplastic anemia treated by syngeneic stem cell transplantations. Am J Hematol 64(4):303–305

Kosaka Y, Yagasaki H, Sano K, Kobayashi R, Ayukawa H, Kaneko T et al (2008) Prospective multicenter trial comparing repeated immunosuppressive therapy with stem-cell transplantation from an alternative donor as second-line treatment for children with severe and very severe aplastic anemia. Blood 111(3):1054–1059

Krell PF, Reuther S, Fischer U, Keller T, Weber S, Gombert M et al (2013) Next-generation-sequencing-spectratyping reveals public T-cell receptor repertoires in pediatric very severe aplastic anemia and identifies a beta chain CDR3 sequence associated with hepatitis-induced pathogenesis. Haematologica 98(9):1388–1396

Kulagin A, Lisukov I, Ivanova M, Golubovskaya I, Kruchkova I, Bondarenko S et al (2014) Prognostic value of paroxysmal nocturnal haemoglobinuria clone presence in aplastic anaemia patients treated with combined immunosuppression: results of two-centre prospective study. Br J Haematol 164(4):546–554

Kulasekararaj AG, Jiang J, Smith AE, Mohamedali AM, Mian S, Gandhi S et al (2014) Somatic mutations identify a subgroup of aplastic anemia patients who progress to myelodysplastic syndrome. Blood 124(17):2698–2704

Kuwatsuka Y, Kanda J, Yamazaki H, Mori T, Miyamura K, Kako S et al (2016) A comparison of outcomes for cord blood transplantation and unrelated bone marrow transplantation in adult aplastic anemia. Biol Blood Marrow Transplant 22(10):1836–1843

Lan Q, Zhang L, Li G, Vermeulen R, Weinberg RS, Dosemeci M et al (2004) Hematotoxicity in workers exposed to low levels of benzene. Science 306(5702):1774–1776

Lane AA, Odejide O, Kopp N, Kim S, Yoda A, Erlich R et al (2013) Low frequency clonal mutations recoverable by deep sequencing in patients with aplastic anemia. Leukemia 27(4):968–971

Li Y, Li X, Ge M, Shi J, Qian L, Zheng Y et al (2011) Long-term follow-up of clonal evolutions in 802 aplastic anemia patients: a single-center experience. Ann Hematol 90(5):529–537

Li J, Lu S, Yang S, Xing W, Feng J, Li W et al (2012) Impaired immunomodulatory ability of bone marrow mesenchymal stem cells on CD4(+) T cells in aplastic anemia. Res Immunol 2:142–147

Li B, Guo L, Zhang Y, Xiao Y, Wu M, Zhou L et al (2016) Molecular alterations in the TCR signaling pathway in patients with aplastic anemia. J Hematol Oncol 9:32

Liang R, Cheng G, Wat MS, Ha SY, Chan LC (1993) Childhood acute lymphoblastic leukaemia presenting with relapsing hypoplastic anaemia: progression of the same abnormal clone. Br J Haematol 83(2):340–342

Libregts SF, Nolte MA (2014) Parallels between immune driven-hematopoiesis and T cell activation: 3 signals that relay inflammatory stress to the bone marrow. Exp Cell Res 329(2):239–247

Linet MS, McCaffrey LD, Morgan WF, Bearden JD III, Szklo M, Sensenbrenner LL et al (1986) Incidence of aplastic anemia in a three county area in South Carolina. Cancer Res 46(1):426–429

Liu CY, Fu R, Wang HQ, Li LJ, Liu H, Guan J et al (2014) Fas/FasL in the immune pathogenesis of severe aplastic anemia. Genet Mol Res 13(2):4083–4088

Liu L, Wang X, Jin S, Hao L, Zhang Y, Zhang X et al (2016) Haploidentical hematopoietic stem cell transplantation for nonresponders to immunosuppressive therapy against acquired severe aplastic anemia. Bone Marrow Transplant 51(3):424–427

Locasciulli A (2002) Acquired aplastic anemia in children: incidence, prognosis and treatment options. Paediatr Drugs 4(11):761–766

Locasciulli A, Arcese W, Locatelli F, Di Bona E, Bacigalupo A (2001) Treatment of aplastic anaemia with granulocyte-colony stimulating factor and risk of malignancy. Italian Aplastic Anaemia Study Group. Lancet 357(9249):43–44

Locasciulli A, Bruno B, Rambaldi A, Saracco P, Dufour C, Finelli C et al (2004) Treatment of severe aplastic anemia with antilymphocyte globulin, cyclosporine and two different granulocyte colony-stimulating factor regimens: a GITMO prospective randomized study. Haematologica 89(9):1054–1061

Locasciulli A, Oneto R, Bacigalupo A, Socie G, Korthof E, Bekassy A et al (2007) Outcome of patients with acquired aplastic anemia given first line bone marrow transplantation or immunosuppressive treatment in the last decade: a report from the European Group for Blood and Marrow Transplantation (EBMT). Haematologica 92(1):11–18

Lu J, Basu A, Melenhorst JJ, Young NS, Brown KE (2004) Analysis of T-cell repertoire in hepatitis-associated aplastic anemia. Blood 103(12):4588–4593

Macartney C, Freilich M, Odame I, Charpentier K, Dror Y (2009) Complete response to tacrolimus in a child with severe aplastic anemia resistant to cyclosporin A. Pediatr Blood Cancer 52(4):525–527

Maciejewski JP, Selleri C (2004) Evolution of clonal cytogenetic abnormalities in aplastic anemia. Leuk Lymphoma 45(3):433–440

Maciejewski J, Selleri C, Anderson S, Young NS (1995) Fas antigen expression on CD34+ human marrow cells is induced by interferon gamma and tumor necrosis factor alpha and potentiates cytokine-mediated hematopoietic suppression in vitro. Blood 85(11):3183–3190

Maciejewski JP, Selleri C, Sato T, Anderson S, Young NS (1996) A severe and consistent deficit in marrow and circulating primitive hematopoietic cells (long-term culture-initiating cells) in acquired aplastic anemia. Blood 88(6):1983–1991

Maciejewski JP, Risitano A, Sloand EM, Nunez O, Young NS (2002) Distinct clinical outcomes for cytogenetic abnormalities evolving from aplastic anemia. Blood 99(9):3129–3135

Maluf E, Hamerschlak N, Cavalcanti AB, Junior AA, Eluf-Neto J, Falcao RP et al (2009) Incidence and risk factors of aplastic anemia in Latin American countries: the LATIN case-control study. Haematologica 94(9):1220–1226

Marsh JC, Mufti GJ (2016) Clinical significance of acquired somatic mutations in aplastic anaemia. Int J Hematol 104(2):159–167

Marsh JC, Chang J, Testa NG, Hows JM, Dexter TM (1990) The hematopoietic defect in aplastic anemia assessed by long-term marrow culture. Blood 76(9):1748–1757

Marsh JC, Gupta V, Lim Z, Ho AY, Ireland RM, Hayden J et al (2011) Alemtuzumab with fludarabine and cyclophosphamide reduces chronic graft-versus-host disease after allogeneic stem cell transplantation for acquired aplastic anemia. Blood 118(8):2351–2357

Marsh JC, Bacigalupo A, Schrezenmeier H, Tichelli A, Risitano AM, Passweg JR et al (2012) Prospective study of rabbit antithymocyte globulin and cyclosporine for aplastic anemia from the EBMT Severe Aplastic Anaemia Working Party. Blood 119(23):5391–5396

Marsh JC, Pearce RM, Koh MB, Lim Z, Pagliuca A, Mufti GJ et al (2014) Retrospective study of alemtuzumab vs ATG-based conditioning without irradiation for unrelated and matched sibling donor transplants in acquired severe aplastic anemia: a study from the British Society for Blood and Marrow Transplantation. Bone Marrow Transplant 49(1):42–48

Marwaha RK, Bansal D, Trehan A, Varma N (2004) Androgens in childhood acquired aplastic anaemia in Chandigarh, India. Trop Doct 34(3):149–152

Mary JY, Baumelou E, Guiguet M (1990) Epidemiology of aplastic anemia in France: a prospective multicentric study. The French Cooperative Group for Epidemiological Study of Aplastic Anemia. Blood 75(8):1646–1653

Mathe G, Amiel JL, Schwarzenberg L, Choay J, Trolard P, Schneider M et al (1970) Bone marrow graft in man after conditioning by antilymphocyte serum. Br Med J 2(5702):131–136

Mather KA, Jorm AF, Parslow RA, Christensen H (2011) Is telomere length a biomarker of aging? A review. J Gerontol A Biol Sci Med Sci 66((2):202–213

McCann SR, Bacigalupo A, Gluckman E, Hinterberger W, Hows J, Ljungman P et al (1994) Graft rejection and second bone marrow transplants for acquired aplastic anaemia: a report from the Aplastic Anaemia Working Party of the European Bone Marrow Transplant Group. Bone Marrow Transplant 13(3): 233–237

McSweeney PA, Carter JM, Green GJ, Romeril KR (1988) Fatal aplastic anemia associated with hepatitis B viral infection. Am J Med 85(2):255–256

Michelozzi IM, Pievani A, Pagni F, Antolini L, Verna M, Corti P et al (2017) Human aplastic anaemia-derived mesenchymal stromal cells form functional haematopoietic stem cell niche in vivo. Br J Haematol 179:669

Mir MA, Geary CG (1980) Aplastic anaemia: an analysis of 174 patients. Postgrad Med J 56(655):322–329

Mishra B, Malhotra P, Ratho RK, Singh MP, Varma S, Varma N (2005) Human parvovirus B19 in patients with aplastic anemia. Am J Hematol 79(2): 166–167

Mizuno S, Aoki K, Ohno Y, Sasaki R, Hamajima N (1982) Time series analysis of age-sex specific death rates from aplastic anemia and the trend in production amount of chloramphenicol. Nagoya J Med Sci 44(3-4):103–115

Moran JL, Siegel D, Sun XM, Ross D (1996) Induction of apoptosis by benzene metabolites in HL60 and CD34+ human bone marrow progenitor cells. Mol Pharmacol 50(3):610–615

Morinet F, Leruez-Ville M, Pillet S, Fichelson S (2011) Concise review: anemia caused by viruses. Stem Cells 29(11):1656–1660

Mortensen BK, Jacobsen N, Heilmann C, Sengelov H (2016) Allogeneic hematopoietic cell transplantation for severe aplastic anemia: similar long-term overall survival after transplantation with related donors compared to unrelated donors. Bone Marrow Transplant 51(2):288–290

Najean Y, Haguenauer O (1990) Long-term (5 to 20 years) evolution of nongrafted aplastic anemias. The Cooperative Group for the Study of aplastic and refractory anemias. Blood 76(11):2222–2228

Nakao S, Lai CJ, Young NS (1989) Dengue virus, a flavivirus, propagates in human bone marrow progenitors and hematopoietic cell lines. Blood 74(4):1235–1240

Nakao S, Takami A, Takamatsu H, Zeng W, Sugimori N, Yamazaki H et al (1997) Isolation of a T-cell clone showing HLA-DRB1*0405-restricted cytotoxicity for hematopoietic cells in a patient with aplastic anemia. Blood 89(10):3691–3699

Narita A, Kojima S (2016) Biomarkers for predicting clinical response to immunosuppressive therapy in aplastic anemia. Int J Hematol 104(2):153–158

Narita A, Muramatsu H, Sekiya Y, Okuno Y, Sakaguchi H, Nishio N et al (2015) Paroxysmal nocturnal hemoglobinuria and telomere length predicts response to immunosuppressive therapy in pediatric aplastic anemia. Haematologica 100(12):1546–1552

Niemeyer CM, Baumann I (2011) Classification of childhood aplastic anemia and myelodysplastic syndrome. Hematology Am Soc Hematol Educ Program 2011:84–89

Nimer SD, Ireland P, Meshkinpour A, Frane M (1994) An increased HLA DR2 frequency is seen in aplastic anemia patients. Blood 84(3):923–927

Nishikawa E, Yagasaki H, Hama A, Yabe H, Ohara A, Kosaka Y et al (2017) Long-term outcomes of 95 children with moderate aplastic anemia treated with horse antithymocyte globulin and cyclosporine. Pediatr Blood Cancer 64(5)

Nishimura J, Murakami Y, Kinoshita T (1999) Paroxysmal nocturnal hemoglobinuria: an acquired genetic disease. Am J Hematol 62(3):175–182

Notta F, Zandi S, Takayama N, Dobson S, Gan OI, Wilson G et al (2016) Distinct routes of lineage development reshape the human blood hierarchy across ontogeny. Science 351(6269):aab2116

Novitzky N, Jacobs P (1995) Immunosuppressive therapy in bone marrow aplasia: the stroma functions normally to support hematopoiesis. Exp Hematol 23(14):1472–1477

Ogawa S (2016) Clonal hematopoiesis in acquired aplastic anemia. Blood 128(3):337–347

Ohara A, Kojima S, Hamajima N, Tsuchida M, Imashuku S, Ohta S et al (1997) Myelodysplastic syndrome and acute myelogenous leukemia as a late clonal complication in children with acquired aplastic anemia. Blood 90(3):1009–1013

Olnes MJ, Scheinberg P, Calvo KR, Desmond R, Tang Y, Dumitriu B et al (2012) Eltrombopag and improved hematopoiesis in refractory aplastic anemia. N Engl J Med 367(1):11–19

Passweg JR, Socie G, Hinterberger W, Bacigalupo A, Biggs JC, Camitta BM et al (1997) Bone marrow transplantation for severe aplastic anemia: has outcome improved? Blood 90(2):858–864

Peffault de Latour R, Purtill D, Ruggeri A, Sanz G, Michel G, Gandemer V et al (2011) Influence of nucleated cell dose on overall survival of unrelated cord blood transplantation for patients with severe acquired aplastic anemia: a study by eurocord and the aplastic anemia working party of the European group for blood and marrow transplantation. Biol Blood Marrow Transplant 17(1):78–85

Pellack-Walker P, Blumer JL (1986) DNA damage in L5178YS cells following exposure to benzene metabolites. Mol Pharmacol 30(1):42–47

Philpott NJ, Scopes J, Marsh JC, Gordon-Smith EC, Gibson FM (1995) Increased apoptosis in aplastic anemia bone marrow progenitor cells: possible pathophysiologic significance. Exp Hematol 23(14):1642–1648

Piao W, Grosse J, Czwalinna A, Ivanyi P, Ganser A, Franzke A (2005) Antigen-recognition sites of micromanipulated T cells in patients with acquired aplastic anemia. Exp Hematol 33(7):804–810

Pitcher LA, Hann IM, Evans JP, Veys P, Chessells JM, Webb DK (1999) Improved prognosis for acquired aplastic anaemia. Arch Dis Child 80(2):158–162

de Planque MM, Bacigalupo A, Wursch A, Hows JM, Devergie A, Frickhofen N et al (1989) Long-term follow-up of severe aplastic anaemia patients treated with antithymocyte globulin. Severe Aplastic Anaemia Working Party of the European Cooperative Group for Bone Marrow Transplantation (EBMT). Br J Haematol 73(1):121–126

Pol S, Thiers V, Driss F, Devergie A, Berthelot P, Brechot C et al (1993) Lack of evidence for a role of HCV in hepatitis-associated aplastic anaemia. Br J Haematol 85(4):808–810

Qian XH, Zhang GC, Jiao XY, Zheng YJ, Cao YH, Xu DL et al (2002) Aplastic anaemia associated with parvovirus B19 infection. Arch Dis Child 87(5):436–437

Quiquandon I, Morel P, Lai JL, Bauters F, Dresch C, Gluckman E et al (1997) Primary Sjogren's syndrome and aplastic anaemia. Ann Rheum Dis 56(7):438

Risitano AM, Maciejewski JP, Green S, Plasilova M, Zeng W, Young NS (2004) In-vivo dominant immune responses in aplastic anaemia: molecular tracking of putatively pathogenetic T-cell clones by TCR beta-CDR3 sequencing. Lancet 364(9431):355–364

Ritchie DS, Underhill C, Grigg AP (2002) Aplastic anemia as a late complication of thymoma in remission. Eur J Haematol 68(6):389–391

Roberts HJ (1990) Pentachlorophenol-associated aplastic anemia, red cell aplasia, leukemia and other blood disorders. J Fla Med Assoc 77(2):86–90

Rosenfeld S, Follmann D, Nunez O, Young NS (2003) Antithymocyte globulin and cyclosporine for severe aplastic anemia: association between hematologic response and long-term outcome. JAMA 289(9):1130–1135

Rugman FP, Cosstick R (1990) Aplastic anaemia associated with organochlorine pesticide: case reports and review of evidence. J Clin Pathol 43(2):98–101

Sagmeister M, Oec L, Gmur J (1999) A restrictive platelet transfusion policy allowing long-term support of outpatients with severe aplastic anemia. Blood 93(9):3124–3126

Sakaguchi H, Nishio N, Hama A, Kawashima N, Wang X, Narita A et al (2014) Peripheral blood lymphocyte telomere length as a predictor of response to immunosuppressive therapy in childhood aplastic anemia. Haematologica 99(8):1312–1316

Samarasinghe S, Steward C, Hiwarkar P, Saif MA, Hough R, Webb D et al (2012) Excellent outcome of matched unrelated donor transplantation in paediatric aplastic anaemia following failure with immunosuppressive therapy: a United Kingdom multicentre retrospective experience. Br J Haematol 157(3):339–346

Samarasinghe S, Marsh J, Dufour C (2014) Immune suppression for childhood acquired aplastic anemia and myelodysplastic syndrome: where next? Haematologica 99(4):597–599

Sanders JE, Storb R, Anasetti C, Deeg HJ, Doney K, Sullivan KM et al (1994) Marrow transplant experience for children with severe aplastic anemia. Am J Pediatr Hematol Oncol 16(1):43–49

Sanders JE, Woolfrey AE, Carpenter PA, Storer BE, Hoffmeister PA, Deeg HJ et al (2011) Late effects among pediatric patients followed for nearly 4 decades after transplantation for severe aplastic anemia. Blood 118(5):1421–1428

Scheinberg P, Nunez O, Young NS (2006) Retreatment with rabbit anti-thymocyte globulin and ciclosporin for patients with relapsed or refractory severe aplastic anaemia. Br J Haematol 133(6):622–627

Scheinberg P, Wu CO, Nunez O, Young NS (2008) Long-term outcome of pediatric patients with severe aplastic anemia treated with antithymocyte globulin and cyclosporine. J Pediatr 153(6):814–819

Scheinberg P, Wu CO, Nunez O, Young NS (2009) Predicting response to immunosuppressive therapy and survival in severe aplastic anaemia. Br J Haematol 144(2):206–216

Scheinberg P, Nunez O, Weinstein B, Scheinberg P, Biancotto A, Wu CO et al (2011) Horse versus rabbit antithymocyte globulin in acquired aplastic anemia. N Engl J Med 365(5):430–438

Schrezenmeier H, Hinterberger W, Hows J (1995) Second immunosuppressive treatment of patients with aplastic anemia not responding to the first course of immunosuppression (IS): a report from the Working Party of Severe Aplastic Anemia for the EBMT. Bone Marrow Transplant 15(Suppl2):65a

Schrezenmeier H, Jenal M, Herrmann F, Heimpel H, Raghavachar A (1996) Quantitative analysis of cobblestone area-forming cells in bone marrow of patients with aplastic anemia by limiting dilution assay. Blood 88(12):4474–4480

Scopes J, Daly S, Atkinson R, Ball SE, Gordon-Smith EC, Gibson FM (1996) Aplastic anemia: evidence for dysfunctional bone marrow progenitor cells and the corrective effect of granulocyte colony-stimulating factor in vitro. Blood 87(8):3179–3185

Shah I, Murthy AK (2005) Aplastic anemia in an HIV infected child. Indian J Pediatr 72(4):359–361

Sharathkumar A, Kirby M, Freedman M, Abdelhaleem M, Chitayat D, Teshima IE et al (2003) Malignant hematological disorders in children with Wolf-Hirschhorn syndrome. Am J Med Genet A 119((2):194–199

Shi J, Ge M, Lu S, Li X, Shao Y, Huang J et al (2012) Intrinsic impairment of CD4(+)CD25(+) regulatory T cells in acquired aplastic anemia. Blood 120(8):1624–1632

Shimamura A (2016) Aplastic anemia and clonal evolution: germ line and somatic genetics. Hematology Am Soc Hematol Educ Program 2016(1):74–82

Siegal D, Xu W, Sutherland R, Kamel-Reid S, Kuruvilla J, Lipton JH et al (2008) Graft-versus-host disease following marrow transplantation for aplastic anemia: different impact of two GVHD prevention strategies. Bone Marrow Transplant 42(1):51–56

Sing GK, Ruscetti FW (1995) The role of human cytomegalovirus in haematological diseases. Bailliere Clin Haematol 8(1):149–163

Sloand E, Kim S, Maciejewski JP, Tisdale J, Follmann D, Young NS (2002) Intracellular interferon-gamma in circulating and marrow T cells detected by flow cytometry and the response to immunosuppressive therapy in patients with aplastic anemia. Blood 100(4):1185–1191

Sloand EM, Yong AS, Ramkissoon S, Solomou E, Bruno TC, Kim S et al (2006) Granulocyte colony-stimulating factor preferentially stimulates proliferation of monosomy 7 cells bearing the isoform IV receptor. Proc Natl Acad Sci U S A 103(39):14483–14488

Socie G, Mary JY, Schrezenmeier H, Marsh J, Bacigalupo A, Locasciulli A et al (2007) Granulocyte-stimulating factor and severe aplastic anemia: a survey by the European Group for Blood and Marrow Transplantation (EBMT). Blood 109(7):2794–2796

Solomou EE, Gibellini F, Stewart B, Malide D, Berg M, Visconte V et al (2007) Perforin gene mutations in patients with acquired aplastic anemia. Blood 109(12):5234–5237

Speck B, Gluckman E, Haak HL, van Rood JJ (1977) Treatment of aplastic anaemia by antilymphocyte globulin with and without allogeneic bone-marrow infusions. Lancet 2(8049):1145–1148

Stanley N, Olson TS, Babushok DV (2017) Recent advances in understanding clonal haematopoiesis in aplastic anaemia. Br J Haematol 177:509

Storb R, Sanders JE, Pepe M, Anasetti C, Appelbaum FR, Buckner CD et al (1991) Graft-versus-host disease prophylaxis with methotrexate/cyclosporine in children with severe aplastic anemia treated with cyclophosphamide and HLA-identical marrow grafts. Blood 78(4):1144–1145

Storb R, Blume KG, O'Donnell MR, Chauncey T, Forman SJ, Deeg HJ et al (2001) Cyclophosphamide and antithymocyte globulin to condition patients with aplastic anemia for allogeneic marrow transplantations: the experience in four centers. Biol Blood Marrow Transplant 7(1):39–44

Teramura M, Kimura A, Iwase S, Yonemura Y, Nakao S, Urabe A et al (2007) Treatment of severe aplastic anemia with antithymocyte globulin and cyclosporin A with or without G-CSF in adults: a multicenter randomized study in Japan. Blood 110(6):1756–1761

Tichelli A, Gratwohl A, Nissen C, Signer E, Stebler Gysi C, Speck B (1992) Morphology in patients with severe aplastic anemia treated with antilymphocyte globulin. Blood 80(2):337–345

Tichelli A, Passweg J, Nissen C, Bargetzi M, Hoffmann T, Wodnar-Filipowicz A et al (1998) Repeated treatment with horse antilymphocyte globulin for severe aplastic anaemia. Br J Haematol 100(2):393–400

Tichelli A, Schrezenmeier H, Socie G, Marsh J, Bacigalupo A, Duhrsen U et al (2011) A randomized controlled study in patients with newly diagnosed severe aplastic anemia receiving antithymocyte globulin (ATG), cyclosporine, with or without G-CSF: a study of the SAA Working Party of the European Group for Blood and Marrow Transplantation. Blood 117(17):4434–4441

Tisdale JF, Dunn DE, Geller N, Plante M, Nunez O, Dunbar CE et al (2000) High-dose cyclophosphamide in severe aplastic anaemia: a randomised trial. Lancet 356(9241):1554–1559

Tisdale JF, Maciejewski JP, Nunez O, Rosenfeld SJ, Young NS (2002) Late complications following treatment for severe aplastic anemia (SAA) with high-dose cyclophosphamide (Cy): follow-up of a randomized trial. Blood 100(13):4668–4670

Torok-Storb B (1990 Winter) Etiological mechanisms in immune-mediated aplastic anemia. Am J Pediatr Hematol Oncol 12(4):396–401

Townsley DM, Dumitriu B, Liu D, Biancotto A, Weinstein B, Chen C et al (2016) Danazol treatment for telomere diseases. N Engl J Med 374(20):1922–1931

Tutelman PR, Aubert G, Milner RA, Dalal BI, Schultz KR, Deyell RJ (2014) Paroxysmal nocturnal haemoglobinuria phenotype cells and leucocyte subset telomere length in childhood acquired aplastic anaemia. Br J Haematol 164(5):717–721

Tzakis AG, Arditi M, Whitington PF, Yanaga K, Esquivel C, Andrews WA et al (1988) Aplastic anemia complicating orthotopic liver transplantation for non-A, non-B hepatitis. N Engl J Med 319(7):393–396

Vassiliou GS, Webb DK, Pamphilon D, Knapper S, Veys PA (2001) Improved outcome of alternative donor bone marrow transplantation in children with severe aplastic anaemia using a conditioning regimen containing low-dose total body irradiation, cyclophosphamide and Campath. Br J Haematol 114(3):701–705

Viale M, Merli A, Bacigalupo A (1991) Analysis at the clonal level of T-cell phenotype and functions in severe aplastic anemia patients. Blood 78(5):1268–1274

Vulliamy TJ, Walne A, Baskaradas A, Mason PJ, Marrone A, Dokal I (2005) Mutations in the reverse transcriptase component of telomerase (TERT) in patients with bone marrow failure. Blood Cells Mol Dis 34(3):257–263

Wagner JL, Deeg HJ, Seidel K, Anasetti C, Doney K, Sanders J et al (1996) Bone marrow transplantation for severe aplastic anemia from genotypically HLA-nonidentical relatives. An update of the Seattle experience. Transplantation 61(1):54–61

Ware RE, Hall SE, Rosse WF (1991) Paroxysmal nocturnal hemoglobinuria with onset in childhood and adolescence. N Engl J Med 325(14):991–996

Williams DA, Bennett C, Bertuch A, Bessler M, Coates T, Corey S et al (2014) Diagnosis and treatment of pediatric acquired aplastic anemia (AAA): an initial survey of the North American Pediatric Aplastic Anemia Consortium (NAPAAC). Pediatr Blood Cancer 61(5):869–874

Xu Y, Takahashi Y, Wang Y, Hama A, Nishio N, Muramatsu H et al (2009) Downregulation of GATA-2 and overexpression of adipogenic gene-PPARgamma in mesenchymal stem cells from patients with aplastic anemia. Exp Hematol 37(12):1393–1399

Yagasaki H, Shichino H, Ohara A, Kobayashi R, Yabe H, Ohga S et al (2014) Immunosuppressive therapy with horse anti-thymocyte globulin and cyclosporine as treatment for fulminant aplastic anemia in children. Ann Hematol 93(5):747–752

Yamaguchi H, Calado RT, Ly H, Kajigaya S, Baerlocher GM, Chanock SJ et al (2005) Mutations in TERT, the gene for telomerase reverse transcriptase, in aplastic anemia. N Engl J Med 352(14):1413–1424

Yamamoto H, Kato D, Uchida N, Ishiwata K, Araoka H, Takagi S et al (2011) Successful sustained engraftment after reduced-intensity umbilical cord blood transplantation for adult patients with severe aplastic anemia. Blood 117(11):3240–3242

Yan L, Fu R, Liu H, Wang H, Liu C, Wang T et al (2015) Abnormal quantity and function of regulatory T cells in peripheral blood of patients with severe aplastic anemia. Cell Immunol 296(2):95–105

Yardley-Jones A, Anderson D, Parke DV (1991) The toxicity of benzene and its metabolism and molecular pathology in human risk assessment. Br J Ind Med 48(7):437–444

Yoshida N, Yagasaki H, Takahashi Y, Yamamoto T, Liang J, Wang Y et al (2008) Clinical impact of HLA-DR15, a minor population of paroxysmal nocturnal haemoglobinuria-type cells, and an aplastic anaemia-associated autoantibody in children with acquired aplastic anaemia. Br J Haematol 142(3):427–435

Yoshimi A, Niemeyer CM, Fuhrer MM, Strahm B (2013) Comparison of the efficacy of rabbit and horse antithymocyte globulin for the treatment of severe aplastic anemia in children. Blood 121(5):860–861

Yoshimi A, van den Heuvel-Eibrink MM, Baumann I, Schwarz S, Simonitsch-Klupp I, de Paepe P et al (2014) Comparison of horse and rabbit antithymocyte globulin in immunosuppressive therapy for refractory cytopenia of childhood. Haematologica 99(4):656–663

Yoshizato T, Dumitriu B, Hosokawa K, Makishima H, Yoshida K, Townsley D et al (2015) Somatic mutations and clonal hematopoiesis in aplastic anemia. N Engl J Med 373(1):35–47

Young NS, Issaragrasil S, Chieh CW, Takaku F (1986) Aplastic anaemia in the Orient. Br J Haematol 62(1):1–6

Zeng W, Maciejewski JP, Chen G, Young NS (2001) Limited heterogeneity of T cell receptor BV usage in aplastic anemia. J Clin Invest 108(5):765–773

Zeng W, Chen G, Kajigaya S, Nunez O, Charrow A, Billings EM et al (2004) Gene expression profiling in CD34 cells to identify differences between aplastic anemia patients and healthy volunteers. Blood 103(1):325–332

Zhang MY, Keel SB, Walsh T, Lee MK, Gulsuner S, Watts AC et al (2015) Genomic analysis of bone marrow failure and myelodysplastic syndromes reveals phenotypic and diagnostic complexity. Haematologica 100(1):42–48

Zhu X, Guan J, Xu J, Wei J, Jiang L, Yin J et al (2014) Pilot study using tacrolimus rather than cyclosporine plus antithymocyte globulin as an immunosuppressive therapy regimen option for severe aplastic anemia in adults. Blood Cells Mol Dis 53(3):157–160

Zonghong S, Meifeng T, Huaquan W, Limin X, Jun W, Rong F et al (2011) Circulating myeloid dendritic cells are increased in individuals with severe aplastic anemia. Int J Hematol 93(2):156–162

Pediatric Myelodysplastic Syndromes

3

Inga Hofmann

Contents

I. Hofmann
Pediatric Hematology/Oncology and Bone Marrow Transplant Program, University of Wisconsin, Madison, WI, USA
e-mail: ihofmann@wisc.edu

G. M. Kupfer et al. (eds.), *Bone Marrow Failure*, Pediatric Oncology,
https://doi.org/10.1007/978-3-319-61421-2_3

3.1 Introduction

The myelodysplastic syndromes (MDS) are a heterogeneous group of clonal hematopoietic stem cell (HSC) disorders characterized by varying degree of cytopenias, ineffective and dysplastic hematopoiesis, and the risk of leukemic transformation. MDS is the most common hematologic malignancy in adults and occurs most frequently in older adults with a median age of >65 years and male predominance.

Pediatric MDS accounts for only ~4% of all pediatric hematologic malignancies (Hasle et al. 1995, 1999a) and has an estimated annual incidence of ~1.8–4 cases per million children. In children the median age of diagnosis is 6.8 years, but the disease can occur in any age group. The male to female distribution of these disorders appears to be equal (Hasle et al. 1999a; Sasaki et al. 2001; Passmore et al. 2003; Luna-Fineman et al. 1999).

Pediatric MDS can occur *de novo* without an apparent underlying cause (*primary MDS*). *Secondary MDS* can develop after chemo- or radiation therapy, in association with an inherited bone marrow failure syndrome (IBMFS) or following an acquired bone marrow failure disorder (BMF), such as idiopathic acquired aplastic anemia (AA). An increasing number of inherited MDS/acute myeloid leukemia (AML) predisposition syndromes have been described and appear to be more common than previously anticipated. This is highlighted by the 2017 revision of the World Health Organization (WHO) classification of myeloid neoplasms and AML, with a new section on "myeloid neoplasms with germline predisposition" (Arber et al. 2016).

Pediatric MDS, IBMFS, and AA represent a spectrum of conditions that share significant clinical, laboratory, and histologic overlap. The majority of cases present with hypocellular bone marrow (BM), making them difficult to distinguish from acquired and inherited BMF disorders (Niemeyer and Baumann 2008). Moreover, BMF disorders can advance to MDS, further complicating diagnosis. Recent advancements in genomics have improved our understanding of clonal events in adult MDS, but little is known about the genetic events that lead to pediatric MDS. As a result, no targeted therapies are available, and hematopoietic stem cell transplantation (HSCT) remains the only curative therapy.

This review will address the current classification system for pediatric MDS and outline differences between pediatric and adult MDS. The clinical presentation, diagnostic work-up, histopathologic features, and recent genetic advances will be discussed. Finally, we review the current available therapies and prognosis of pediatric MDS.

3.2 Classification of MDS in Pediatric Patients

3.2.1 Historical Background

In 1976 the French-American-British Cooperative Group (FAB) introduced the first MDS classification system called "dysmyelopoietic syndromes." Until then the disease had been called "preleukemia" or "smoldering leukemia." In 1982 the modern term "myelodysplastic syndromes" (MDS) was introduced. The FAB classification contained five categories of MDS: (1) refractory anemia (RA), (2) refractory anemia with ringed sideroblasts (RARS), (3) refractory anemia with excess blasts (RAEB), (4) RAEB in transformation (RAEB-T), and (5) chronic myelomonocytic leukemia (CMML). This classification system established the basis for the first WHO classification introduced in 2000, which has undergone several updates to accommodate additional diagnostic criteria such as blast count, degree of dysplasia, cytogenetic changes, and most recently molecular changes. The most recent update to the WHO classification occurred in 2017 and incorporated an increasing number of molecular genetic changes into the classification, which will be discussed in this review as it pertains to pediatric cases (Arber et al. 2016).

3.2.2 Differences Between Adult and Pediatric MDS

Over the years, several significant differences between pediatric and adult MDS have been recognized. First, pediatric patients frequently present with hypocellular BM in contrast to adults who typically present with hypercellular BM. Second, pediatric patients more commonly present with thrombocytopenia and neutropenia, as opposed to isolated anemia (Kardos et al. 2003). Therefore, the term refractory cytopenia (RC) is used to describe this condition rather than the term refractory anemia (RA), which has been used in adults. Third, RARS and deletions in 5q are rare in children (Hasle et al. 1995; Sasaki et al. 2001; Luna-Fineman et al. 1999; Hasle et al. 1999b; Passmore et al. 1995; Antillon et al. 1998; Hasle et al. 2003; Shikano et al. 1992; Uyttebroeck et al. 1995). In fact, ringed sideroblasts in a pediatric patient are usually indicative of other etiologies such as nutritional deficiencies, drug toxicity, or congenital sideroblastic anemias, including Pearson marrow-pancreas syndrome, and should be considered in the differential diagnosis (Knerr et al. 2003; Fleming 2011).

In response to the differences between adult and pediatric MDS and the limited literature on pediatric patients, a pediatric classification scheme was proposed by Hasle and colleagues in 2003 (Hasle et al. 2003). These guidelines built on the 2000 WHO classification and established the first diagnostic criteria for pediatric MDS, requiring the presence of at least two of the following: (1) sustained unexplained cytopenia, (2) at least bilineage morphologic myelodysplasia, (3) acquired clonal cytogenetic abnormality in hematopoietic cells, or (4) increased BM blasts (>5%) (Hasle et al. 2003). In addition, juvenile myelomonocytic leukemia (JMML) and MDS associated with Down syndrome were recognized as distinct entities.

This separate pediatric MDS classification was crafted to address two challenges: (1) to differentiate MDS with a low blast count from acquired and inherited BMF conditions (AA and IBMFS) and (2) to segregate MDS with excess blasts (RAEB) from *de novo* AML. The first pediatric classification scheme divided pediatric MDS into three main categories: refractory cytopenia (RC), RAEB, and RAEB-T (Table 3.1).

Table 3.1 Original WHO classification of childhood MDS

Diagnostic category	PB blasts%	BM blasts%
Refractory cytopenia of childhood (RCC)	<2	<5
Refractory anemia with excess blasts (RAEB)	2–19	5–19
RAEB in transformation (RAEB-T)	20–29	20–29

Adapted from WHO Classification of Tumours of Haematopoietic and Lymphoid Tissues. Baumann et al. (2008)

3.2.3 Current Classification of Pediatric MDS

In 2008, the WHO classification introduced a pediatric MDS classification for the first time (Kardos et al. 2003). The pediatric classification was built on the basis of the earlier proposal by Hasle and colleagues brought forth in 2003 (Hasle et al. 2003). The 2008 WHO classification of pediatric MDS is largely based on the peripheral blood (PB) and BM blast percentage and is outlined in Table 1 (Baumann et al. 2008). The major difference between the proposal by Hasle et al. and the WHO classification is that the term RC was updated to refractory cytopenia of childhood (RCC).

Table 3.2 Revised 2016 WHO classification of adult and pediatric MDS and associated PB and BM findings and cytogenetics

Diagnostic category	Dysplastic lineages	Cytopenias[a]	BM blasts[b]	PB blasts[b]	Ring sideroblasts	Karyotype
MDS with single lineage dysplasia (MDS-SLD)	1	1–2	<5%	<1%	<15% or <5% if Sf3b1 mutated	Any[c]
MDS with multilineage dysplasia (MDS-MLD)	2–3	1–3	<5%	<1%	<15% or <5% if Sf3b1 mutated	Any[c]
MDS with ring sideroblasts (MDS-RS)						
MDS-RS with single lineage dysplasia (MDS-RS-SLD)	1	1–2	<5%	<1%	≥15% or ≥5% if Sf3b1 mutated	Any[c]
MDS-RS with multilineage dysplasia (MDS-RS-MLD)	2–3	1–3	<5%	<1%	≥15% or ≥5% if Sf3b1 mutated	Any[c]
MDS with isolated del(5q)	1–3	1–2	<5%	<1%	None or any	del(5q) alone or with 1 additional abnormality except −7 or del(7q)
MDS with excess blasts (MDS-EB)						
MDS-EB-1	0–3	1–3	5–9%	2–4%	None or any	Any
MDS-EB-2	0–3	1–3	10–19%	5–19%	None or any	Any
MDS, unclassifiable (MDS-U)						
With 1% PB blasts	1–3	1–3	<5%	1%[d]	None or any	Any
With single lineage dysplasia and pancytopenia	1	3	<5%	<1%	None or any	Any
Based on defining cytogenetic abnormality	0	1–3	<5%	<1%	<15%[e]	MDS-defining abnormality
Refractory cytopenia of childhood (RCC)[f]	1–3	1–3	<5%	<2%	None	Any

Adopted from Arber et al. (2016) and WHO Classification of Tumours of Haematopoietic and Lymphoid Tissues (revised 4th edition). Swerdlow et al. (2017)

[a]Cytopenias defined as hemoglobin <10 g/dL; platelet count <100 × 10^9/L, absolute neutrophil count <1.8 × 10^9/L, PB monocyte count <1 × 10^9/L

[b]Typically no Auer rods present except MDS-EB-2 may have Auer rods

[c]Any cytogenetic abnormality by conventional karyotype analysis unless it fulfills all the criteria for MDS with isolated del(5q)

[d]1% PB blasts must be recorded in at least two separate occasions

[e]Cases with ≥15% ring sideroblasts by definition have significant erythroid dysplasia and are classified as MDS-RS-SLD

[f]RCC remains a provisional entity

The 2017 revision to the WHO classification of myeloid neoplasms and acute leukemia included several changes to the classification of adult MDS (Table 3.2). These included modifications that reflect that the diagnosis of MDS largely relies on the degree of dysplasia and blast percentage with less emphasis on the magnitude of a specific cytopenia. Therefore, the terminology for adult MDS has changed from using terms such as "refractory anemia" to "myelodysplastic syndrome" followed by appropriate modifiers such as single versus multilineage dysplasia, ring sideroblasts, excess blasts, or del(5q). Furthermore, the recent revision seeks to address the rapidly evolving field of genetics and genomics in MDS. Targeted gene sequencing can detect somatic mutations in 80–90% of MDS patients, but the presence of an MDS-associated somatic mutation alone is not considered diagnostic of MDS in the current WHO classification (Arber et al. 2016).

A number of specific mutations are associated with disease outcomes in adult MDS and are specifically mentioned in the revised classification. For example, *TP53* mutations are associated with aggressive disease, predict a poor response to lenalidomide in patients with del(5q), and confer a poor prognosis in all subtypes of MDS. MDS patients with ring sideroblasts (MDS-RS) have recurrent mutations in the spliceosome gene *SF3B1*, which confers a favorable prognosis. The updated classification now includes a category of MDS-RS with single or multilineage dysplasia (lacking excess blasts) or with isolated del(5q) (Table 3.2). Furthermore, the requirement of at least 15% ring sideroblasts was removed for all cases with a *SF3B1* mutation.

While these recent changes in the revised WHO classification reflect advances in the understanding of MDS in adults, many of these changes do not affect classification of MDS in children since MDS with del(5q) and MDS-RS are rarely seen. How somatic mutations impact the clinical course and outcome of pediatric MDS patients remain uncertain and more data are needed to determine the clinical and prognostic significance of somatic mutations in children with MDS.

Over the last few years, an increasing number of inherited MDS/AML predisposition syndromes have been described and appear to be more common than previously anticipated. This is highlighted by the 2017 revision of the WHO classification of myeloid neoplasms and AML, with a new section on "myeloid neoplasms with germline predisposition" (Arber et al. 2016) (Table 3.3). This is a separate category within

Table 3.3 Inherited conditions associated with myelodysplastic syndrome (MDS)

Myeloid neoplasms with germline predisposition to MDS
Myeloid neoplasms with germline predisposition without preexisting disorder or organ dysfunction (non-syndromic)
AML with germline *CEBPA* mutation
Myeloid neoplasms with germline *DDX41* mutation[a#]
Myeloid neoplasms with germline predisposition and preexisting platelet disorders
Myeloid neoplasms with germline *RUNX1* mutation[a]
Myeloid neoplasms with germline *ANKRD26* mutation[a]
Myeloid neoplasms with germline *ETV6* mutation[a]
Myeloid neoplasms with germline predisposition and other organ dysfunction (syndromic)
Myeloid neoplasms with germline *GATA2* mutation
Myeloid neoplasms associated with IBMFS (e.g., FA, SDS, SNC, DBA)
Myeloid neoplasms associated with telomere biology disorders (DC)
JMML associated with neurofibromatosis, Noonan syndrome
Noonan syndrome-like disorders
Myeloid neoplasms associated with Down syndrome[a]
Others
Familial MDS (at least one first degree relative with MDS/AML) without identified genetic cause[b]

Adapted from Arber et al. (2016) and WHO Classification of Tumours of Haematopoietic and Lymphoid Tissues (revised 4th edition). Swerdlow et al. (2017)

FA = Fanconi anemia, SDS = Shwachman-Diamond syndrome, SCN = severe congenital neutropenia, DBA = Diamond-Blackfan anemia, # typically not seen in children

[a]Myeloid and lymphoid neoplasms have been reported

[b]Familial cases of MDS not due to genetic causes listed above

the WHO classification and not restricted to MDS, but applicable to all myeloid neoplasms (MDS and AML). Germline predispositions are more frequent in pediatric MDS; therefore this new category is highly applicable and a valuable tool for the diagnosis of children with MDS and myeloid disease.

It is important to note that the 2017 revision of the 2008 WHO classification made no significant changes to the classification of childhood MDS, RCC remains a provisional entity within this group. The revised edition clarifies that pediatric MDS cases with increased blasts (2–19% blasts in PB or 5–19% blasts in BM) should be classified using the same criteria as for adult MDS with excess blasts. Therefore RAEB is now called MDS-EB. The 2008 WHO classification held on to the RAEB-T (20–29% blasts) used on the older FAB classificaton system. Based on the 2017 revision the term AML with myelodysplasia-related changes (AML-MRC) should now be used.

3.3 Refractory Cytopenia of Childhood

RCC is the most frequent subtype of pediatric MDS accounting for at least 50% of cases (Passmore et al. 2003; Niemeyer and Baumann 2008). Most patients with RCC present with hypocellular BM making the differential diagnosis to acquired or inherited BMF conditions challenging (Niemeyer and Baumann 2011). The presence of a clonal cytogenetic marker is helpful in confirming the diagnosis; however, about 61–67% of patients with RCC have normal cytogenetics (Niemeyer and Baumann 2011).

RCC remains a provisional entity in the 2017 revision of the WHO classification. RCC includes a wide range of phenotypes, ranging from hypo- to hypercellular RCC with limited unilineage dysplasia to overt multilineage dysplasia, which remains one of the challenges with the current pediatric MDS classification. RCC with multilineage dysplasia (RCMD) is easily appreciated as unequivocal MDS. In contrast, hypocellular RCC with minimal or unilineage dysplasia can be difficult to differentiate from acquired AA and IBMFS. The clinical and prognostic implications of unilineage versus multilineage dysplasia in pediatric MDS remain uncertain (Hasle et al. 2003; Cantu Rajnoldi et al. 2005). Therefore, the recommendation was made to group all pediatric MDS without excess blasts into the RCC category, regardless of the degree of dysplasia and cellularity. One study presents an opposing view and suggests that patients with RCC and multilineage dysplasia have a significantly higher incidence of disease progression (Hasegawa et al. 2014), which would favor the use of RCMD as a separate category.

3.3.1 Differentiating Severe Aplastic Anemia from Hypocellular Refractory Cytopenia of Childhood

The diagnosis of RCC remains controversial due to the limitations in the reproducibility of the diagnostic criteria and limited data on the clinical implications (Hasegawa et al. 2014; Yang et al. 2012). While some studies suggest that the classification of RCC is valuable and reproducible (Baumann et al. 2012), others suggest that the diagnosis is difficult to establish with certainty (Forester et al. 2015) and does not accurately predict response and outcomes after immunosuppressive therapy (Hasegawa et al. 2014; Forester et al. 2015). The revised WHO classification has not added clarification, additional criteria, or data to support or reject this classification scheme. Therefore, RCC remains to be defined as (1) dysplasia in one or more hematopoietic lineages or in at least 10% of cells in one cell line and (2) <5% blasts in the marrow (Baumann et al. 2008). Differentiating hypocellular RCC from severe aplastic anemia (SAA) remains difficult. For this reason, the WHO outlined key histological differences between the two disorders (Table 3.4; Fig. 3.1), which heavily rely on a topographic diagnosis with certain histologic patterns.

It is critical to remember that patients with IBMFS (e.g., Fanconi anemia (FA), dyskerato-

Table 3.4 Histopathologic criteria of hypocellular RCC and SAA as outlined in the WHO classification

Lineage characteristics	RCC	SAA
Erythroid	Patchy, left-shifted erythropoiesis with increased mitoses	Lacking foci or left-shifted erythroid cells or only showing single small focus of <10 cells of erythroid cells with maturation
Myeloid	Markedly decreased, left-shifted myelopoiesis	Lacking or markedly decreased myelopoiesis with very few small foci of granulopoiesis with maturation
Megakaryocytes	Markedly decreased megakaryopoiesis Dysplastic changes (micromegakaryocytes)[a]	Lacking or only very few megakaryocytes present No dysplastic changes or micromegakaryocytes[a]
Lymphoid	Lymphocytes, PC, and MC may be focally increased or dispersed	Lymphocytes, PC, and MC may be focally increased or dispersed
CD34+ cells	Not increased	Not increased

Adapted from the 2008 WHO classification and Hofmann (2015)
PC = plasma cells, MC = mast cells
[a]Immunohistochemistry with CD61 staining is required for the detection of micromegakaryocytes

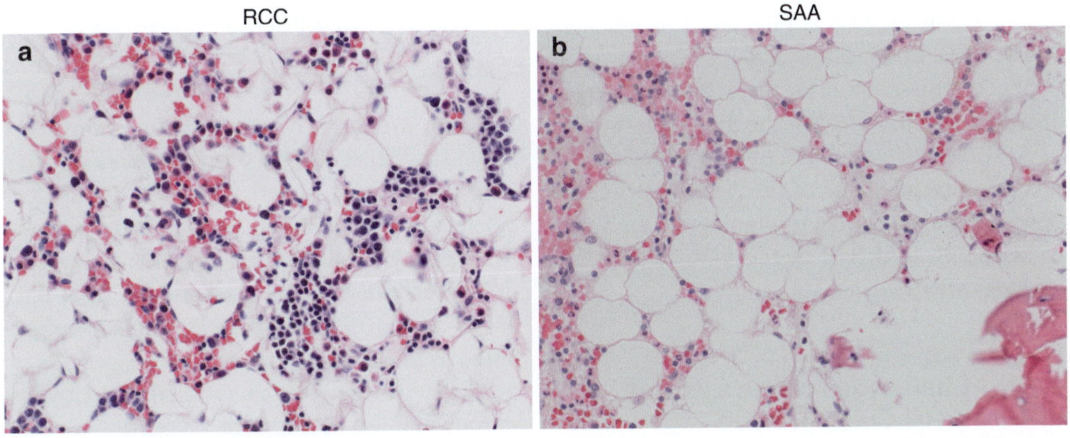

Fig. 3.1 Histology of hypocellular refractory anemia of childhood (RCC) compared to severe aplastic anemia (SAA). (**a**) The image shows an example of a child's marrow with hypocellular RCC (left) and illustrates a hypocellular marrow with patches of erythroid predominant hematopoiesis (BM). Erythroid islands show increased early forms, mitosis, and occasional nuclear contour abnormalities. Scattered mildly left-shifted myeloid elements are noted in the background. Megakaryocytes are not present. (**b**) In contrast, an image of marrow from a child with severe aplastic anemia (SAA) (right) shows a severely hypocellular, adipose-rich marrow with scattered lymphocytes and fully maturing myeloid cells including segmented neutrophils. Clusters of immature erythroid cells are not seen. Megakaryocytes are absent. Magnification 400× [Images Hofmann (2015) Pediatric myelodysplastic syndromes, with permission]

sis congenita (DC), or Shwachman-Diamond syndrome (SDS)) show histologic features consistent with RCC (Hasle et al. 2003; Yoshimi et al. 2013; Elghetany 2007). Therefore, these conditions must be excluded by molecular testing. For patients with IBMFS that progressed to overt MDS or AML, the disease should be categorized according to the new WHO classification of "myeloid neoplasms with germline predisposition."

3.4 Advanced MDS

Advanced MDS is characterized by morphologic dysplasia and increased blast count in the BM. Historically the blast cutoff for the diagnosis of AML was set at 30% and had been lowered to 20% for pediatric and adult *de novo* AML. For this reason, the category of RAEB-T was omitted in the 2008 WHO classification of adult MDS, and these cases are now regarded as AML-MRC.

In contrast, the 2008 WHO classification for advanced pediatric MDS retained the old FAB classification system and recognized two categories: (1) RAEB-1 (5–10% blasts) or RAEB-2 (11–20% blasts) and (2) RAEB-T (20–29% blasts). This recommendation was made based on limited evidence in the pediatric literature that a blast cutoff of 20% is of clinical significance (Hasle et al. 2003; Hasle 2007; Niemeyer et al. 2005). The blast cutoff for the definition of AML is arbitrary, and, in reality, the transition of MDS to AML is likely a continuum. The recent 2017 revision retained much of the 2008 classification system but updated the terminology from RAEB to MDS-EB. RAEB-T should now be classified as AML-MRC.

3.5 Challenges of the Current WHO Classification

The WHO classification is the current standard for diagnosis of pediatric MDS. While these guidelines allow for accurate classification of most pediatric MDS (Elghetany 2007), there are several limitations that need to be addressed in future editions.

First, classification based on blast count alone is a crude method of distinguishing clinical phenotypes. With the rapid advancement of sequencing technologies, additional inherited predisposition syndromes may be identified that will aid in the classification and characterization of pediatric MDS. Second, the provisional entity of RCC includes a wide range of phenotypes ranging from hypocellular conditions with limited dysplasia to overt MDS with unequivocal or trilineage dysplasia and hypercellular marrow. The lack of better-defined subcategories, like those used in the adult classification system (e.g., such as differentiation between uni- versus multilineage dysplasia—RCMD) makes it difficult to interpret clinical studies. Third, the different terminologies and definitions used in pediatric and adult MDS patients cause confusion. Another complicating factor is that the pediatric MDS classification schemes are not universally applied in the literature of pediatric MDS further confounding the interpretation of clinical outcomes. For this reason, the use of consistent contemporary terms for pediatric and adult MDS subtypes would be helpful.

3.6 Primary Versus Secondary MDS

Pediatric MDS can be classified into primary or secondary MDS. Primary MDS occurs *de novo* with no apparent underlying cause and is considered idiopathic in nature. Secondary pediatric MDS can result from a number of acquired conditions or inherited predispositions (Table 3.3). MDS related to underlying germline predisposition is increasingly recognized, especially in pediatric patients, which is highlighted by the introduction of a separate category "myeloid neoplasms with germline predisposition" and discussed in detail below.

Patients with AA treated with immunosuppressive therapy (IST) can develop secondary MDS and clonal evolution. Conventionally AA has been regarded as an acquired cause of secondary MDS (Hasle et al. 2003; Elghetany 2007) although it is possible that these patients have an underlying inherited genetic predisposition, which could explain the poor outcomes of some AA patients with clonal progression to MDS.

Therapy-related myeloid neoplasms (t-MNs) is a distinct category in the WHO classification, which contains therapy-related MDS (t-MDS) and AML (t-AML). T-MDS occurs following chemo- or radiation therapy. The most frequently involved cytogenetic changes involve chromosomes 7, 5, and 11q23, which are observed in more than 90% of the cases (Tsurusawa et al. 2005). Increasing evidence shows that some patients with t-MNs carry germline mutations in cancer predisposition genes—therefore a careful family history and possible genetic testing should be considered (Churpek et al. 2016).

3.7 MDS Due to Germline Predisposition

Familial MDS has long been recognized as a unique disease entity in the literature, but it was not until recently that we have gained a better understanding of the molecular genetic underpinnings of these disorders. Novel sequencing technologies have allowed for a rapid advancement in the field with an increasing number of MDS predisposition genes described over the last few years. This accumulation of genetic information in cases of familial MDS and AML is now reflected in the 2017 revision of the WHO classification of myeloid neoplasms and leukemia with the introduction of the new category "myeloid neoplasms with germline predisposition." Germline predispositions to MDS/AML can be syndromic, involving other organ systems (e.g., *GATA2*, *SAMD9*, *SBDS*, *TERC*, *TERT*) (Kirwan et al. 2009; Liew and Owen 2011; Nagamachi et al. 2013; Churpek et al. 2013; Hahn et al. 2011; Hsu et al. 2011; Ostergaard et al. 2011; Spinner et al. 2014; Vinh et al. 2010; Wlodarski et al. 2016; Narumi et al. 2016), non-syndromic (e.g., *CEBPA*, *DDX41*) (Owen et al. 2008; Smith et al. 2004; Cardoso et al. 2016; Lewinsohn et al. 2016; Li et al. 2016; Polprasert et al. 2015), or associated with preexisting platelet disorders (e.g., *RUNX1*, *ANKRD26*, *ETV6*) (Buijs et al. 2012; Churpek et al. 2010; Michaud et al. 2002; Zhang et al. 2015; Noris et al. 2013) (Table 3.3). These germline predispositions can occur de novo in the proband or passed down from the parents and are inherited following gene-specific patterns.

The line between an IBMFS, such as FA, SDS, or DC, and transformation to an overt MDS is often blurry. Patients with BM failure due to an inherited predisposition frequently show some degree of background dysplasia at baseline and typically present with a morphological picture of hypocellular RCC (Yoshimi et al. 2013). For example, patients with marrow failure due to SDS often show dysmyelopoiesis (in particular in the neutrophil series) at baseline without overt progression to MDS (Wong et al. 2010). Patients with GATA2 haploinsufficiency show unique megakaryocytic dysplasia with large separated, "pulled apart" appearing nuclei that often precedes the development of MDS (Spinner et al. 2014; Calvo et al. 2011). Therefore, minimal diagnostic criteria for secondary MDS following an underlying IBMFS have been developed (Hasle et al. 2003) and include increased BM blast count, development of hypercellular marrow in presence of persistent PB cytopenias, and acquired clonal chromosomal abnormalities. It is important to note that not all clonal cytogenetic abnormalities are associated with disease progression and poor outcomes. Some patients with FA and SDS have persistent cytogenetic changes for years without evolution to MDS/AML (Alter 2003; Alter et al. 1993; Maarek et al. 1996).

3.7.1 MDS Due to Germline Mutations in *GATA2*

Autosomal-dominant germline *GATA2* mutations cause a spectrum of disorders ranging from low-grade MDS to high-grade MDS/AML with poor prognosis (Wlodarski et al. 2016; Hofmann et al. 2013a; Hofmann et al. 2013b). The disease can occur in pediatric and adult patients but appears to be more common in children and the younger adult population. When first discovered in 2011, four entities were described: (1) autosomal-dominant familial MDS/AML (Hahn et al. 2011); (2) Emberger syndrome, characterized by lymphedema, warts, and predisposition to MDS/AML (Ostergaard et al. 2011); (3) MonoMac syndrome, comprised of monocytopenia and nontuberculous mycobacterial infection (Hsu et al. 2011; Vinh et al. 2010); and (4) dendritic cell, monocyte, and B and natural killer cell lymphoid deficiency (DCML) (Bigley and Collin 2011; Bigley et al. 2011; Dickinson et al. 2011).

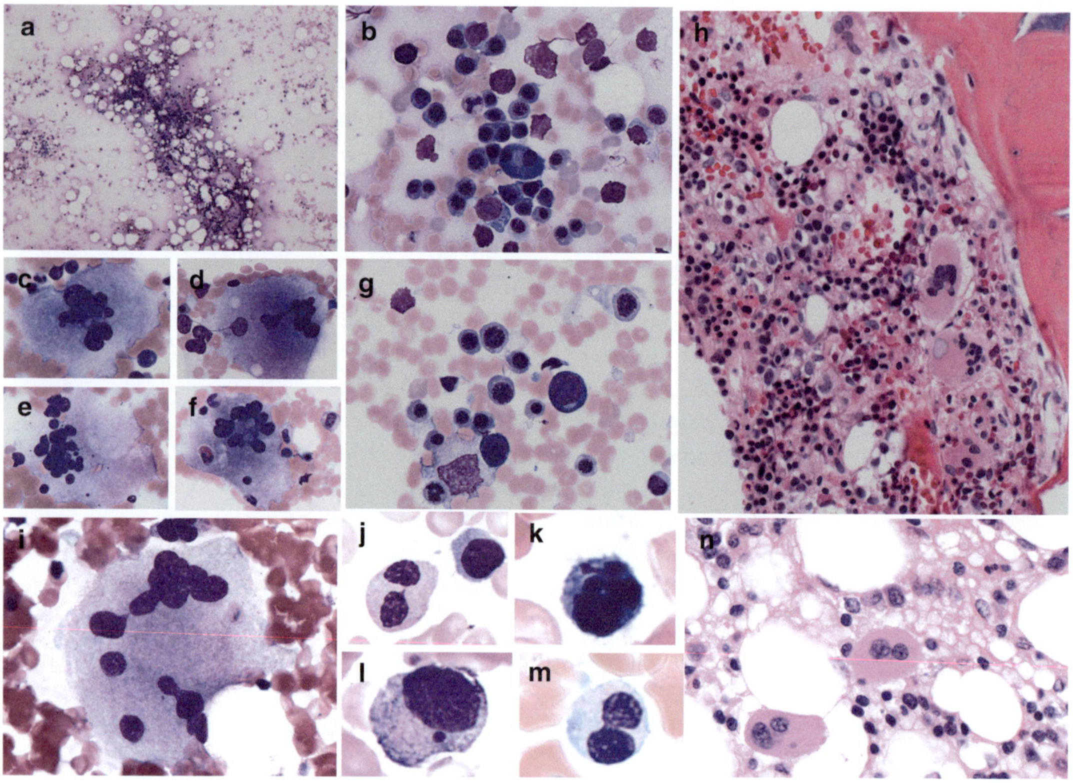

Fig. 3.2 Unique histopathology in pediatric MDS due to *GATA2* mutation. (**a–g**) Representative images from the marrow of a 17-year-old male with fevers, lymphadenopathy, and splenomegaly secondary to primary EBV infection. He eventually developed persistent pancytopenia (absolute neutrophil count (ANC) 400 cells/μL, absolute monocyte count (AMC) 0 cells/μL, platelet count 44 cells/μL) with morphological dysplasia, despite normalizing EBV titers and negative laboratory and molecular work-up for hemophagocytic lymphohistiocytosis. The BM aspirate was hypocellular (**a**) (200×) with a relative erythroid hyperplasia with megaloblastoid changes and dyserythropoiesis (**b**, **g**) (400×). Megakaryocytes displayed marked dysplasia with hyperlobated pulled apart nuclei (**c–f**) (1000×). The biopsy showed a hypocellular marrow with erythroid hyperplasia and dysplastic megakaryocytes appearing in loose clusters (**h**) (400×). Images (**i**)–(**n**) are from an 18-year-old young male with a hydrocele and an incidental finding of pancytopenia (WBC 1.9 cells/μL, Hgb 10.2 g/dL, MCV 106, platelet count 134 cells/μL). The subsequent BM aspirate shows characteristic dysplastic megakaryocytes (**i**), myeloid and erythroid dysplasia with pseudo-Pelger-Huet forms (**j**), erythroid nuclear contour abnormalities (**k**) nuclear satellites (**l**), and hypogranular myeloid cells (**m**), and erythroid dysplasia with nuclear contour abnormalities (**k**) (**i–m** 1000×). The biopsy showed a hypocellular marrow with erythroid hyperplasia and dysplastic megakaryocytes (**n**) (400×). Both patients were ultimately diagnosed with MDS due to mutations in *GATA2* [Images Hofmann (2015) Pediatric myelodysplastic syndromes, with permission]

It is now recognized that these conditions represent a spectrum of hematopoietic, lymphatic, and immune system disorders. The reasons for the wide phenotypic spectrum remain enigmatic (Fig. 3.2).

Mutations in *GATA2* can occur sporadically in the proband or as familial MDS (Hsu et al. 2011; Vinh et al. 2010). *GATA2* mutations include missense mutations and in-frame deletions involving the zinc fingers, nonsense mutations, frameshifts and deletions predicted to yield null alleles, and *cis*-element mutations at the +9.5 intronic enhancer (Hsu et al. 2013; Johnson et al. 2012). In pediatric MDS patients, mutations in the coding region impair DNA binding or prevent full-length GATA2 synthesis, while enhancer mutations decrease GATA2 expression—both disrupting GATA2-dependent genetic networks, thus yielding pathologies (Hahn et al. 2011; Hsu et al. 2011; Ostergaard et al. 2011; Spinner et al. 2014; Dickinson et al.

2011; Hsu et al. 2013; Johnson et al. 2012; Kazenwadel et al. 2012; Pasquet et al. 2013).

To date, a wide spectrum of clinical phenotypic features have been described which include immunodeficiency, predisposition to MDS/AML, pulmonary alveolar proteinosis (PAP), congenital lymphedema, sensorineural hearing loss, thrombotic events, panniculitis/erythema nodosum, increased incidence of miscarriages, infections (e.g., fungal, Epstein-Barr virus (EBV), *Clostridium difficile*), and human papillomavirus (HPV) and EBV-driven tumors (Spinner et al. 2014). The clinical presentation, specifically onset and severity of the disease, can be very heterogeneous. Some patients are asymptomatic at the time of diagnosis, while others present with life-threatening infections or MDS/AML. Varying severity of phenotypes can even be observed within a single family. Genotype-phenotype associations have failed to fully explain the spectrum in the disease phenotype (Spinner et al. 2014).

It is important to note that the clinical presentation of patients with GATA2-related BMF can overlap with acquired AA. Routine laboratory values, flow cytometry, BM morphology, and cytogenetic studies can aid in the differential diagnosis and identify patients at high risk of carrying a *GATA2* mutation for whom GATA2 sequencing is indicated (Ganapathi et al. 2015). For example, hemoglobin levels and platelet and absolute neutrophil counts (ANC) are typically lower in AA patients compared to GATA2 patients. In contrast, the monocyte and lymphocyte counts are often severely decreased in GATA2 patients, but only mildly reduced in patients with AA (Ganapathi et al. 2015).

Flow cytometry of BM from GATA2-mutated patients typically shows a reduced number of monocytes, although the number of monocytes can be increased in advanced MDS. Decreased B cells and NK cells and a complete loss of B-cell precursors/hematogones (CD19+, CD10+, CD20−) are usually observed. Furthermore, an expansion of T cells with an inverted CD4:CD8 ratio, and an increase in large granular lymphocytes (CD3+, CD16+, CD56+) cells can be seen. Increased myeloid blasts are often noted, in particular in advanced disease (Vinh et al. 2010; Calvo et al. 2011; Ganapathi et al. 2015).

The majority of patients with a *GATA2* mutation (84%) meet histomorphologic criteria for MDS, most commonly classified as MDS with multilineage dysplasia and <5% blasts (Spinner et al. 2014). GATA2 patients show unique BM morphology characteristics. The most common finding is a unique megakaryocytic dysplasia, observed in ~90% of patients (Spinner et al. 2014; Calvo et al. 2011; Ganapathi et al. 2015). Megakaryocytes are often large and show separated “pulled apart” and peripherally placed nuclear lobes, which can be seen prior to or without overt progression to MDS/AML. Micromegakaryocytes have been observed as well (Ganapathi et al. 2015). Features of erythroid (megaloblastoid changes, nuclear contour irregularities, and bi-nucleation) or myeloid dysplasia (maturation dyssynchrony and hypogranulation) occur less frequently (in about 50% of the cases). The myeloid-to-erythroid ratio is frequently reversed. Reticulin fibrosis is a common feature of GATA2-mediated MDS seen in about 50% of the cases (Ganapathi et al. 2015). A subset of patients shows clinical and histologic features of chronic myelomonocytic leukemia (CMML), which typically indicates disease progression to a proliferative state with increased myelomonocytic cells (Spinner et al. 2014).

Monosomy 7 is the most common cytogenetic abnormality in GATA2-mutated MDS, suggesting an association between monosomy 7 and *GATA2* (Wlodarski et al. 2016). Other cytogenetic abnormalities include trisomy 8, gain of 1q, and deletions of parts or the entire chromosome 6 (Spinner et al. 2014; Ganapathi et al. 2015).

The association with monosomy 7 is intriguing. The historic literature reports on pediatric patients with “monosomy 7 syndrome,” a disease characterized by a leukoerythroblastic anemia and thrombocytopenia associated with loss of one copy of chromosome 7. The BM typically showed an increase in blasts and reticulin fibrosis in a background of a dysplastic marrow (Sieff et al. 1981). A subset of these cases was familial in origin (Hasle et al. 1999b) and showed significant clinical and histologic overlap with the features observed in contemporary pediatric patients’ MDS due to *GATA2* mutation. We can now presume that a subset of the patients that were historically described as “monosomy 7 syn-

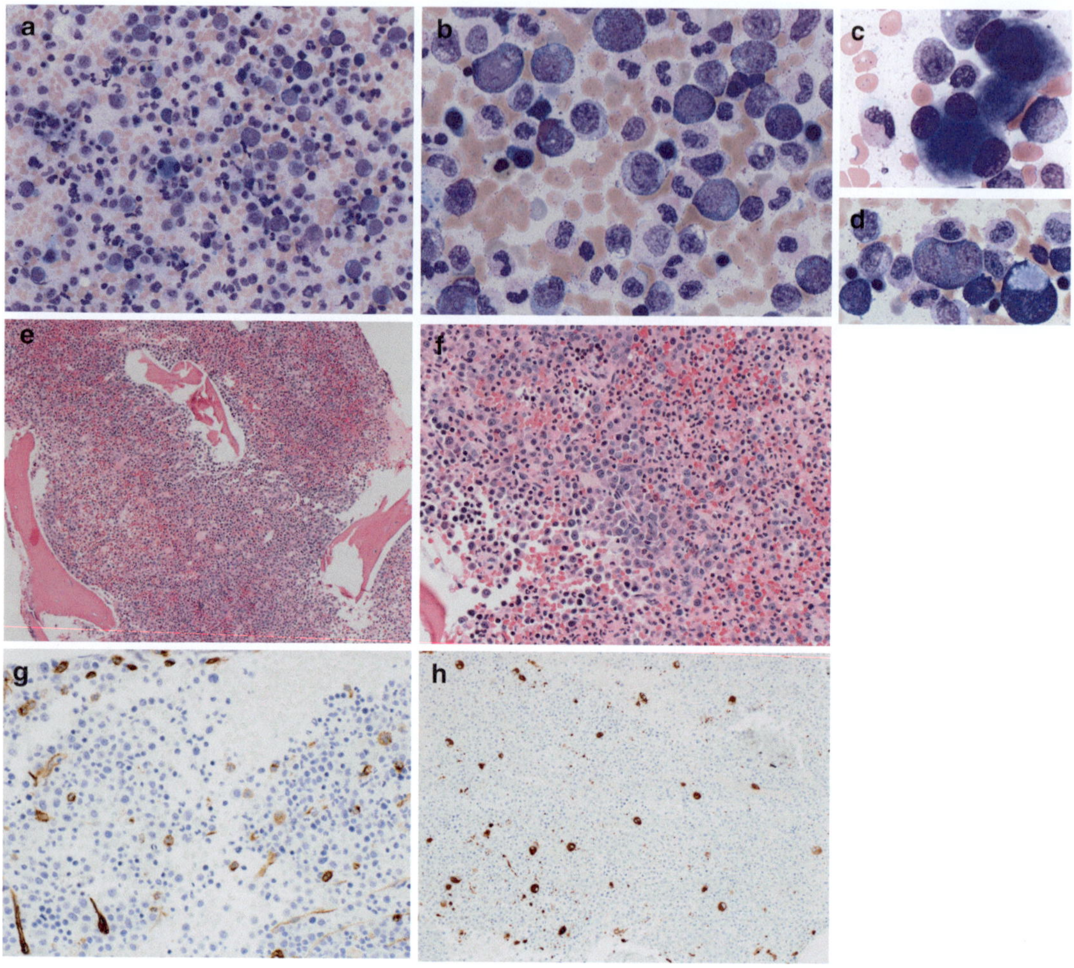

Fig. 3.3 Monosomy 7 syndrome. Representative bone marrow (BM) aspirate and biopsy images of the marrow from a 19-year-old male with "monosomy 7 syndrome." The patient presented with easy bruising and a leukocytosis of 39.0 cells/μL with 2% circulating blasts and the presence of metamyelocytes and myelocytes on the peripheral blood smear. The absolute monocyte count was 2.15 cells/μL. The hemoglobin (Hgb) was 10.0 g/dL and the platelet count was 76 × 10^3/μL. Cytogenetic studies showed monosomy 7 in 20 out of 20 metaphases. (**a**, **b**) BM aspirate (200× and 400×) showed a hypercellular myeloid predominant marrow. The myeloid elements were left shifted and dysplastic with hypolobated forms. The erythroid series showed megaloblastoid maturation. Megakaryocytes showed frequent dysplastic forms. (**c**) High power view (1000×) of two dysplastic megakaryocytes with separated nuclear lobes. (**d**) Illustration of dysplastic early promonocyte to monocyte with two nuclei and nuclear satellite. (**e**) BM biopsy (100×) showed a hypercellular marrow with (**f**) myeloid predominance and clusters of early myeloid forms (200×). (**g**) Immunohistochemistry (IHC) for CD34 showed scattered blasts comprising <5% of the overall cellularity (200×). (**h**) ICH for CD61 highlighted increased and often smaller sized megakaryocytes, including micromegakaryocytes, small hypolobated forms, and dysplastic forms with separated nuclear lobes (100×) [Images Hofmann (2015) Pediatric myelodysplastic syndromes, with permission]

drome" or MDS/AML with monosomy 7 is likely due to *GATA2* mutation (Fig. 3.3).

In summary, patients with GATA2-related MDS show unique clinical and histologic features that should be carefully evaluated in any pediatric patient with suspected MDS or BMF. The histopathology, in particular the megakaryocytic dysplasia, is striking enough to provide instant pattern recognition. Because of the significant clinical and genetic implications for patients with *GATA2* mutation, genetic testing is mandatory on all patients that display phenotypic features of familial MDS, Emberger syndrome, and MonoMac syndrome. Genetic testing should be considered in all pediatric patients with MDS or BMF and in those patients with a hematologic malignancy and monosomy 7. Testing of family members and genetic counseling should be offered to all patients with documented *GATA2* mutation but is obligatory for any related HSCT donors.

3.7.2 MDS Due to Germline Mutations in *SAMD9*

Recently two other syndromes with germline predisposition to myeloid malignancy have been described. MIRAGE syndrome is characterized by myelodysplasia, infection, restriction of growth, adrenal hypoplasia, genital phenotypes, and enteropathy (Narumi et al. 2016). Ataxia-pancytopenia (AP) syndrome, initially described in 1978 by Frederick Pei Li (Li et al. 1978), is characterized by cerebellar ataxia, variable cytopenias, and predisposition to BMF and myeloid leukemia. Both syndromes have been found to be due to heterozygous germline mutations in sterile alpha motif (SAM) domain gene (*SAMD9*). The autosomal-dominant inheritance and phenotype suggest *SAMD9* variants are activating mutations.

Interestingly, *SAMD9* resides in the common microdeletion cluster in 7q21.3 (Asou et al. 2009). Haploinsufficiency of *SAMD9*L, a mouse *SAMD9* ortholog, causes myeloid malignancy with monosomy 7 that resembles monosomy 7-linked human disease (Nagamachi et al. 2013). The initial description of MIRAGE syndrome included two patients with mosaic monosomy 7 that was present at the time of the genetic diagnosis. Subsequently both patients developed MDS with monosomy 7 between age 2 and 3 years (Narumi et al. 2016). Similar findings were observed in patients with AP syndrome (Chen et al. 2016). The association with monosomy 7 is intriguing. Mosaic monosomy 7 occurred before the onset of clinical overt MDS thereby removing the *SAMD9* mutant allele in a subset of cells. SAMD9 mutant cells showed a growth-restricted phenotype in several tissues. This suggests that deletion of chromosome 7 provides an escape mechanism and growth and survival advantage by eliminating *SAMD9* mutant cells (Chen et al. 2016) and is the first human disease example of "adaptation by aneuploidy".

3.8 Somatic Mutations in MDS

The advent of novel sequencing technologies has accelerated the pace of discovery in adult MDS. Since the early genetic studies that lead to discovery of somatic mutations in oncogenes (*NRAS*/*KRAS*) and tumor suppressor genes (*TP53*, *RUNX1*) (Kaneko et al. 1995; Pedersen-Bjergaard et al. 2002a; Pedersen-Bjergaard et al. 2002b), over 40 MDS-associated gene mutations have been discovered in the last several years, including identification of epigenetic regulators (*TET2*, *ASXL1*, *EZH2*, *DNMT3A*, *IDH1*/*IDH2*) and, most recently, genes in the splicing machinery (*SFRB1*, *U2AF1*, *ZRSR2*) and cohesion complex genes (*STAG2*, *SMC3*, *RAD21*). In adult MDS, somatic mutations in splicing factors and epigenetic regulators are present in about 75% of cases, followed by isolated TP53 mutations and mutations in a variety of other genes including transcription factors (*RUNX1*, *ETV6*, *GATA2*, *PHF6*), kinase signaling (*NRAS*, *KRAS*, *JAK2*, *CBL*), and cohesion complex genes (Papaemmanuil et al. 2011; Visconte et al. 2012; Yoshida et al. 2011). Interestingly, the majority of these changes—in particular those of splicing factors and epigenetic regulation—do not appear to be present in children (Hirabayashi et al. 2012), suggesting that pediatric MDS is indeed a distinct disorder that is more commonly due to genetic predisposition to MDS rather than acquisition of somatic clonal events. A recent large-scale whole-exome sequencing study on DNA samples from over 17,000 individuals showed that patients under the age of 40 years rarely had somatic mutations in adult MDS-associated genes. The most common mutations identified were *DNMT3A*, *TET2*, and *ASXL1* disease-associated variants, suggesting that mutations in epigenetic pathways accumulate with age and likely play a less prominent role in children (Jaiswal et al. 2014).

The precise role and clinical implications of secondary somatic mutations in pediatric MDS remain uncertain and are a field of active investigation. A recent study by Lindsley et al. in collaboration with the Center for International Blood and Marrow Transplant Research (CIBMTR) evaluated the association of somatic mutations with HSCT outcomes such as overall survival (OS), relapse rate, and transplant-related mortality (TRM) (Lindsley et al. 2017). The study included pediatric and adult MDS patients with de novo (primary) MDS and a subset of patients with inherited predisposition due to germline mutations in MDS or IBMFS-causing genes. Somatic mutations in *TET2*, *DNMT3A*, *SRSF2*, *SF3B1*, and *PPM1D* were significantly more common in older adults than in children and adults <40 years of age. In contrast, mutations in *GATA2* (presumed germline), *PIGA* (somatic), and compound heterozygous mutations in *SBDS* (presumed germline) were significantly more common in children and young adults. Patients with biallelic *SBDS* mutations had associated somatic TP53 mutations and showed poor survival, suggesting that the presence of TP53 indicates disease progression from a marrow failure state to MDS (Lindsley et al. 2017).

TP53 was uniformly associated with poor prognosis in all patients regardless of age and intensity of the conditioning regimen. In adults, RAS pathway mutations were associated with inferior outcomes and shorter survival usually due to high relapse rate. However, this adverse effect was only observed in the patients that received a reduced intensity-conditioning regimen, suggesting that some molecular markers might require more intensive therapy (Lindsley et al. 2017).

3.9 Clinical Presentation

The clinical presentation in pediatric MDS patients can be highly variable. Symptoms are usually related to type and degree of cytopenia. In contrast to adult MDS, most pediatric MDS patients present with bleeding due to thrombocytopenia or infection secondary to neutropenia. Isolated anemia is less frequently seen in children. If anemia is present, it is usually macrocytic and accompanied by thrombocytopenia or neutropenia. Organomegaly is infrequently present and usually associated with advanced disease. Some patients, especially those with RCC, come to medical attention because of an incidental finding of cytopenia during a routine health checkup (Kardos et al. 2003).

Special attention should be given to involvement of other organ systems, in particular in patients with a suspected genetic predisposition syndrome. For example, pediatric MDS patients with *GATA2* mutation can present with signs of immunodeficiency, infections, lymphedema, hearing loss, and warts long before a diagnosis of MDS is made. Patients with MDS related to SDS may present with failure to thrive or pancreatic insufficiency.

The clinical course in children with MDS can be highly variable and range from a low-grade MDS and BM failure with an indolent course and stable disease for years to an aggressive disease with rapid progression to AML. The reasons for this disease spectrum remain uncertain.

3.10 Diagnostic Work-Up

3.10.1 Laboratory Evaluation

Pediatric MDS is often a diagnosis of exclusion; therefore the work-up of patients with suspected disease requires a comprehensive laboratory evaluation to rule out secondary causes and evaluate for the presence of an underlying inherited predisposition (Table 3.5).

A number of non-hematologic disorders can cause low blood counts and/or hypoplastic marrow in children and must be ruled out by ancillary laboratory tests. Those disorders include vitamin (e.g., B12, folate) and mineral (e.g., copper) deficiencies and zinc toxicity (Gabreyes et al. 2013), viral infections and toxin or drug exposure (Bowen 2013), rheumatologic disorders (juvenile idiopathic arthritis), mitochondrial disorders (Pearson syndrome), metabolic disorders (meva-

Table 3.5 Suggested diagnostic work-up for pediatric patients with suspected MDS

Diagnostic checklist	
Basic laboratory	CBC with differential (ANC, AMC) Reticulocyte count Basic chemistry studies (electrolytes, LDH, uric acid) Renal and liver function tests Hemoglobin F (hemoglobin electrophoresis)
Immunology	Lymphocyte subsets (B- and T-cell subsets)
Other laboratory	High-resolution HLA typing[a] Nutritional deficiencies (folate, B12, copper) Infectious studies (CMV, EBV, HSV, parvovirus B19, VZV, HIV, leishmaniasis, etc.)
Bone marrow failure/ genetic predisposition work-up	Fanconi anemia (chromosomal breakage with DEB from PB) Dyskeratosis congenita (telomere length in lymphocyte subsets, gene sequencing as indicated[b]) Shwachman-Diamond syndrome (*SBDS* gene sequencing, isoamylase, stool elastase) *GATA2* (on all cases) *CEBPA*, *DDX41*, *RUNX1/AML1*, *ANKRD26*, *ETV6*, *SAMD9* based on clinical suspicion or in cases of familial MDS Other IBMFS based on clinical index of suspicion PNH clone on PB by flow cytometry
Histopathology	Peripheral blood smear review Bone marrow aspirate for morphology Bone marrow biopsy for histology IHC staining (at minimum CD34 and CD61 suggested) Reticulin stain Iron stain on aspirate
Additional studies	Flow cytometry Karyotype on BM FISH on BM (1q, 3q, −5, 5q−, −7, 7q−, +8, 20q−)

ANC = absolute neutrophil count, AMC = absolute monocyte count; DEB = diepoxybutane, PB = peripheral blood; BM = bone marrow

[a]High-resolution HLA typing should be performed on the patient and any potential related donors once diagnosis is confirmed

[b]Gene sequencing should be performed if telomere length shows very short telomeres diagnostic for DC [adopted from Hofmann (2015), with permission]

lonate kinase deficiency), and inherited anemias (e.g., CDA). In addition, a comprehensive molecular work-up to rule out the presence of an underlying IBMFS should be performed (Niemeyer and Baumann 2011). At a minimum, the work-up for an underlying IBMFS should include testing for Fanconi anemia, Shwachman-Diamond syndrome, and dyskeratosis congenita since it would significantly change the management of the patient, in particular if HSCT were indicated.

3.10.2 Histopathology

The careful evaluation of the PB smear to assess morphological abnormalities and the presence of circulating blasts is a first important step in the evaluation of cytopenia. In addition, a high-quality BM aspirate and biopsy are required for an accurate assessment of dysplasia, cellularity, and marrow architecture. The aspirate allows for assessment of cytologic dysplasia and accurate blast count, while the biopsy is essential to determine cellularity, the presence of reticulin fibrosis, and the marrow architecture. The biopsy also facilitates the identification of dysplastic megakaryocytes, in particular with the aid of immunohistochemistry (IHC). The biopsy is critically important for the assessment of pediatric MDS as most patients present with hypocellular marrow and patchy hematopoiesis that may be missed on a suboptimal, hypospicular aspirate.

In addition, a number of ancillary IHC and special stains are often needed to facilitate the diagnostic work-up. The WHO classification for pediatric MDS mandates the addition of a CD61 or CD41 stain to identify micromegakaryocytes, which are supportive of the diagnosis of RCC and important in the differentiation from acquired AA. Other lineage- or stage-specific IHC markers (CD34, CD117 (C-KIT), CD71, glycophorin A, MPO, and lysozyme) can also be helpful. CD3, CD20, CD79a, and TdT are helpful in the assessment of lymphoid populations, in particular when increased lymphocytes are noted, which can often be seen in younger children or in a reactive process. A reticulin stain can highlight background fibrosis, which can be seen in association with monosomy 7 and germline *GATA2* mutations (Spinner et al. 2014; Calvo et al. 2011; Ganapathi et al. 2015).

3.10.3 Cytogenetics and Molecular Studies

Cytogenetic and molecular testing is an essential component for the work-up of a patient with suspected marrow failure or MDS. Although many pediatric MDS patients have a normal karyotype, the identification of a clonal cytogenetic marker can aid in the diagnosis. Routine karyotype and fluorescence in situ hybridization (FISH) should be performed in all patients with suspected MDS. Specific probes should be used to detect the following abnormalities: gain of 1q or 3q, monosomy 5 or deletion of 5q, monosomy 7 or deletion of 7q, trisomy 8, monosomy 20 or deletion of 20q, and MLL (11q23).

The complete loss of chromosome 7 (−7), or partial deletion of its long arm (7q−), is the most common cytogenetic abnormality in myeloid malignancies, including de novo and therapy-related AML and MDS (10–20% of the cases) (Luna-Fineman et al. 1999; Hasle et al. 1999b; Hasle et al. 2007; Johnson and Cotter 1997; Slovak et al. 2000). Monosomy 7 is associated with rapid disease progression to AML, high relapse rate, and poor prognosis (Hasle et al. 2007; Slovak et al. 2000; Germing et al. 2005; Gohring et al. 2010; Greenberg et al. 1997). Monosomy 7 is the most common cytogenetic abnormality in pediatric MDS (~30% of cases) (Gohring et al. 2010), followed by trisomy 8. A complex karyotype involving three or more cytogenetic changes occurs infrequently but is associated with a poor prognosis (Gohring et al. 2010). In contrast to adults, abnormalities in chromosome 5, in particular the MDS with isolated del(5q), and loss of 20q or chromosome X are infrequently seen in children.

An underlying IBMFS, such as FA, DC, or SDS, should be ruled out by molecular or functional testing, as these diseases can have cryptic presentations and their presence will significantly impact clinical management. Germline mutations in myeloid neoplasm predisposition genes (e.g., *GATA2*, *RUNX1*, *ETV6*, *ANKRD26*, *CEBPA*) can occur in patients with sporadic and familial MDS and should be assessed in pediatric MDS patients as well as any potential related HSCT donors (Hahn et al. 2011; Hsu et al. 2011; Ostergaard et al. 2011; Spinner et al. 2014; Calvo et al. 2011; Hsu et al. 2013; Kazenwadel et al. 2012).

Pediatric MDS and BMF disorders, in particular those due to *GATA2* mutations, can present with features of immunodeficiency. A lymphocyte subset analysis of B- and T-cell subsets can provide helpful insights into the disease process.

3.10.4 Flow Cytometry

Flow cytometry to assess blast count, aberrant immunophenotypic markers, and the presence of a paroxysmal nocturnal hemoglobinuria (PNH) clone should also be conducted. Small subclinical PNH clones can be found in patients with RCC (Aalbers et al. 2014). Overt PNH disease with thrombosis and hemolysis is an unusual finding in children (van den Heuvel-Eibrink 2007).

Evidence in adult patients with MDS demonstrates that immunophenotypic abnormalities in the myelomonocytic, erythroid, and myeloid blast cells can provide complementary data aiding in the diagnosis of MDS and differentiating it from other non-clonal cytopenias (Westers et al.

2012). However, studies assessing the value of flow cytometry analysis in pediatric patients are limited. Immunophenotypic characterization of advanced MDS in pediatric patients can help in distinguishing from *de novo* AML (Veltroni et al. 2009) and identify aberrant expression of surface markers such as CD7 that are associated with poor outcomes (Veltroni et al. 2009; Font and Subira 2008; Font et al. 2006; Ogata et al. 2002; Ogata and Yoshida 2005; van de Loosdrecht et al. 2008).

Flow cytometric scoring systems are increasingly incorporated into the hematopathology evaluation of adult MDS (Della Porta et al. 2012; Ogata et al. 2009). However, the diagnostic utility of flow cytometry scoring in low-grade pediatric MDS remains uncertain. Flow cytometry assessment in MDS requires a highly standardized approach and specialized expertise that is not uniformly available.

3.11 Treatment Options in Pediatric MDS

HSCT remains the only curative therapy for pediatric MDS. High-resolution human leukocyte antigen (HLA) typing should be performed early to expedite the search for a matched related donor (MRD) or unrelated donor (URD). Because of the high incidence of germline predisposition to MDS in children, any MRD should be carefully evaluated for a cryptic presentation of an underlying IBMFS or genetic predisposition to MDS. The work-up of a MRD should include a CBC with differential and PB smear review. A BM aspirate and biopsy, and cytogenetic and FISH studies should be strongly considered to rule out familial MDS. For patients with a known germline predisposition to pediatric MDS (e.g., *GATA2*, *ETV6*, *RUNX1*, *ANKRD26*, *DDX41*, *CEBPA*, or MDS secondary to an IBMFS), the respective gene should be ruled out by molecular testing in any possible MRD.

The literature on HSCT outcomes for pediatric MDS is limited and includes mostly small retrospective studies with a wide range of MDS-related diagnoses, varying pre-transplant therapies and conditioning regimens, stem cell sources, and graft-versus-host disease (GVHD) prophylaxis. Traditionally a myeloablative conditioning regimen approach has been used in pediatric MDS in an attempt to fully irradiate the clonal disease. A myeloablative approach is usually associated with increased toxicity and transplant related mortality, and perhaps some patients with lower-grade disease (e.g., hypocellular RCC without monosomy 7) might need less intensive therapy. Indeed, a reduced intensity-conditioning (RIC) approach has successfully been employed in patients with low-grade MDS (Strahm et al. 2007).

The referral to an experienced HSCT center should occur immediately after diagnosis to promote early discussions with the family about treatment options and timing and facilitate donor identification. Several studies indicate that transplanting pediatric MDS patients with RCC prior to disease progression is associated with improved outcomes (Woodard et al. 2011; Smith et al. 2013). Pediatric patients with advanced MDS should be transplanted as quickly as feasible after confirmation of the diagnosis.

The use of pre-HSCT chemotherapy to reduce the blast count for advanced MDS patients remains controversial. Historically, pediatric MDS patients with advanced disease (RAEB, RAEB-T) were often included in AML treatment protocols and therefore were treated with induction chemotherapy (Fleming 2011). However, recent data suggest that intensive chemotherapy before HSCT does not improve outcomes or relapse incidence (RI) in most patients with advanced MDS. The only exception is those patients with pediatric MDS that show progression to AML with more than 30% blasts (Smith et al. 2013; Strahm et al. 2011). Based on the data available, expedited HSCT should be considered in most patients with RAEB, particularly if a donor can be accessible immediately. Induction chemotherapy would uniformly be recommended for patients with MDS with progression to AML (>30% blasts). Giving induction cycles of chemotherapy might reduce the blast count and perhaps decrease relapse rate, but it also carries the risk of delaying definitive curative therapy with HSCT as infectious complications or lack of treatment response might delay cellular therapy. For patients with advanced MDS, the treatment plan is often determined on a case-by-case basis and is dependent on patient disease status, risk assessment, and donor availability, all of which need to be carefully discussed with the family.

More recently alternative cellular therapies, in particular α-β-depleted haploidentical HSCT from a parent, have opened up new treatment strategies for pediatric patients that lack a suitable matched related or unrelated donor or a donor that can be available on an urgent timeline.

The use of hypomethylating agents is frequently utilized in adult patients with MDS and has been shown to improve OS (Fenaux et al. 2009). However, these agents have some limitations since the response can take several months (Sekeres and Cutler 2014) and are associated with a risk of febrile neutropenia (Fenaux et al. 2009; Lubbert et al. 2011; Silverman et al. 2006). The use of hypomethylating agents has not been systematically evaluated in children and to date is not part of standard of care for pediatric MDS. Isolated cases, particularly in patients that have failed standard of care therapy with HSCT, might benefit from those agents. In general their use should be carefully considered on an individual basis and be limited to clinical trials and compassionate use.

3.12 Prognosis

The phenotypic spectrum and prognosis of pediatric patients with MDS vary widely. Some patients with low-grade pediatric MDS, in particular RCC without high-risk cytogenetic abnormalities, need for transfusions, or risk of neutropenia have relatively stable disease for weeks to years. In this setting, a careful "watch and wait" strategy is often a reasonable first approach to help understand the individual patient's disease biology and clinical course. Refraining from more intensive therapies in this patient group early in the diagnosis will help avoid unnecessary treatments for those rare patients that might have a spontaneous resolution of the disease or perhaps show evidence of an IBMFS or acquired AA that would be treated differently. If cytopenias worsen or clonal cytogenetics develop, a more intensive treatment approach, usually in the form of HSCT, is indicated.

All pediatric MDS patients, even those with hypocellular RCC, remain at risk for clonal transformation and progression to leukemia that is estimated at about 30% for patients with RCC over 5 years. While monosomy 7 and complex karyotype (≥3 abnormalities) are known to be associated with increased risk for disease progression to leukemia, it is difficult to predict when this will occur (Kardos et al. 2003; Hasle et al. 2003; Gohring et al. 2010). Given the clinical heterogeneity and lack of precise prognostic factors, the optimal timing for HSCT and the need for upfront chemotherapy in advanced MDS remain uncertain.

Reported outcomes of pediatric MDS after HSCT vary. Earlier studies showed a 3-year OS between 18% and 74% depending on stage, with RAEB-T having the worst outcomes (Yusuf et al. 2004). A recent large study from the Center of International Blood and Marrow Transplant Research showed an 8-year disease-free survival rate of 40–65% for RCC and 28–48% for RAEB/RAEB-T and a 1-year transplant-related mortality of 13–42% (Hsu et al. 2013). The European Working Group of Childhood MDS reported more favorable outcomes for children with advanced MDS with a 5-year OS of 63% and with a TRM and RI of 21%, each (Strahm et al. 2011).

Recent evidence supports the hypothesis that somatic clonal evolution in the context of an underlying inherited predisposition to MDS and BMF may indicate clinical disease progression. For example, acquired somatic *ASXL1* mutations have been identified in patients with GATA2 haploinsufficiency and were associated with progression from MDS to leukemia (West et al. 2014). Furthermore, *TP53* mutations in patients with SDS have been linked to a poor prognosis (Lindsley et al. 2017). *RAS* kinase pathway mutations are reported to be a late somatic event in advanced MDS. Deep sequencing technologies enable us to identify small subclones in BM of MDS patients, which may equip us to identify patients at risk for leukemic transformation prior to overt clinical leukemia. Identifying specific clonal markers that are associated with poor prognosis in pediatric MDS might allow us to tailor therapies, such as favoring a more intensive myeloablative conditioning regimen or the addition of hypomethylating agents post-HSCT to reduce relapse risk. Personalized approaches in pediatric MDS that are based on the patient's individual genetics and disease biology will help us to improve outcomes of those children.

Conclusions

Pediatric MDS is a rare and heterogeneous group of clonal hematopoietic stem cell disorders that remains difficult to diagnosis. Accurate diagnosis of pediatric MDS requires careful analysis by a team of experienced pediatric hematologists and hematopathologists, in conjunction with multiple molecular studies. Pediatric MDS is diagnosed using the 2008 WHO classification system. The 2017 revision to the classification system has not brought forth any significant changes to the pediatric approach to MDS. Within this classification scheme, RCC remains a provisional entity and its clinical implications are still uncertain and under active debate. Increasing data supports that an underlying genetic predisposition is the cause for pediatric MDS in many cases. The functional molecular mechanisms for the varying disease phenotypes in pediatric MDS remain poorly understood in many cases. Ongoing advancements in NGS technologies will continue to be important to help diagnose and characterize pediatric MDS more precisely. Many questions about the pediatric MDS classification system, the functional mechanisms of germline and somatic mutations, and optimal treatment strategies remain. In a disease as rare as pediatric MDS, meaningful rapid progress to the outcomes of these patients will depend upon global collaborative efforts, which will allow us to collectively analyze clinical, genomic, and treatment outcomes.

Acknowledgment *Conflict of Interest*: Author IH declares that she has no conflict of interest.

Ethical Approval: This article does not contain any studies with human participants or animals performed by the author.

References

Aalbers AM, van der Velden VH, Yoshimi A et al (2014) The clinical relevance of minor paroxysmal nocturnal hemoglobinuria clones in refractory cytopenia of childhood: a prospective study by EWOG-MDS. Leukemia 28(1):189–192

Alter BP (2003) Cancer in Fanconi anemia, 1927-2001. Cancer 97(2):425–440

Alter BP, Scalise A, McCombs J, Najfeld V (1993) Clonal chromosomal abnormalities in Fanconi's anaemia: what do they really mean? Br J Haematol 85(3):627–630

Antillon F, Raimondi SC, Fairman J et al (1998) 5q- in a child with refractory anemia with excess blasts: similarities to 5q- syndrome in adults. Cancer Genet Cytogenet 105(2):119–122

Arber DA, Orazi A, Hasserjian R et al (2016) The 2016 revision to the World Health Organization classification of myeloid neoplasms and acute leukemia. Blood 127(20):2391–2405

Asou H, Matsui H, Ozaki Y et al (2009) Identification of a common microdeletion cluster in 7q21.3 subband among patients with myeloid leukemia and myelodysplastic syndrome. Biochem Biophys Res Commun 383(2):245–251

Baumann I, Niemeyer CM, Bennett JM (2008) Childhood myelodysplastic syndrome. In: Swerdlow SH, Harris NL, Jaffe ES, Pileri SA, Stein H, Thiele J, Vardimaan JW (eds) WHO classification of tumours of haematopoietic and lymphoid tissues. IARC, Lyon, pp 104–107

Baumann I, Fuhrer M, Behrendt S et al (2012) Morphological differentiation of severe aplastic anaemia from hypocellular refractory cytopenia of childhood: reproducibility of histopathological diagnostic criteria. Histopathology 61(1):10–17

Bigley V, Collin M (2011) Dendritic cell, monocyte, B and NK lymphoid deficiency defines the lost lineages of a new GATA-2 dependent myelodysplastic syndrome. Haematologica 96(8):1081–1083

Bigley V, Haniffa M, Doulatov S et al (2011) The human syndrome of dendritic cell, monocyte, B and NK lymphoid deficiency. J Exp Med 208(2):227–234

Bowen DT (2013) Occupational and environmental etiology of MDS. Best Pract Res Clin Haematol 26(4):319–326

Buijs A, Poot M, van der Crabben S et al (2012) Elucidation of a novel pathogenomic mechanism using genome-wide long mate-pair sequencing of a congenital t(16;21) in a series of three RUNX1-mutated FPD/AML pedigrees. Leukemia 26(9):2151–2154

Calvo KR, Vinh DC, Maric I et al (2011) Myelodysplasia in autosomal dominant and sporadic monocytopenia immunodeficiency syndrome: diagnostic features and clinical implications. Haematologica 96(8):1221–1225

Cantu Rajnoldi A, Fenu S, Kerndrup G et al (2005) Evaluation of dysplastic features in myelodysplastic syndromes: experience from the morphology group of the European Working Group of MDS in Childhood (EWOG-MDS). Ann Hematol 84(7):429–433

Cardoso SR, Ryan G, Walne AJ et al (2016) Germline heterozygous DDX41 variants in a subset of familial myelodysplasia and acute myeloid leukemia. Leukemia 30(10):2083–2086

Chen DH, Below JE, Shimamura A et al (2016) Ataxia-pancytopenia syndrome is caused by missense mutations in SAMD9L. Am J Hum Genet 98(6):1146–1158

Churpek JE, Garcia JS, Madzo J, Jackson SA, Onel K, Godley LA (2010) Identification and molecular characterization of a novel 3′; mutation in RUNX1 in a family with familial platelet disorder. Leuk Lymphoma 51(10):1931–1935

Churpek JE, Lorenz R, Nedumgottil S et al (2013) Proposal for the clinical detection and management of patients and their family members with familial myelodysplastic syndrome/acute leukemia predisposition syndromes. Leuk Lymphoma 54(1):28–35

Churpek JE, Marquez R, Neistadt B et al (2016) Inherited mutations in cancer susceptibility genes are common among survivors of breast cancer who develop therapy-related leukemia. Cancer 122(2):304–311

van de Loosdrecht AA, Westers TM, Westra AH, Drager AM, van der Velden VH, Ossenkoppele GJ (2008) Identification of distinct prognostic subgroups in low- and intermediate-1-risk myelodysplastic syndromes by flow cytometry. Blood 111(3):1067–1077

Della Porta MG, Picone C, Pascutto C et al (2012) Multicenter validation of a reproducible flow cytometric score for the diagnosis of low-grade myelodysplastic syndromes: results of a European LeukemiaNET study. Haematologica 97(8):1209–1217

van den Heuvel-Eibrink MM (2007) Paroxysmal nocturnal hemoglobinuria in children. Paediatr Drugs 9(1):11–16

Dickinson RE, Griffin H, Bigley V et al (2011) Exome sequencing identifies GATA-2 mutation as the cause of dendritic cell, monocyte, B and NK lymphoid deficiency. Blood 118(10):2656–2658

Elghetany MT (2007) Myelodysplastic syndromes in children: a critical review of issues in the diagnosis and classification of 887 cases from 13 published series. Arch Pathol Lab Med 131(7):1110–1116

Fenaux P, Mufti GJ, Hellstrom-Lindberg E et al (2009) Efficacy of azacitidine compared with that of conventional care regimens in the treatment of higher-risk myelodysplastic syndromes: a randomised, open-label, phase III study. Lancet Oncol 10(3):223–232

Fleming MD (2011) Congenital sideroblastic anemias: iron and heme lost in mitochondrial translation. Hematology Am Soc Hematol Educ Program 2011:525–531

Font P, Subira D (2008) Expression of CD7 in myelodysplastic syndromes (MDS): is this a truly prognostic factor? Leuk Res 32(1):185–186

Font P, Subira D, Mtnez-Chamorro C et al (2006) Evaluation of CD7 and terminal deoxynucleotidyl transferase (TdT) expression in CD34+ myeloblasts from patients with myelodysplastic syndrome. Leuk Res 30(8):957–963

Forester CM, Sartain SE, Guo D et al (2015) Pediatric aplastic anemia and refractory cytopenia: a retrospective analysis assessing outcomes and histomorphologic predictors. Am J Hematol 90:320

Gabreyes AA, Abbasi HN, Forbes KP, McQuaker G, Duncan A, Morrison I (2013) Hypocupremia associated cytopenia and myelopathy: a national retrospective review. Eur J Haematol 90(1):1–9

Ganapathi KA, Townsley DM, Hsu AP et al (2015) GATA2 deficiency-associated bone marrow disorder differs from idiopathic aplastic anemia. Blood 125(1):56–70

Germing U, Hildebrandt B, Pfeilstocker M et al (2005) Refinement of the international prognostic scoring system (IPSS) by including LDH as an additional prognostic variable to improve risk assessment in patients with primary myelodysplastic syndromes (MDS). Leukemia 19(12):2223–2231

Gohring G, Michalova K, Beverloo HB et al (2010) Complex karyotype newly defined: the strongest prognostic factor in advanced childhood myelodysplastic syndrome. Blood 116(19):3766–3769

Greenberg P, Cox C, LeBeau MM et al (1997) International scoring system for evaluating prognosis in myelodysplastic syndromes. Blood 89(6):2079–2088

Hahn CN, Chong CE, Carmichael CL et al (2011) Heritable GATA2 mutations associated with familial myelodysplastic syndrome and acute myeloid leukemia. Nat Genet 43(10):1012–1017

Hasegawa D, Chen X, Hirabayashi S et al (2014) Clinical characteristics and treatment outcome in 65 cases with refractory cytopenia of childhood defined according to the WHO 2008 classification. Br J Haematol 166(5):758–766

Hasle H (2007) Myelodysplastic and myeloproliferative disorders in children. Curr Opin Pediatr 19(1):1–8

Hasle H, Kerndrup G, Jacobsen BB (1995) Childhood myelodysplastic syndrome in Denmark: incidence and predisposing conditions. Leukemia 9(9):1569–1572

Hasle H, Wadsworth LD, Massing BG, McBride M, Schultz KR (1999a) A population-based study of childhood myelodysplastic syndrome in British Columbia, Canada. Br J Haematol 106(4):1027–1032

Hasle H, Arico M, Basso G et al (1999b) Myelodysplastic syndrome, juvenile myelomonocytic leukemia, and acute myeloid leukemia associated with complete or partial monosomy 7. European Working Group on MDS in Childhood (EWOG-MDS). Leukemia 13(3):376–385

Hasle H, Niemeyer CM, Chessells JM et al (2003) A pediatric approach to the WHO classification of myelodysplastic and myeloproliferative diseases. Leukemia 17(2):277–282

Hasle H, Alonzo TA, Auvrignon A et al (2007) Monosomy 7 and deletion 7q in children and adolescents with acute myeloid leukemia: an international retrospective study. Blood 109(11):4641–4647

Hirabayashi S, Flotho C, Moetter J et al (2012) Spliceosomal gene aberrations are rare, coexist with oncogenic mutations, and are unlikely to exert a driver effect in childhood MDS and JMML. Blood 119(11):e96–e99

Hofmann I (2015) Pediatric myelodysplastic syndromes. J Hematopathol 8(3):127–141

Hofmann I, Krasker J, Campagna D, Kierstead D, Schmitz-Abe K, Markianos K, Lee M, Sieff C, Williams DA, Fleming MD (2013a) GATA2 mutations in pediatric myelodysplastic syndrome and bone marrow failure disorders. Leuk Res 37:S20

Hofmann I, Krasker J, Campagna D, Kierstead D, Schmitz-Abe K, Markianos K, Lee M, Sieff C, Williams DA, Fleming MD (2013b) GATA2 mutations in pediatric myelodysplastic syndrome and bone marrow failure disorders. Pediatr Blood Cancer 60:S2

Hsu AP, Sampaio EP, Khan J et al (2011) Mutations in GATA2 are associated with the autosomal dominant and sporadic monocytopenia and mycobacterial infection (MonoMAC) syndrome. Blood 118(10): 2653–2655

Hsu AP, Johnson KD, Falcone EL et al (2013) GATA2 haploinsufficiency caused by mutations in a conserved intronic element leads to MonoMAC syndrome. Blood 121(19):3830–3837. S3831-3837.

Jaiswal S, Fontanillas P, Flannick J et al (2014) Age-related clonal hematopoiesis associated with adverse outcomes. N Engl J Med 371(26):2488–2498

Johnson E, Cotter FE (1997) Monosomy 7 and 7q--associated with myeloid malignancy. Blood Rev 11(1):46–55

Johnson KD, Hsu AP, Ryu MJ et al (2012) Cis-element mutated in GATA2-dependent immunodeficiency governs hematopoiesis and vascular integrity. J Clin Invest 122(10):3692–3704

Kaneko H, Misawa S, Horiike S, Nakai H, Kashima K (1995) TP53 mutations emerge at early phase of myelodysplastic syndrome and are associated with complex chromosomal abnormalities. Blood 85(8):2189–2193

Kardos G, Baumann I, Passmore SJ et al (2003) Refractory anemia in childhood: a retrospective analysis of 67 patients with particular reference to monosomy 7. Blood 102(6):1997–2003

Kazenwadel J, Secker GA, Liu YJ et al (2012) Loss-of-function germline GATA2 mutations in patients with MDS/AML or MonoMAC syndrome and primary lymphedema reveal a key role for GATA2 in the lymphatic vasculature. Blood 119(5):1283–1291

Kirwan M, Vulliamy T, Marrone A et al (2009) Defining the pathogenic role of telomerase mutations in myelodysplastic syndrome and acute myeloid leukemia. Hum Mutat 30(11):1567–1573

Knerr I, Metzler M, Niemeyer CM et al (2003) Hematologic features and clinical course of an infant with Pearson syndrome caused by a novel deletion of mitochondrial DNA. J Pediatr Hematol Oncol 25(12):948–951

Lewinsohn M, Brown AL, Weinel LM et al (2016) Novel germ line DDX41 mutations define families with a lower age of MDS/AML onset and lymphoid malignancies. Blood 127(8):1017–1023

Li FP, Potter NU, Buchanan GR, Vawter G, Whang-Peng J, Rosen RB (1978) A family with acute leukemia, hypoplastic anemia and cerebellar ataxia: association with bone marrow C-monosomy. Am J Med 65(6):933–940

Li R, Sobreira N, Witmer PD, Pratz KW, Braunstein EM (2016) Two novel germline DDX41 mutations in a family with inherited myelodysplasia/acute myeloid leukemia. Haematologica 101(6):e228–e231

Liew E, Owen C (2011) Familial myelodysplastic syndromes: a review of the literature. Haematologica 96(10):1536–1542

Lindsley RC, Saber W, Mar BG et al (2017) Prognostic mutations in myelodysplastic syndrome after stem-cell transplantation. N Engl J Med 376(6):536–547

Lubbert M, Suciu S, Baila L et al (2011) Low-dose decitabine versus best supportive care in elderly patients with intermediate- or high-risk myelodysplastic syndrome (MDS) ineligible for intensive chemotherapy: final results of the randomized phase III study of the European Organisation for Research and Treatment of Cancer Leukemia Group and the German MDS Study Group. J Clin Oncol 29(15):1987–1996

Luna-Fineman S, Shannon KM, Atwater SK et al (1999) Myelodysplastic and myeloproliferative disorders of childhood: a study of 167 patients. Blood 93(2):459–466

Maarek O, Jonveaux P, Le Coniat M, Derre J, Berger R (1996) Fanconi anemia and bone marrow clonal chromosome abnormalities. Leukemia 10(11):1700–1704

Michaud J, Wu F, Osato M et al (2002) In vitro analyses of known and novel RUNX1/AML1 mutations in dominant familial platelet disorder with predisposition to acute myelogenous leukemia: implications for mechanisms of pathogenesis. Blood 99(4):1364–1372

Nagamachi A, Matsui H, Asou H et al (2013) Haploinsufficiency of SAMD9L, an endosome fusion facilitator, causes myeloid malignancies in mice mimicking human diseases with monosomy 7. Cancer Cell 24(3):305–317

Narumi S, Amano N, Ishii T et al (2016) SAMD9 mutations cause a novel multisystem disorder, MIRAGE syndrome, and are associated with loss of chromosome 7. Nat Genet 48(7):792–797

Niemeyer CM, Baumann I (2008) Myelodysplastic syndrome in children and adolescents. Semin Hematol 45(1):60–70

Niemeyer CM, Baumann I (2011) Classification of childhood aplastic anemia and myelodysplastic syndrome. Hematology Am Soc Hematol Educ Program 2011:84–89

Niemeyer CM, Kratz CP, Hasle H (2005) Pediatric myelodysplastic syndromes. Curr Treat Options Oncol 6(3):209–214

Noris P, Favier R, Alessi MC et al (2013) ANKRD26-related thrombocytopenia and myeloid malignancies. Blood 122(11):1987–1989

Ogata K, Yoshida Y (2005) Clinical implications of blast immunophenotypes in myelodysplastic syndromes. Leuk Lymphoma 46(9):1269–1274

Ogata K, Nakamura K, Yokose N et al (2002) Clinical significance of phenotypic features of blasts in patients with myelodysplastic syndrome. Blood 100(12):3887–3896

Ogata K, Della Porta MG, Malcovati L et al (2009) Diagnostic utility of flow cytometry in low-grade myelodysplastic syndromes: a prospective validation study. Haematologica 94(8):1066–1074

Ostergaard P, Simpson MA, Connell FC et al (2011) Mutations in GATA2 cause primary lymphedema associated with a predisposition to acute myeloid leukemia (Emberger syndrome). Nat Genet 43(10): 929–931

Owen C, Barnett M, Fitzgibbon J (2008) Familial myelodysplasia and acute myeloid leukaemia--a review. Br J Haematol 140(2):123–132

Papaemmanuil E, Cazzola M, Boultwood J et al (2011) Somatic SF3B1 mutation in myelodysplasia with ring sideroblasts. N Engl J Med 365(15):1384–1395

Pasquet M, Bellanne-Chantelot C, Tavitian S et al (2013) High frequency of GATA2 mutations in patients with mild chronic neutropenia evolving to MonoMac syndrome, myelodysplasia, and acute myeloid leukemia. Blood 121(5):822–829

Passmore SJ, Hann IM, Stiller CA et al (1995) Pediatric myelodysplasia: a study of 68 children and a new prognostic scoring system. Blood 85(7):1742–1750

Passmore SJ, Chessells JM, Kempski H, Hann IM, Brownbill PA, Stiller CA (2003) Paediatric myelodysplastic syndromes and juvenile myelomonocytic leukaemia in the UK: a population-based study of incidence and survival. Br J Haematol 121(5):758–767

Pedersen-Bjergaard J, Andersen MK, Christiansen DH, Nerlov C (2002a) Genetic pathways in therapy-related myelodysplasia and acute myeloid leukemia. Blood 99(6):1909–1912

Pedersen-Bjergaard J, Christiansen DH, Andersen MK, Skovby F (2002b) Causality of myelodysplasia and acute myeloid leukemia and their genetic abnormalities. Leukemia 16(11):2177–2184

Polprasert C, Schulze I, Sekeres MA et al (2015) Inherited and somatic defects in DDX41 in myeloid neoplasms. Cancer Cell 27(5):658–670

Sasaki H, Manabe A, Kojima S et al (2001) Myelodysplastic syndrome in childhood: a retrospective study of 189 patients in Japan. Leukemia 15(11):1713–1720

Sekeres MA, Cutler C (2014) How we treat higher-risk myelodysplastic syndromes. Blood 123(6):829–836

Shikano T, Ishikawa Y, Anakura M (1992) Myelodysplastic syndrome with partial deletion of the long arm of chromosome 5: first report of a case in a child. Acta Paediatr Jpn 34(5):539–542

Sieff CA, Chessells JM, Harvey BA, Pickthall VJ, Lawler SD (1981) Monosomy 7 in childhood: a myeloproliferative disorder. Br J Haematol 49(2):235–249

Silverman LR, McKenzie DR, Peterson BL et al (2006) Further analysis of trials with azacitidine in patients with myelodysplastic syndrome: studies 8421, 8921, and 9221 by the Cancer and Leukemia Group B. J Clin Oncol 24(24):3895–3903

Slovak ML, Kopecky KJ, Cassileth PA et al (2000) Karyotypic analysis predicts outcome of preremission and postremission therapy in adult acute myeloid leukemia: a Southwest Oncology Group/ Eastern Cooperative Oncology Group Study. Blood 96(13):4075–4083

Smith ML, Cavenagh JD, Lister TA, Fitzgibbon J (2004) Mutation of CEBPA in familial acute myeloid leukemia. N Engl J Med 351(23):2403–2407

Smith AR, Christiansen EC, Wagner JE et al (2013) Early hematopoietic stem cell transplant is associated with favorable outcomes in children with MDS. Pediatr Blood Cancer 60(4):705–710

Spinner MA, Sanchez LA, Hsu AP et al (2014) GATA2 deficiency: a protean disorder of hematopoiesis, lymphatics, and immunity. Blood 123(6):809–821

Strahm B, Locatelli F, Bader P et al (2007) Reduced intensity conditioning in unrelated donor transplantation for refractory cytopenia in childhood. Bone Marrow Transplant 40(4):329–333

Strahm B, Nollke P, Zecca M et al (2011) Hematopoietic stem cell transplantation for advanced myelodysplastic syndrome in children: results of the EWOG-MDS 98 study. Leukemia 25(3):455–462

Swerdlow SH, Campo E, Harris NL, Jaffe ES, Pileri SA, Stein H, Thiele J (eds) (2017) WHO classification of tumours of haematopoietic and lymphoid tissues, 4th edn. IARC, Lyon

Tsurusawa M, Manabe A, Hayashi Y et al (2005) Therapy-related myelodysplastic syndrome in childhood: a retrospective study of 36 patients in Japan. Leuk Res 29(6):625–632

Uyttebroeck A, Brock P, De Groote B et al (1995) 5q- syndrome in a child. Cancer Genet Cytogenet 80(2):121–123

Veltroni M, Sainati L, Zecca M et al (2009) Advanced pediatric myelodysplastic syndromes: can immunophenotypic characterization of blast cells be a diagnostic and prognostic tool? Pediatr Blood Cancer 52(3):357–363

Vinh DC, Patel SY, Uzel G et al (2010) Autosomal dominant and sporadic monocytopenia with susceptibility to mycobacteria, fungi, papillomaviruses, and myelodysplasia. Blood 115(8):1519–1529

Visconte V, Makishima H, Jankowska A et al (2012) SF3B1, a splicing factor is frequently mutated in refractory anemia with ring sideroblasts. Leukemia 26(3):542–545

West RR, Hsu AP, Holland SM, Cuellar-Rodriguez J, Hickstein DD (2014) Acquired ASXL1 mutations are common in patients with inherited GATA2 mutations and correlate with myeloid transformation. Haematologica 99(2):276–281

Westers TM, Ireland R, Kern W et al (2012) Standardization of flow cytometry in myelodysplastic syndromes: a report from an international consortium and the European LeukemiaNet Working Group. Leukemia 26(7):1730–1741

Wlodarski MW, Hirabayashi S, Pastor V et al (2016) Prevalence, clinical characteristics, and prognosis of GATA2-related myelodysplastic syndromes in children and adolescents. Blood 127(11):1387–1397. quiz 1518.

Wong TE, Calicchio ML, Fleming MD, Shimamura A, Harris MH (2010) SBDS protein expression patterns in the bone marrow. Pediatr Blood Cancer 55(3):546–549

Woodard P, Carpenter PA, Davies SM et al (2011) Unrelated donor bone marrow transplantation for myelodysplastic syndrome in children. Biol Blood Marrow Transplant 17(5):723–728

Yang W, Zhang P, Hama A, Ito M, Kojima S, Zhu X (2012) Diagnosis of acquired bone marrow failure syndrome during childhood using the 2008 World Health Organization classification system. Int J Hematol 96(1):34–38

Yoshida K, Sanada M, Shiraishi Y et al (2011) Frequent pathway mutations of splicing machinery in myelodysplasia. Nature 478(7367):64–69

Yoshimi A, Niemeyer C, Baumann I et al (2013) High incidence of Fanconi anaemia in patients with a morphological picture consistent with refractory cytopenia of childhood. Br J Haematol 160(1): 109–111

Yusuf U, Frangoul HA, Gooley TA et al (2004) Allogeneic bone marrow transplantation in children with myelodysplastic syndrome or juvenile myelomonocytic leukemia: the Seattle experience. Bone Marrow Transplant 33(8):805–814

Zhang MY, Churpek JE, Keel SB et al (2015) Germline ETV6 mutations in familial thrombocytopenia and hematologic malignancy. Nat Genet 47(2):180–185

Fanconi Anemia: A Pathway of Hematopoiesis and Cancer Predisposition

4

Ali Suliman, Franklin O. Smith, and Gary M. Kupfer

Contents

A. Suliman
Section of Hematology-Oncology, Department of Pediatrics, Yale Cancer Center, Yale University, New Haven, CT, USA

F. O. Smith
Medpace, Cincinnati, OH, USA

University of Cincinnati College of Medicine, Cincinnati, OH, USA

G. M. Kupfer (✉)
Section of Hematology-Oncology, Department of Pediatrics, Yale Cancer Center, Yale University, New Haven, CT, USA

Department of Pathology, Yale University, New Haven, CT, USA
e-mail: gary.kupfer@yale.edu

G. M. Kupfer et al. (eds.), *Bone Marrow Failure*, Pediatric Oncology,
https://doi.org/10.1007/978-3-319-61421-2_4

Fanconi anemia (FA) is a rare genetic disorder, inherited as an autosomal recessive disease (except in the case of the rare X-linked FA-B form). It is a complex, multi-system, and chronic disorder requiring precise diagnosis, careful and judicious treatment delivered as multidisciplinary care across several medical and surgical specialties, and lifetime, close monitoring. The Fanconi anemia name is misleading; while the first manifestation of the disorder is often hematologic, this is not the sole nor the most important clinical problem for many patients. The disorder phenotype may be quite variable, leading to mistaken or delayed diagnosis. The patient evaluation must include a complete history, physical examination, laboratory testing, hearing evaluation, endocrine system evaluation, gastrointestinal and renal imaging, and cancer surveillance, in addition to bone marrow aspiration and biopsy. While bone marrow failure is ultimately treated with bone marrow transplant, continued monitoring for squamous cell carcinoma and other cancer types is crucial due to the manyfold increased incidence of solid tumors in these patients.

At the cellular level, cells derived from FA patients display hypersensitivity to DNA cross-linking agents resulting in genomic instability in the form of broken and radial chromosomes upon cross-linker exposure and metaphase arrest (Bagby and Alter 2006). An emerging picture of dysfunctional DNA repair appears to account for the pathophysiology of FA, although large gaps in the complete elucidation of the mechanism remain. Currently, biallelic mutations in at least 20 genes account for the FA phenotype (Ceccaldi et al. 2016).

This chapter reviews the current clinical aspects of FA including presentation, diagnosis, and management, followed by a review of the molecular aspects of FA as they are currently understood.

4.1 Clinical Presentation

FA was described first by Dr. Guido Fanconi in 1927 (Ceccaldi et al. 2016; Shimamura and Alter 2010). FA is classically described by skeletal birth defects, bone marrow failure, and progression to acute myeloid leukemia (AML). Physical abnormalities are present in approximately two-thirds of patients, including short stature, café au lait spots, malformations of the thumbs and forearms, microphthalmia, kidney and urinary tract malformations, abnormal ears, gastrointestinal atresias, microcephaly, endocrine dysfunction, and developmental delay. A diagnosis of FA should be considered in any newborn with abnormalities of the thumbs and forearms, especially if macrocytic changes are seen on the child's CBC. In striking contrast, some patients with FA have none of these physical anomalies and are phenotypically normal. Hematological manifestations are the most frequent presenting problem in children with FA, with bone marrow failure presenting at a median of 8 years of age (Butturini et al. 1994). Patients with FA have an increased risk of myelodysplastic syndrome (MDS), and AML (Alter and Kupfer 1993; Rosenberg et al. 2003). They also have an increased risk of solid tumor development of the head and neck, esophagus, vulva, cervix, and liver tumors. These tumors often present at an earlier age than is observed in patients without FA. The inclusion of FA as a possible diagnosis should be a part of the differential diagnosis for any patient presenting at a young age, especially if the clinical and laboratory stigmata of FA are present. An accurate diagnosis of FA in these patients is critical for safe and effective treatment since standard doses of chemotherapy and radiation therapy have the potential to produce life-threatening toxicity as a result of the FA patient's defects in DNA repair. Along the same line, FA should be suspected in patients who experience excessive toxicity in the aftermath of chemotherapy or radiation (Alter and Kupfer 1993; D'Andrea 2010; Fanconi Anemia Research Fund, Inc. 2014).

4.2 Diagnosis

A diagnosis of FA should be considered when a child presents with a clinical history, including family history, physical exam (Table 4.1), and initial clinical laboratory testing suggestive

Table 4.1 Physical abnormalities seen in FA patients (D'Andrea 2010)

Physical abnormality	Percent of FA patients
Short stature	51
Skin abnormalities	55
Arm abnormalities	43
Head abnormalities	26
Eye abnormalities	23
Kidney abnormalities	21
Ear abnormalities	11
Developmental disability	11

of FA. Pancytopenia or isolated cytopenias in these patients should prompt examination of the bone marrow to assess cellularity and evidence for MDS and AML (Shimamura and Alter 2010; Tischkowitz and Dokal 2004). In addition to conventional analysis that include morphology and flow cytometry, mononuclear cells from the bone marrow are stimulated to grow in the presence of a tubulin blocker such as colchicine, with or without a DNA cross-linking agent such as diepoxybutane (DEB) or mitomycin C (MMC), and the subsequent metaphase spreads are quantified for chromosomal breakage as compared to a normal control or known FA patient (Auerbach 2009, 2015). Analysis of the cell cycle by DNA flow cytometry reveals a characteristic elevation of the G2/M peak in the presence of DNA cross-linking agents.

After confirmation of a diagnosis FA, identification of the complementation group and specific gene mutation is important to individualize treatment for the patient and provide genetic counseling to the family. For example, a child with the BRCA2/FANCD1 variant of FA means that each parent is a carrier of these gene mutations and is at increased risk of associated cancers, including cancers of the breast, ovaries, and prostate. In addition, there are some groups of FA patients in whom a genotype/phenotype relationship exists. For example, FA patients with a BRCA2 mutation have a more severe clinical course with earlier onset of marrow failure and progression to AML, as compared to the other complementation groups of FA. On the other hand, most FA subtypes are not associated with phenotype severity, making prediction of disease progression difficult.

In years past, complementation group assignment was traditionally accomplished by transduction of wild-type cDNAs into cells with subsequent analysis of cell survival in the presence of a DNA cross-linking agent. Using current technology, exome sequencing is now performed to provide this critical information.

About 25% of the patients with FA have evidence of somatic mosaicism manifested as decreased sensitivity to DNA cross-linking agent-treated hematopoietic cells, accounted for by a compensatory mutation in another region of the germane FA gene. Interestingly, this phenomenon is only seen in hematopoietic cells, presumably due to the fact that the bone marrow is under selective pressure to keep up with hematopoietic demands. In situations where somatic mosaicism is suspected, a skin biopsy is necessary to provide skin fibroblasts for culture and subsequent DEB testing (Butturini et al. 1994; Lo Ten Foe et al. 1997; Soulier et al. 2005).

4.3 Acute Myeloid Leukemia/Myelodysplastic Syndrome

Typically, MDS and AML in FA are often preceded by bone marrow failure. MDS usually presents as refractory cytopenia with multilineage dysplasia (World Health Organization 2016 classification), with or without excess of blasts (Scheinberg and Young 2012; Cioc et al. 2010; Arber et al. 2016). These cases of AML are typically FAB M1–M4 subtypes (Velez-Ruelas et al. 2006). As noted above, there is a higher risk of developing AML/MDS and solid tumors at an earlier age in patients with the FAND1/BRAC2 FA subtype (Alter 2014).

4.4 Solid Tumor

The estimated cumulative probability of solid tumor in FA patients is 80% by the age of 45 years (Rosenberg et al. 2003; Alter et al. 2010). The most common solid tumors are head and neck squamous cell carcinomas, esophagus, or vulva, even after HCT (Rosenberg et al. 2005). A group from France looked at the database to identify solid tumors occurring in patients registered with or determined to have FA during childhood in France between 1986 and 2012. Their cases were diagnosed with FA after they presented with solid tumor initially, one of the cases was fetus with brain tumor. They found predominance of BRCA2 mutation in FA with childhood solid tumors (Malric et al. 2015). In general, any solid tumor in childhood that associated with increased sensitivity and side effect of alkylating agent may rise the suspicion of FA diagnosis. These solid tumors are hard to treat mainly due to the patients' hypersensitivity to chemoradiotherapy.

4.5 Treatment of Patients with Fanconi Anemia

4.5.1 Androgens

The treatment of patients with FA is profoundly impacted by their inability to tolerate standard chemotherapy, radiation therapy, and HCT. Standard doses of chemotherapy and radiation result in excessive toxicity and death in patients with FA, a result of defects in DNA repair pathways. Bone marrow failure is often treated with androgens. Synthetic androgens have been widely used for the treatment of cytopenias in patients with FA for more than 50 years. The beneficial effects of androgens are most pronounced in the red cells and platelets, but neutrophil counts may also improve (Shahidi and Diamond 1961; Diamond and Shahidi 1967). The mechanism of action by which androgens improve blood counts is unclear. A transient improvement in blood counts after treatment with androgens is seen in approximately 50% of patients. This transient response has a variable time course, but ultimately, all patients will lose this response and become refractory to androgen therapy. However, it appears as if as many as 10–20% of patients receiving continuous low-dose androgen therapy might never need a transplant, unless MDS/AML develops. Thus, androgen treatment may delay the need for HCT to treat marrow failure for months and even years, in androgen-responsive patients. This is particularly important for patients and families who decline immediate HCT, for patients without a suitable allogeneic donor, and for patients for whom HCT would be associated with excessive risk. However, one risk of delaying HCT is the development of risk of developing MDS/AML while on androgen therapy.

Side effects of androgens include virilization, increased growth with premature closure of the epiphyses with resulting exacerbation of short adult stature, hyperactivity and behavioral changes including aggression, hepatic adenoma (benign) or hepatocellular carcinoma, peliosis hepatis, and hypertension (Fanconi Anemia Research Fund, Inc. 2014; Shahidi and Diamond 1961; Diamond and Shahidi 1967). The most commonly used androgen since 1961 is oxymetholone, although prospective clinical trials to establish the optimal dose have never been conducted in patients with FA. The commonly used starting dose of oxymetholone is ~2 mg/kg/day (but doses as high as 5 mg/kg may be required). Most patients who will have an androgen response will respond within 3 months with a stabilization or an increase in the hemoglobin and/or platelet levels. If a response occurs, then the general strategy is to slowly taper the daily dose of oxymetholone in 10–20% decrements every 3–4 months until an effective dose that minimizes side effects is obtained (Fanconi Anemia Research Fund, Inc. 2014; Shahidi and Diamond 1961; Diamond and Shahidi 1967).

Another synthetic androgen that produces less virilization than oxymetholone is danazol. A recent retrospective study demonstrated the effectiveness of danazol in seven of eight patients with FA (starting dose 3.5–7.7 mg/kg/day): Three patients (two females and one male) were treated successfully for more than 3 years and one female for more than 10 years without exhibiting progressive marrow failure requiring stem cell transplantation (Scheckenbach et al. 2012). Oxandrolone was evaluated in single-arm, phase I/II study with escalation dose if no toxicities; nine patients completed the study. This study showed that oxandrolone is well tolerated and has less side effect in treatment of BMF (Rose et al. 2014).

4.5.2 Hematopoietic Cell Transplantation

Hematopoietic cell transplant is the only curative treatment for bone marrow failure associated with FA. Historically, FA patients undergoing HCT have had significant morbidity and mortality due to graft failure, conditioning regimen-related toxicity, and graft-versus-host disease (GVHD) (Myers and Davies 2009). HCT conditioning regimens are modified for patients with FA because of the defects in DNA repair that result in chromosomal instability in all FA cells, including the non-hematopoietic tissues and organs. However, with the identification of conditioning regimens that are tolerated in these patients, children with FA who receive transplants from HLA-matched related donors for bone marrow failure, MDS, and AML have excellent outcomes. Despite this improvement in outcome for recipients of matched related donor transplants, the outcome for patients receiving transplants from unrelated donor remained poor, until the addition of fludarabine to the conditioning regimen. In recent years, fludarabine-based reduced-intensity conditioning regimens, with or without T-cell depletion, have resulted in a much lower risk of graft failure and GVHD and dramatically improved patient outcomes for patients receiving unrelated donor HCT (Tan et al. 2006). This has led to greater use of unrelated donors for FA patients who do not have an available matched sibling donor (Fanconi Anemia Research Fund, Inc. 2014; MacMillan and Wagner 2010; Stepensky et al. 2011).

Patients with FA are at increased risk of malignancy following HCT. This was especially true when total body irradiation (TBI) was used (Rosenberg et al. 2008) and when GVHD was excessive. These patients were noted to have a 4.4-fold higher risk of squamous cell carcinoma (SSC) compared with patients with FA of the same age who have not received an HCT (Rosenberg et al. 2005). Thus, post-HCT screening for SSC and other solid tumors requires intensive surveillance (Eiler et al. 2008). Also, residual FA cells that survive the conditioning may give a rise to AML as late as 10 years after HCT (Farzin et al. 2007).

Taken together, HCT has been shown be potentially curative of bone marrow failure, MDS, and AML, although it does not prevent the occurrence of solid tumors. The decision to proceed to HCT is always a difficult one, given the potential for HCT-associated morbidity and mortality (Khan et al. 2016).

4.5.3 Supportive Care

Improvements in supportive care also contribute to better outcomes in patients with FA. Improvements in blood banking result in safer blood products for the treatment of thrombocytopenia and anemia. Cytokines and growth factors have reduced infections and bleeding, although some worry remains about the long-term risk of exposing patients with FA to filgrastim that may have the potential for clonal outgrowth (Scheinberg and Young 2012; Eiler et al. 2008; Wagner et al. 2007).

4.5.4 Gene Therapy

Gene therapy is a promising future direction for treating FA patients. There have been a number of preclinical studies showing correction of FA phenotype after in vitro gene delivery by viral vector (Noll et al. 2001; Adair et al. 2012; Molina-Estevez et al. 2015). These studies and the successes in other conditions and diseases like adrenoleukodystrophy (Cartier et al. 2009), beta thalassemia (Negre et al. 2016), and Wiskott-Aldrich syndrome (Singh et al. 2017), using lentiviral vector, lead to the start of clinical trials using gene therapy. However, the collection of the hematopoietic stem cells in FA patients remains a big challenge since the BMF is the main manifestation of the disease (Kelly et al. 2007). Moreover, these cells are very fragile and respond poorly to manipulations required for successful gene transfer. The first two trials that failed to achieve sustained engraftment may be due to the controversial lack of conditioning chemoablative therapy and the low cell dose infused after modification (Kelly et al. 2007; Liu et al. 1999). This modality still needs the development of more efficient ways to collect stem cell and safe and effective therapeutic vector technologies.

4.6 Molecular Biology of Fanconi Anemia

At the cellular level, cells derived from patients with FA display hypersensitivity to DNA cross-linking agents, including MMC and DEB. Treatment with these agents induces an abnormally prolonged S phase and cell cycle arrest in G2 (Akkari et al. 2001). As the result of this response, one function of the FA pathway has long been hypothesized to function in sensing DNA damage and initiating repair. This hypothesis has been confirmed by work elucidating the interactions of FA proteins with established DNA repair proteins and by the identification of DNA repair genes as bona fide FA genes. A significant body of work has identified a role for the FA pathway in cell signaling in response to stress stimuli and in apoptosis in the cytoplasm, thereby affecting maintenance of the hematopoietic machinery.

The FA proteins have been grouped into three broad categories: the upstream FA core complex, which contains FANC A, FANCB, FANCC, FANCE, FANCF, FANCG, FANCM, and FANCL, and the E3 ligase along with FA-associated proteins FAAP20 and FAAP100; the ID2 complex which is the substrate of the E3 ubiquitin ligase activity of the core complex and, by virtue of the name, contains FANCD2 and FANCI; and the downstream proteins, including BRCA2/FANCD1, BACH1/FANJ, PLAB2/FANCN, RAD51C/FANCO, SLX4/FANCP, XPF/FANCQ, RAD51/FANCR, BRCA1/FANCS, UBE2T/FANCT, and XRCC2/FANCU (Ceccaldi et al. 2016). The FA pathway is implicated in a number of cancer patients without FA, including breast cancer (Table 4.2).

4.6.1 Fanconi Anemia Core Complex Proteins (Upstream Proteins)

The nuclear "core" complex is composed of 8 of the 20 FA proteins, whose chromatin localization is mediated by FANCM binding to DNA after damage or during S phase and coalescing into foci upon chromatin. The core complex's chief function is the monoubiquitination of FANCD2 and FANCI at K561 and K523 sites, respectively. This is mediated by the FANCL protein, which contains E3 ubiquitin ligase activity, and its E2 partner protein UBE2T/FANCT. This putative E3 ligase activity is the purported enzyme that modifies the downstream heterodimer FANCD2-FANCI, placing a monoubiquitin on each in response to DNA damage or during S phase (Ceccaldi et al. 2016; Meetei et al. 2005; Joenje and Patel 2001; Garcia-Higuera et al. 2001; Sato et al. 2012). Thus, biallelic mutations in any one of the core complex FA genes (with the exception of the FANCB gene, an X-linked gene) as well as FANCD2 and FANCI result in the absence of monoubiquitinated FANCD2. Immunoblotting demonstrating the absence or reduction of monoubiquitinated FANCD2 has been proposed as a surrogate marker for a large majority of FA patients.

Several of the core complex proteins, including FANCA, FANCB, and FANCE, contain nuclear localization signals supporting the idea that the core complex fully assembles in the nucleus (Lightfoot et al. 1999; Meetei et al. 2004; de Winter et al. 2000). FANCM heterodimerizes with FA-associated protein 24 (FAAP24) (Ciccia et al. 2007; Kim et al. 2008), and depletion of FAAP24 has been shown to disrupt the chromatin association of FANCM and to destabilize FANCM, leading to failure of the core complex to localize to chromatin (Kim et al. 2008). Additionally, FANCM facilitates activation of the ATR-mediated DNA damage checkpoint response. The ATPase activity of FANCM is located within the amino-terminal DEAH helicase-like domain, responsible for translocase and branch migration activities (Collis et al. 2008; Gari et al. 2008). This ATPase activity is generally found to be dispensable for core complex targeting and FANCD2 ubiquitination but is required for replication fork stability and efficient checkpoint response (Collis et al. 2008; Blackford et al. 2012; Huang et al. 2010). Several of the core complex proteins including FANCA, FANCG, and FANCM are also regulated by phosphorylation and dephosphorylation throughout the cell cycle (Kim et al.

Table 4.2 The 20 Fanconi anemia genes

Complementation group	Responsible gene	Chromosome location	Protein molecular weight (kD)	Known motifs	Necessary for FANCD2 monoubiquitinated
A	FANCA	16q24.3	163	2NLSs, NESs	Yes
B	FANCB	Xp22.31	95	NLS	Yes
C	FANCC	9q22.3	63	None	Yes
D1	FANCD1/BRCA2	13q12.13	380	8 BRC repeats, HD, 3 OBs, TD	No
D2	FANCD2	3p25.3	155, 162	None	Yes
E	FANCE	6p21-22	60	2 NLSs	Yes
F	FANCF	11p15	42	None	Yes
G	FANCG/XRCC9	9p13	68	7 TPRs	Yes
I	FANCI/KIAA1794	15q25-26	146	None	Yes
J	FANCJ/BRIP1/ BACH1	17q22-24	130	ATPase, 7 helicase-specific motifs	No
L	FANCL/PHF9	2p16.1	43	3 WD40s, PHD	Yes
M	FANCM	14q21.2	250	7 helicase-specific motifs, degenerate endonuclease domain, ATPase	Yes
N	FANCN/PALB2	16p12	130	2 WD40s	No
O	FANCO/RAD51C	17q22	42.1		No
P	FANCP/SLX4	16q13.3	200		
Q	ERCC4, XPF; RAD1; FANCQ; XFEPS; ERCC11	16p13.12	104	ERCC1 and XPF/ ERCC4	No
R	RECA; BRCC5; FANCR; MRMV2; HRAD51; RAD51A; HsRad51; HsT16930	15q15.1	37		
S	FANCS BRCA1				
T	FANCT, UBE2T	1q32.1			
U	FANCU, XRCC2	7q36	32		

2008; Gari et al. 2008; Yamashita et al. 1998; Qiao et al. 2004; Mi et al. 2004). These modifications also seem to be necessary for intact FA pathway function. For example, FANCA is phosphorylated on S1449, induced by DNA damage during S phase by ataxia telangiectasia and Rad3-related protein kinase (ATR) (Collins et al. 2009). ATR also interacts with other members of the FA pathway, such as being responsible for the phosphorylation of FANCG on serine 7, necessary for the interaction of FANCG with FANCD1/BRCA2, XRCC2, and FANCD2 (Wilson et al. 2008).

Although evidence has shown that an intact core complex is unequivocally necessary for activation of the FA pathway, FA core complex proteins interact among themselves to form subcomplexes. FANCB and FANCL directly interact and have been found to interact with FANCA. The interaction between FANCA and FANCL is dependent on FANCB, FANCG, and FANCM but independent of FANCC, FANCE, and FANCF. Although the function of these subcomplexes remains elusive, the FANCA protein has been shown directly to interact with a central portion of the BRCA1 protein in a DNA damage-independent manner

(Folias et al. 2002). The FANCG protein has been shown to interact with XRCC3 and FANCD1/BRCA2 (Hussain et al. 2003). These findings provide a framework for the protein interactions that occur "upstream" in the FA pathway and suggest that besides the FA core complex, different subcomplexes exist that may have specific functions other than the monoubiquitination of FANCD2 (Medhurst et al. 2006; Rajendra et al. 2014). FANCE mediates the interaction of the core complex with FANCD2, because FANCE has been demonstrated to interact with FANCD2 both in vitro and in vivo (Pace et al. 2002; Bouffard et al. 2015). FANCE phosphorylation by CHK1 in two highly conserved sequences sites (threonine 346 and serine 374) is required for proper FA pathway function, although FANCD2 ubiquitination and foci formation are intact in T346A/S374A double-mutant FA-E cells. Further experiments showed that T346-phosphorylated FANCE colocalized with FANCD2 in discrete nuclear foci following UV irradiation (Wang et al. 2007; Enders 2008). Also FANCL was found to form a subcomplex with FANCB and FAAP100, which is absolutely required for the E3 ligase activity, as well as FANCC-FANCE-FANCF subcomplex that helps bind at sites of DNA damage along with FANCA-FANCG-FAAP20 subcomplex (Huang et al. 2014).

In noncanonical fashion, FANCC binds and facilitates activation of STAT1 when induced by INF-γ and hematopoietic growth factors (Pang et al. 2000), and rescuing FA-C cells with WT-FANCC suppresses the expression of INF-γ-inducible genes (Fagerlie et al. 2001). This finding is supported by animal studies, which found that FANCC$^{-/-}$ mice have impaired type1 IFN receptor-induced JAK/STAT signaling and abnormal cell differentiation (Fagerlie et al. 2004), yet another implication of FA pathway in cell signaling and differentiation.

4.6.2 FANCD2-FANCI

Following treatment with DNA cross-linker agents (Garcia-Higuera et al. 2001) or during the S phase of the cell cycle (Taniguchi et al. 2002a), the FANCD2-FANCI heterodimer becomes monoubiquitinated. These modifications result in translocation of the two proteins to chromatin and recruitment of downstream effector FA proteins at the site of DNA damage (Wang et al. 2004). FANCI, identified by a screen for phosphopeptides corresponding to consensus substrates of ATM/ATR (Dorsman et al. 2007), is also monoubiquitinated by FANCL on lysine 523. ATR has also been shown to phosphorylate FANCI on serines 730 and 1121 and threonine 952 (Smogorzewska et al. 2007).

FANCD2 is ubiquitinated at lysine 561, and together both of these modifications are required for binding to chromatin, DNA repair, and normal progression of the cell cycle (Wang et al. 2004; Dorsman et al. 2007; Smogorzewska et al. 2007; Sims et al. 2007). Structural analysis of the ID2 complex suggested that there are conformational changes inducible by interaction with the DNA (Longerich et al. 2014) as well as core complex subcomplexes, such as FANCB/FANCL/FAAP100 subcomplex (Joo et al. 2011). FANCD2-FANCI is also regulated by phosphorylation, as ATM was shown to phosphorylate FANCD2 on serine 222 in normal cells in response to IR, but not ICL, and this phosphorylation event was shown to be necessary for proper cellular response to double-strand breaks (Taniguchi et al. 2002b). On the other hand, additional phosphorylation events at S691, T717, and S331 have all been demonstrated to be responsible for resistance to ICLs (Ho et al. 2006; Zhi et al. 2009).

The removal of ubiquitin from the ID2 complex is catalyzed by ubiquitin-specific protease-1 and USP1-associated factor-1 (USP1-UAF1) deubiquitinase, which also targets other proteins, such as ubiquitinated PCNA, and this reaction happens upon completion of replication fork repair and restart (Smogorzewska et al. 2007; Nijman et al. 2005). USP1 is activated by heterodimerization in concert with UAF1 (Cohn et al. 2007; Villamil et al. 2012). ID2 complex deubiquitination is suppressed by USP gene silencing and cleavage and proteolytic degradation of USPI protein (Huang et al. 2006; Piatkov et al. 2012). USP1-UAF1 is now a target of developing inhibitor development to either potentiate chemotherapeutic effect of ICL or overcome resistance of some cancer cells to DNA cross-linker therapy (Liang et al. 2014; Kim et al. 2009; Park et al. 2013).

Fanconi anemia-associated nuclease 1 (FAN1) was identified using an shRNA screen to identify genes responsible for ICL resistance. It colocalizes with ID2 complex at the site of DNA damage through a ubiquitin-binding domain and contains intrinsic 5′–3′ exonuclease and endonuclease activity (Smogorzewska et al. 2010). Although FAN1 participates in the FA pathway, mutations in its gene have not been shown to be causative in FA but have been found to cause karyomegalic interstitial nephritis (Zhou et al. 2012), a kidney abnormality not found in FA typically, even though it does exhibit renal findings.

4.6.3 FANCD1/BRCA2, FANCP/SLX4, FANCQ/ERCC4, FANCJ/BACH1, and FANCN/PALB2 (Downstream Proteins)

Biallelic mutations in these genes do not affect FANCD2 ubiquitination but cause an FA phenotype, hence termed the "downstream" part of the FA pathway (Ceccaldi et al. 2016; Deans and West 2011).

The FANCD1 gene is identical to the familial breast-ovarian cancer susceptibility gene BRCA2, and biallelic mutations of the FANCD1/BRCA2 gene result in the FA phenotype, whereas monoallelic mutation result in increased breast and ovarian cancer susceptibility (Howlett et al. 2002; Hirsch et al. 2004). The FANCD1/BRCA2 protein consists of eight BRC repeats that have been shown to bind the RAD51 recombinase (Wong et al. 1997; Yang et al. 2002, 2005) and five C-terminal domains consisting of a helical domain, three oligonucleotide/oligosaccharide-binding folds, and a tower domain. The oligosaccharide-binding domains bind ssDNA, and the tower domain participates in dsDNA binding, and thus the FANCD1/BRCA2 protein recruits RAD51 to both ssDNA/dsDNA junctions of a processed DNA break to promote HR (Yang et al. 2002). BRCA1/FANCS, on the other hand, in combination with BRCA1-associated RING domain protein 1 (BARD1), which exhibits ubiquitin ligase activity (Wu-Baer et al. 2003), is necessary for proper localization of RAD51 to the ssDNA and promotes the strand invasion step in HR. FANCN/PALB2 was identified first as colocalizing with BRCA2 and required for its function (Xia et al. 2006). Cells lacking PALB2 lack chromatin-bound BRCA2 and are completely unable to form RAD51 foci and thus exhibit HR defects (Xia et al. 2007). PALB2 is also a breast and ovarian cancer susceptibility gene.

The FANCJ gene is identical to the BRIP1 (BRCA1 interacting protein C-terminal helicase 1) and BACH1 (BRCA1-associated C-terminal helicase genes) (Levitus et al. 2005; Levran et al. 2005; Cantor et al. 2001). As the names of BRIP1 and BACH1 imply, the FANCJ/BRIP1/BACH1 protein directly binds to the BRCT domain of BRCA1. The BRCT domain is a phosphoprotein-binding domain, and phosphorylation of FANCJ/BRIP1/BACH1 on serine 990 is required for this interaction (Yu et al. 2003). This protein is also a DNA-dependent ATPase and a 5′ to 3′ DNA helicase, which contains seven helicase-specific motifs. FANCJ has been shown to be a structure-specific helicase, dissociating guanine quadruplex DNA in vitro (Wu et al. 2008). FANCJ/BACH1/BRIP1 has been linked to the DNA mismatch repair through its interaction with the MLH1 protein (Peng et al. 2007; Williams et al. 2011). FANCJ also regulates and is required for efficient loading of FANCD2 on the chromatin following DNA damage in a manner independent to the ubiquitination step of FANCD2 (Chen et al. 2014).

Ubiquitinated FANCD2 recruits FANCP/SLX4, which has a ubiquitin-recognizing motif (ubiquitin-binding zinc finger 4) that is required for this interaction (Yamamoto et al. 2011; Crossan et al. 2011). FANCP/SLX4 also binds to and thus acts as a scaffold for the structure-specific endonucleases, XPF-ERCC1, MUS81, EME1, and SLX1 (Klein Douwel et al. 2014; Cybulski and Howlett 2011), which are comprised of two N-terminal C2HC zinc finger domains, related to the UBZ4 family of ubiquitin-binding domains (UBDs) (Hofmann 2009).

While FANCP/SLX4 interacts directly with the MUS81-EME1 heterodimer, which leads to initial incision of the ICL, FANCP/SLX4 does not seem to be required for ICL-induced DSB formation as robust and persistent levels of γH2AX nuclear foci are observed in FANCP-/SLX4-deficient cells (Stoepker et al. 2011).

FANCQ/ERCC4 is activated by FANCP/SLX4 and has endonuclease activity that helps release the ICL (Klein Douwel et al. 2014; Hodskinson et al. 2014). The catalytic component of a structure-specific DNA repair endonuclease is responsible for the 5-prime incision during DNA repair involved in homologous recombination (Svendsen et al. 2009). FANCQ /ERCC4 protein sits at the crossroads of several repair pathways, including nucleotide excision repair, ICL repair, alternative end joining, and single-strand annealing (Bogliolo et al. 2013; Kashiyama et al. 2013; Soltys et al. 2013). RAD51C/FANCO, a paralog of RAD51, also a familial breast cancer gene, was found to form multiple complexes with defined roles in HR (Somyajit et al. 2010; Dray et al. 2010). Studies have shown that biallelic mutations in RAD51C/FANCO lead to FA phenotype (Vaz et al. 2010).

Replication restart after replication stress requires BLM helicase, which is deficient in Bloom's syndrome. The interaction between the BLM protein and the FA pathway was first elucidated through the purification composed of multiple FA proteins mediated by FANCA pulldown and known BLM-interacting proteins, since called the BRAFT complex. This complex shows in vivo activity on branched DNA structures, such as Holliday junctions, which can occur during the repair of stalled or collapsed replication forks by HR (Seki et al. 2006; Meetei et al. 2003). In addition, FANCD2 and BLM demonstrate colocalization in nuclear foci and coimmunoprecipitation following DNA damage, providing further evidence linking the FA pathway to the HR (Pichierri et al. 2004).

Translesion (TLS) polymerases replicate through sites of DNA damage, which typically obstruct the replicative DNA fork. Each TLS polymerase, such as PolH, PolK, and REV1, is specialized to operate through a specific type of DNA lesion and keep the replication fork moving regardless of DNA damage (McCulloch and Kunkel 2008). The protein proliferating cell nuclear antigen (PCNA) functions as a polymerase clamp, tethering a polymerase to DNA in need of replication to increase processivity (Andersen et al. 2008). An interaction between PCNA and FA proteins was first suggested by studies indicating that PCNA colocalizes with FANCD1/BRCA2, BRCA1/FANCD2, and RAD51 in nuclear foci following treatment with ultraviolet irradiation and hydroxyurea (Chen et al. 1998). It was later discovered that PCNA also colocalizes in foci containing FANCD2 in cells treated with hydroxyurea (Hussain et al. 2004; Lehmann 2006; Chen et al. 2016). Monoubiquitinated PCNA recruits REV1, a TLS polymerase that fills the gap and catalyzes the insertion of the random nucleotides in the double-strand breaks created by ICL adduct (Long et al. 2011). REV1 interacts with FAAP20, an FA core complex member, promotes formation, and colocalizes with REV1 foci (Kim et al. 2012). Further studies in FA-A, FA-G, and FA-D2 patient-derived cell lines show that the core complex proteins FANCA and FANCG are required for REV1 nuclear foci formation, whereas FANCD2 is not (Mirchandani et al. 2008). Additionally, REV7/FANCV has recently been characterized as a new FA gene (Bluteau et al. 2016).

4.7 The Fanconi Anemia Pathway, Oxidative Stress, and Cytokine Sensitivity

Cells from patients with FA are, as has been known for many years, highly sensitive to oxidative stress (Joenje et al. 1981; Nordenson 1977; Dallapiccola et al. 1985). Others have argued that the main function of the FA pathway is to regulate oxidative stress, because reactive oxygen species have been documented to be involved in bone marrow failure (Gordon-Smith and Rutherford 1989; Bornman et al. 1999), cancer (Kovacic and Jacintho 2001), endocrinopathies (Evans et al. 2000), abnormalities in skin pigmentation (Memoli et al. 1997), and malformations

(Wells et al. 1997), all well-defined features of FA. FANCC was shown to bind and interact with NADPH cytochrome P450 reductase and glutathione S-transferase P1-1 (GSTP1) (Kruyt et al. 1998; Cumming et al. 2001), two proteins with redox regulatory function. Microarray studies comparing mRNA expression levels found that nuclear factor-1, heat shock protein 70, and cyclooxygenase 2 were consistently overexpressed in FANCC-deficient cells as compared with their corrected counterparts (Zanier et al. 2004). The FANCG protein has been shown to interact with cytochrome P-450 2E1, which has been shown to be involved in metabolism of xenobiotics, such as MMC (Futaki et al. 2002). Finally, both FANCA and FANCG have been shown to be redox-sensitive proteins that multimerize following H_2O_2 treatment, lending plausibility to the hypothesis that the FA pathway may function in oxidative stress management in cells (Park et al. 2004). Among several interactors, ATM and forkhead box O3 (FOXO3a) were reported to exert oxidative stress-specific coordinated actions with FANCD2 (Li et al. 2010; Castillo et al. 2011), and both ATM and FOXO3a have established functions in response to oxidative DNA damage (Watters 2003; Yalcin et al. 2008).

There is increasing body of evidence implicating FA phenotype with premature aging and oxidative stress. One study showed that the production of hydroxyl radicals from FA leukocytes is elevated, and FA cells also display mitochondrial dysfunction and elevated levels of reactive oxygen species (ROS) (Kumari et al. 2014). DNA from FA patients shows higher levels of 8-oxo-deoxyguanosine (8-oxo-dG), a marker of base oxidation, than in DNA from aged-matched normal controls (Degan et al. 1995; Pagano et al. 2004, 2012). FA cells also exhibit altered expression levels of some growth factors and cytokines, including unusually high levels of intracellular tumor necrosis factor-a (TNF-a), a cytokine capable of initiating the apoptotic pathway (Schultz and Shahidi 1994). This may be mediated through multiple interactions with several effectors, including, among others, mitogen-activated protein kinase, nuclear factor-κB (NF-κB) (two major stress-signaling pathways), interleukin-6, and the c-Jun NH2-terminal kinase pathway (Briot et al. 2008; Ibanez et al. 2009; Saadatzadeh et al. 2009). The interactions between TNF-α and its receptors (TNF-ARI, TNF-ARII) enhance intracellular events as nuclear factor-κB (NF-κB) activation and transcriptional activity that are enhanced in FA cells compared to normal cells (Ibanez et al. 2009).

Animal studies utilizing FA mouse models found that *Fancc*$^{-/-}$ mice underwent excess inflammatory response as a result of hematopoietic suppression that was corrected by wild-type *Fancc* gene, suggesting a potential role of the FANCC protein in innate immunity. The lipopolysaccharide-mediated hematopoietic suppression was elicited by TNF-α and triggered reactive oxygen species formation, along with overexpression of the stress kinase p38 (Sejas et al. 2007). Another study showed that administration of nitroxide antioxidant (Tempol) in *Fancd2*$^{-/-}$ mice results in a significant delay in the onset of epithelial tumors (Zhang et al. 2008), while others found that using resveratrol, a polyphenol with antioxidant properties, in *Fancc*$^{-/-}$ mice, partially corrected hematopoietic defects (Zhang et al. 2010).

A new report also showed that the FA pathway plays a central role in mitochondria hemostasis, both in antiviral defense and clearance of damaged mitochondria and decreases mitochondrial ROS production. Interestingly this function is genetically distinct from its role in DNA repair. For example, the FANCC c.67delG containing cells are sensitive to DNA cross-linker but not to cytokines like TNF-α and IFN-γ, in contrast to WT-FANCC, which rescues both (Sumpter et al. 2016).

4.8 FA and Reactive Aldehydes

Aldehydes are naturally formed by-products of cellular metabolism endogenously as well as available to the cell through exogenous exposure (Shen et al. 2014). Acetaldehyde is a by-product of ethanol oxidation and an intermediate of carbohydrate metabolism, and it forms ICLs, mainly by reacting with guanines (Matsuda et al. 1998; Wang et al. 2000). Both are highly reactive and found to form DNA adducts in vivo (Garcia et al. 2011; Langevin et al. 2011). FA cells show hypersensitivity to both formaldehyde and acetaldehyde and accumulate dsDNA breaks (Ridpath et al. 2007; Rosado et al. 2011), thus suggesting that both may act as a source of DNA damage. A recent study from the Patel group found that acetaldehyde-catabolizing enzyme Aldh2 is essential for the development of mouse *Fancd2*$^{-/-}$ embryos. Nevertheless, acetaldehyde-catabolism-competent mothers (*Aldh2*$^{(+/-)}$)) can support the development of double-mutant (Aldh2$(^{-/-})$ Fancd2$(^{-/-})$) mice, but these mice developed BMF rapidly when exposed to ethanol. Lastly, *Fancd2*$^{-/-}$ *Aldh2*$^{-/-}$ mice spontaneously develop acute leukemia in the first 6 months of life (Langevin et al. 2011). The aged double-knockout mice that did not develop leukemia spontaneously go on to develop aplastic anemia, with the concomitant accumulation of damaged DNA within the hematopoietic stem and progenitor cell (HSPC) pool (Garaycoechea et al. 2012). This finding is suggestive of broader role of the endogenous metabolic by-products in causation of the FA phenotype.

Conclusion

Knowledge about the biology of FA, the disease manifestations of abnormalities in the FA pathway, and better approaches to the care of these patients has increased dramatically over the past several decades. At least twenty FA and FA-associated causative genes have now been identified. The role of these resulting proteins in DNA repair, signal transduction, and oxidative damage regulation is increasingly defined. However, despite this expansion of knowledge, there are many unanswered questions about the complex biology of this critical pathway that will form the basis for future research:

What are the functions of individual proteins and the subcomplexes composed by core complex proteins?

How are the downstream effector FA proteins recruited to these nuclear foci?

How do the various processes governed by the FA pathway interrelate?

What further disease genes remain to be discovered?

How can knowledge about the biology of the FA pathway translate to better therapies for patients with FA and in patients without FA who also have abnormalities in the FA pathway?

References

Adair JE et al (2012) Cyclophosphamide promotes engraftment of gene-modified cells in a mouse model of Fanconi anemia without causing cytogenetic abnormalities. J Mol Med (Berl) 90(11):1283–1294

Akkari YM et al (2001) The 4N cell cycle delay in Fanconi anemia reflects growth arrest in late S phase. Mol Genet Metab 74(4):403–412

Alter BP (2014) Fanconi anemia and the development of leukemia. Best Pract Res Clin Haematol 27(3–4):214–221

Alter BP, Kupfer G (1993) Fanconi anemia. In: Pagon RA et al (eds) GeneReviews(R). University of Washington, Seattle, WA

Alter BP et al (2010) Malignancies and survival patterns in the National Cancer Institute inherited bone marrow failure syndromes cohort study. Br J Haematol 150(2):179–188

Andersen PL, Xu F, Xiao W (2008) Eukaryotic DNA damage tolerance and translesion synthesis through covalent modifications of PCNA. Cell Res 18(1): 162–173

Arber DA et al (2016) The 2016 revision to the World Health Organization classification of myeloid neoplasms and acute leukemia. Blood 127(20): 2391–2405

Auerbach AD (2009) Fanconi anemia and its diagnosis. Mutat Res 668(1–2):4–10

Auerbach AD (2015) Diagnosis of Fanconi anemia by diepoxybutane analysis. Curr Protoc Human Genet 85:8.7.1–8.7.17

Bagby GC, Alter BP (2006) Fanconi anemia. Semin Hematol 43(3):147–156

Blackford AN et al (2012) The DNA translocase activity of FANCM protects stalled replication forks. Hum Mol Genet 21(9):2005–2016

Bluteau D et al (2016) Biallelic inactivation of REV7 is associated with Fanconi anemia. J Clin Invest 126:3580

Bogliolo M et al (2013) Mutations in ERCC4, encoding the DNA-repair endonuclease XPF, cause Fanconi anemia. Am J Hum Genet 92(5):800–806

Bornman L et al (1999) Differential regulation and expression of stress proteins and ferritin in human monocytes. J Cell Physiol 178(1):1–8

Bouffard F et al (2015) Analysis of a FANCE splice isoform in regard to DNA repair. J Mol Biol 427(19):3056–3073
Briot D et al (2008) Aberrant activation of stress-response pathways leads to TNF-alpha oversecretion in Fanconi anemia. Blood 111(4):1913–1923
Butturini A et al (1994) Hematologic abnormalities in Fanconi anemia: an International Fanconi Anemia Registry study. Blood 84(5):1650–1655
Cantor SB et al (2001) BACH1, a novel helicase-like protein, interacts directly with BRCA1 and contributes to its DNA repair function. Cell 105(1):149–160
Cartier N et al (2009) Hematopoietic stem cell gene therapy with a lentiviral vector in X-linked adrenoleukodystrophy. Science 326(5954):818–823
Castillo P, Bogliolo M, Surralles J (2011) Coordinated action of the Fanconi anemia and ataxia telangiectasia pathways in response to oxidative damage. DNA Repair (Amst) 10(5):518–525
Ceccaldi R, Sarangi P, D'Andrea AD (2016) The Fanconi anaemia pathway: new players and new functions. Nat Rev Mol Cell Biol 17(6):337–349
Chen J et al (1998) Stable interaction between the products of the BRCA1 and BRCA2 tumor suppressor genes in mitotic and meiotic cells. Mol Cell 2(3): 317–328
Chen X et al (2014) The Fanconi anemia proteins FANCD2 and FANCJ interact and regulate each other's chromatin localization. J Biol Chem 289(37):25774–25782
Chen X et al (2016) A novel role for non-ubiquitinated FANCD2 in response to hydroxyurea-induced DNA damage. Oncogene 35(1):22–34
Ciccia A et al (2007) Identification of FAAP24, a Fanconi anemia core complex protein that interacts with FANCM. Mol Cell 25(3):331–343
Cioc AM et al (2010) Diagnosis of myelodysplastic syndrome among a cohort of 119 patients with fanconi anemia: morphologic and cytogenetic characteristics. Am J Clin Pathol 133(1):92–100
Cohn MA et al (2007) A UAF1-containing multisubunit protein complex regulates the Fanconi anemia pathway. Mol Cell 28(5):786–797
Collins NB et al (2009) ATR-dependent phosphorylation of FANCA on serine 1449 after DNA damage is important for FA pathway function. Blood 113(10):2181–2190
Collis SJ et al (2008) FANCM and FAAP24 function in ATR-mediated checkpoint signaling independently of the Fanconi anemia core complex. Mol Cell 32(3):313–324
Crossan GP et al (2011) Disruption of mouse Slx4, a regulator of structure-specific nucleases, phenocopies Fanconi anemia. Nat Genet 43(2):147–152
Cumming RC et al (2001) Fanconi anemia group C protein prevents apoptosis in hematopoietic cells through redox regulation of GSTP1. Nat Med 7(7): 814–820
Cybulski KE, Howlett NG (2011) FANCP/SLX4: a Swiss army knife of DNA interstrand crosslink repair. Cell Cycle 10(11):1757–1763
D'Andrea AD (2010) Susceptibility pathways in Fanconi's anemia and breast cancer. N Engl J Med 362(20):1909–1919
Dallapiccola B et al (1985) Effect of oxidants and antioxidants on chromosomal breakage in Fanconi anemia lymphocytes. Hum Genet 69(1):62–65
de Winter JP et al (2000) Isolation of a cDNA representing the Fanconi anemia complementation group E gene. Am J Hum Genet 67(5):1306–1308
Deans AJ, West SC (2011) DNA interstrand crosslink repair and cancer. Nat Rev Cancer 11(7):467–480
Degan P et al (1995) In vivo accumulation of 8-hydroxy-2′-deoxyguanosine in DNA correlates with release of reactive oxygen species in Fanconi's anaemia families. Carcinogenesis 16(4):735–741
Diamond LK, Shahidi NT (1967) Treatment of aplastic anemia in children. Semin Hematol 4(3):278–288
Dorsman JC et al (2007) Identification of the Fanconi anemia complementation group I gene, FANCI. Cell Oncol 29(3):211–218
Dray E et al (2010) Enhancement of RAD51 recombinase activity by the tumor suppressor PALB2. Nat Struct Mol Biol 17(10):1255–1259
Eiler ME, Frohnmayer D, Lynn Frohnmayer M, Larsen K, Joyce Owen P (2008) Fanconi anemia guidelines for diagnosis and management. Fanconi Anemia Research Fund, Inc, Eugene, OR
Enders GH (2008) Expanded roles for Chk1 in genome maintenance. J Biol Chem 283(26):17749–17752
Evans LM et al (2000) The effect of GH replacement therapy on endothelial function and oxidative stress in adult growth hormone deficiency. Eur J Endocrinol 142(3):254–262
Fagerlie SR et al (2001) Functional correction of FA-C cells with FANCC suppresses the expression of interferon gamma-inducible genes. Blood 97(10):3017–3024
Fagerlie SR et al (2004) Impaired type I IFN-induced Jak/STAT signaling in FA-C cells and abnormal CD4+ Th cell subsets in Fancc−/− mice. J Immunol 173(6):3863–3870
Fanconi Anemia Research Fund, Inc. (2014) Fanconi anemia: guidelines for diagnosis and management. Fanconi Anemia Research Fund, Inc, Eugene, OR
Farzin A et al (2007) Matched sibling donor haematopoietic stem cell transplantation in Fanconi anaemia: an update of the Cincinnati Children's experience. Br J Haematol 136(4):633–640
Folias A et al (2002) BRCA1 interacts directly with the Fanconi anemia protein FANCA. Hum Mol Genet 11(21):2591–2597
Futaki M et al (2002) The FANCG Fanconi anemia protein interacts with CYP2E1: possible role in protection against oxidative DNA damage. Carcinogenesis 23(1):67–72
Garaycoechea JI et al (2012) Genotoxic consequences of endogenous aldehydes on mouse haematopoietic stem cell function. Nature 489(7417):571–575
Garcia CC et al (2011) [13C2]-Acetaldehyde promotes unequivocal formation of 1,N2-propano-2′-

deoxyguanosine in human cells. J Am Chem Soc 133(24):9140–9143
Garcia-Higuera I et al (2001) Interaction of the Fanconi anemia proteins and BRCA1 in a common pathway. Mol Cell 7(2):249–262
Gari K et al (2008) The Fanconi anemia protein FANCM can promote branch migration of Holliday junctions and replication forks. Mol Cell 29(1):141–148
Gordon-Smith EC, Rutherford TR (1989) Fanconi anaemia--constitutional, familial aplastic anaemia. Baillieres Clin Haematol 2(1):139–152
Hirsch B et al (2004) Association of biallelic BRCA2/FANCD1 mutations with spontaneous chromosomal instability and solid tumors of childhood. Blood 103(7):2554–2559
Ho GP et al (2006) Phosphorylation of FANCD2 on two novel sites is required for mitomycin C resistance. Mol Cell Biol 26(18):7005–7015
Hodskinson MR et al (2014) Mouse SLX4 is a tumor suppressor that stimulates the activity of the nuclease XPF-ERCC1 in DNA crosslink repair. Mol Cell 54(3):472–484
Hofmann K (2009) Ubiquitin-binding domains and their role in the DNA damage response. DNA Repair (Amst) 8(4):544–556
Howlett NG et al (2002) Biallelic inactivation of BRCA2 in Fanconi anemia. Science 297(5581):606–609
Huang TT et al (2006) Regulation of monoubiquitinated PCNA by DUB autocleavage. Nat Cell Biol 8(4):339–347
Huang M et al (2010) The FANCM/FAAP24 complex is required for the DNA interstrand crosslink-induced checkpoint response. Mol Cell 39(2):259–268
Huang Y et al (2014) Modularized functions of the Fanconi anemia core complex. Cell Rep 7(6):1849–1857
Hussain S et al (2003) Direct interaction of the Fanconi anaemia protein FANCG with BRCA2/FANCD1. Hum Mol Genet 12(19):2503–2510
Hussain S et al (2004) Direct interaction of FANCD2 with BRCA2 in DNA damage response pathways. Hum Mol Genet 13(12):1241–1248
Ibanez A et al (2009) Elevated levels of IL-1beta in Fanconi anaemia group A patients due to a constitutively active phosphoinositide 3-kinase-Akt pathway are capable of promoting tumour cell proliferation. Biochem J 422(1):161–170
Joenje H, Patel KJ (2001) The emerging genetic and molecular basis of Fanconi anaemia. Nat Rev Genet 2(6):446–457
Joenje H et al (1981) Oxygen-dependence of chromosomal aberrations in Fanconi's anaemia. Nature 290(5802):142–143
Joo W et al (2011) Structure of the FANCI-FANCD2 complex: insights into the Fanconi anemia DNA repair pathway. Science 333(6040):312–316
Kashiyama K et al (2013) Malfunction of nuclease ERCC1-XPF results in diverse clinical manifestations and causes Cockayne syndrome, xeroderma pigmentosum, and Fanconi anemia. Am J Hum Genet 92(5):807–819
Kelly PF et al (2007) Stem cell collection and gene transfer in Fanconi anemia. Mol Ther 15(1):211–219
Khan NE, Rosenberg PS, Alter BP (2016) Preemptive bone marrow transplantation and event-free survival in Fanconi anemia. Biol Blood Marrow Transplant 22(10):1888–1892
Kim JM et al (2008) Cell cycle-dependent chromatin loading of the Fanconi anemia core complex by FANCM/FAAP24. Blood 111(10):5215–5222
Kim JM et al (2009) Inactivation of murine Usp1 results in genomic instability and a Fanconi anemia phenotype. Dev Cell 16(2):314–320
Kim H et al (2012) Regulation of Rev1 by the Fanconi anemia core complex. Nat Struct Mol Biol 19(2):164–170
Klein Douwel D et al (2014) XPF-ERCC1 acts in unhooking DNA interstrand crosslinks in cooperation with FANCD2 and FANCP/SLX4. Mol Cell 54(3):460–471
Kovacic P, Jacintho JD (2001) Mechanisms of carcinogenesis: focus on oxidative stress and electron transfer. Curr Med Chem 8(7):773–796
Kruyt FA et al (1998) Abnormal microsomal detoxification implicated in Fanconi anemia group C by interaction of the FAC protein with NADPH cytochrome P450 reductase. Blood 92(9):3050–3056
Kumari U et al (2014) Evidence of mitochondrial dysfunction and impaired ROS detoxifying machinery in Fanconi anemia cells. Oncogene 33(2):165–172
Langevin F et al (2011) Fancd2 counteracts the toxic effects of naturally produced aldehydes in mice. Nature 475(7354):53–58
Lehmann AR (2006) Translesion synthesis in mammalian cells. Exp Cell Res 312(14):2673–2676
Levitus M et al (2005) The DNA helicase BRIP1 is defective in Fanconi anemia complementation group J. Nat Genet 37(9):934–935
Levran O et al (2005) The BRCA1-interacting helicase BRIP1 is deficient in Fanconi anemia. Nat Genet 37(9):931–933
Li J et al (2010) Oxidative stress-specific interaction between FANCD2 and FOXO3a. Blood 115(8):1545–1548
Liang Q et al (2014) A selective USP1-UAF1 inhibitor links deubiquitination to DNA damage responses. Nat Chem Biol 10(4):298–304
Lightfoot J et al (1999) Characterization of regions functional in the nuclear localization of the Fanconi anemia group A protein. Hum Mol Genet 8(6):1007–1015
Liu JM et al (1999) Engraftment of hematopoietic progenitor cells transduced with the Fanconi anemia group C gene (FANCC). Hum Gene Ther 10(14):2337–2346
Lo Ten Foe JR et al (1997) Somatic mosaicism in Fanconi anemia: molecular basis and clinical significance. Eur J Hum Genet 5(3):137–148
Long DT et al (2011) Mechanism of RAD51-dependent DNA interstrand cross-link repair. Science 333(6038):84–87
Longerich S et al (2014) Regulation of FANCD2 and FANCI monoubiquitination by their interaction and by DNA. Nucleic Acids Res 42(9):5657–5670

MacMillan ML, Wagner JE (2010) Haematopoeitic cell transplantation for Fanconi anaemia - when and how? Br J Haematol 149(1):14–21

Malric A et al (2015) Fanconi anemia and solid malignancies in childhood: a national retrospective study. Pediatr Blood Cancer 62(3):463–470

Matsuda T et al (1998) Specific tandem GG to TT base substitutions induced by acetaldehyde are due to intrastrand crosslinks between adjacent guanine bases. Nucleic Acids Res 26(7):1769–1774

McCulloch SD, Kunkel TA (2008) The fidelity of DNA synthesis by eukaryotic replicative and translesion synthesis polymerases. Cell Res 18(1):148–161

Medhurst AL et al (2006) Evidence for subcomplexes in the Fanconi anemia pathway. Blood 108(6):2072–2080

Meetei AR et al (2003) A multiprotein nuclear complex connects Fanconi anemia and Bloom syndrome. Mol Cell Biol 23(10):3417–3426

Meetei AR et al (2004) X-linked inheritance of Fanconi anemia complementation group B. Nat Genet 36(11):1219–1224

Meetei AR et al (2005) A human ortholog of archaeal DNA repair protein Hef is defective in Fanconi anemia complementation group M. Nat Genet 37(9):958–963

Memoli S et al (1997) Diffusible melanin-related metabolites are potent inhibitors of lipid peroxidation. Biochim Biophys Acta 1346(1):61–68

Mi J et al (2004) FANCG is phosphorylated at serines 383 and 387 during mitosis. Mol Cell Biol 24(19):8576–8585

Mirchandani KD, McCaffrey RM, D'Andrea AD (2008) The Fanconi anemia core complex is required for efficient point mutagenesis and Rev1 foci assembly. DNA Repair (Amst) 7(6):902–911

Molina-Estevez FJ et al (2015) Lentiviral-mediated gene therapy in Fanconi anemia-A mice reveals long-term engraftment and continuous turnover of corrected HSCs. Curr Gene Ther 15(6):550–562

Myers KC, Davies SM (2009) Hematopoietic stem cell transplantation for bone marrow failure syndromes in children. Biol Blood Marrow Transplant 15(3):279–292

Negre O et al (2016) Gene therapy of the β-hemoglobinopathies by lentiviral transfer of the β(A(T87Q))-globin gene. Hum Gene Ther 27(2):148–165

Nijman SM et al (2005) The deubiquitinating enzyme USP1 regulates the Fanconi anemia pathway. Mol Cell 17(3):331–339

Noll M et al (2001) Preclinical protocol for in vivo selection of hematopoietic stem cells corrected by gene therapy in Fanconi anemia group C. Mol Ther 3(1):14–23

Nordenson I (1977) Effect of superoxide dismutase and catalase on spontaneously occurring chromosome breaks in patients with Fanconi's anemia. Hereditas 86(2):147–150

Pace P et al (2002) FANCE: the link between Fanconi anaemia complex assembly and activity. EMBO J 21(13):3414–3423

Pagano G et al (2004) Gender- and age-related distinctions for the in vivo prooxidant state in Fanconi anaemia patients. Carcinogenesis 25(10):1899–1909

Pagano G et al (2012) Oxidative stress in Fanconi anaemia: from cells and molecules towards prospects in clinical management. Biol Chem 393(1–2):11–21

Pang Q et al (2000) The Fanconi anemia protein FANCC binds to and facilitates the activation of STAT1 by gamma interferon and hematopoietic growth factors. Mol Cell Biol 20(13):4724–4735

Park SJ et al (2004) Oxidative stress/damage induces multimerization and interaction of Fanconi anemia proteins. J Biol Chem 279(29):30053–30059

Park E et al (2013) Inactivation of Uaf1 causes defective homologous recombination and early embryonic lethality in mice. Mol Cell Biol 33(22):4360–4370

Peng M et al (2007) The FANCJ/MutLα interaction is required for correction of the cross-link response in FA-J cells. EMBO J 26(13):3238–3249

Piatkov KI et al (2012) The auto-generated fragment of the Usp1 deubiquitylase is a physiological substrate of the N-end rule pathway. Mol Cell 48(6): 926–933

Pichierri P, Franchitto A, Rosselli F (2004) BLM and the FANC proteins collaborate in a common pathway in response to stalled replication forks. EMBO J 23(15):3154–3163

Qiao F et al (2004) Phosphorylation of Fanconi anemia (FA) complementation group G protein, FANCG, at serine 7 is important for function of the FA pathway. J Biol Chem 279(44):46035–46045

Rajendra E et al (2014) The genetic and biochemical basis of FANCD2 monoubiquitination. Mol Cell 54(5):858–869

Ridpath JR et al (2007) Cells deficient in the FANC/BRCA pathway are hypersensitive to plasma levels of formaldehyde. Cancer Res 67(23):11117–11122

Rosado IV et al (2011) Formaldehyde catabolism is essential in cells deficient for the Fanconi anemia DNA-repair pathway. Nat Struct Mol Biol 18(12): 1432–1434

Rose SR et al (2014) Oxandrolone for the treatment of bone marrow failure in Fanconi anemia. Pediatr Blood Cancer 61(1):11–19

Rosenberg PS, Greene MH, Alter BP (2003) Cancer incidence in persons with Fanconi anemia. Blood 101(3):822–826

Rosenberg PS et al (2005) Risk of head and neck squamous cell cancer and death in patients with Fanconi anemia who did and did not receive transplants. Blood 105(1):67–73

Rosenberg PS, Alter BP, Ebell W (2008) Cancer risks in Fanconi anemia: findings from the German Fanconi Anemia Registry. Haematologica 93(4):511–517

Saadatzadeh MR et al (2009) Distinct roles of stress-activated protein kinases in Fanconi anemia-type C-deficient hematopoiesis. Blood 113(12):2655–2660

Sato K et al (2012) DNA robustly stimulates FANCD2 monoubiquitylation in the complex with FANCI. Nucleic Acids Res 40(10):4553–4561

Scheckenbach K et al (2012) Treatment of the bone marrow failure in Fanconi anemia patients with danazol. Blood Cells Mol Dis 48(2):128–131

Scheinberg P, Young NS (2012) How I treat acquired aplastic anemia. Blood 120(6):1185–1196

Schultz JC, Shahidi NT (1994) Detection of tumor necrosis factor-alpha in bone marrow plasma and peripheral blood plasma from patients with aplastic anemia. Am J Hematol 45(1):32–38

Sejas DP et al (2007) Inflammatory reactive oxygen species-mediated hematopoietic suppression in Fancc-deficient mice. J Immunol (Baltimore, Md.: 1950) 178(8):5277–5287

Seki M, Tada S, Enomoto T (2006) Function of recQ family helicase in genome stability. Subcell Biochem 40:49–73

Shahidi NT, Diamond LK (1961) Testosterone-induced remission in aplastic anemia of both acquired and congenital types. N Engl J Med 264(19):953–967

Shen L et al (2014) Mechanism and function of oxidative reversal of DNA and RNA methylation. Annu Rev Biochem 83(1):585–614

Shimamura A, Alter BP (2010) Pathophysiology and management of inherited bone marrow failure syndromes. Blood Rev 24(3):101–122

Sims AE et al (2007) FANCI is a second monoubiquitinated member of the Fanconi anemia pathway. Nat Struct Mol Biol 14(6):564–567

Singh S et al (2017) Safe and effective gene therapy for murine Wiskott-Aldrich syndrome using an insulated lentiviral vector. Mol Ther Methods Clin Dev 4:1–16

Smogorzewska A et al (2007) Identification of the FANCI protein, a monoubiquitinated FANCD2 paralog required for DNA repair. Cell 129(2):289–301

Smogorzewska A et al (2010) A genetic screen identifies FAN1, a Fanconi anemia-associated nuclease necessary for DNA interstrand crosslink repair. Mol Cell 39(1):36–47

Soltys DT et al (2013) Novel XPG (ERCC5) mutations affect DNA repair and cell survival after ultraviolet but not oxidative stress. Hum Mutat 34(3):481–489

Somyajit K, Subramanya S, Nagaraju G (2010) RAD51C: a novel cancer susceptibility gene is linked to Fanconi anemia and breast cancer. Carcinogenesis 31(12):2031–2038

Soulier J et al (2005) Detection of somatic mosaicism and classification of Fanconi anemia patients by analysis of the FA/BRCA pathway. Blood 105(3):1329–1336

Stepensky P et al (2011) Bone marrow transplantation for Fanconi anemia using fludarabine-based conditioning. Biol Blood Marrow Transplant 17(9):1282–1288

Stoepker C et al (2011) SLX4, a coordinator of structure-specific endonucleases, is mutated in a new Fanconi anemia subtype. Nat Genet 43(2):138–141

Sumpter R Jr et al (2016) Fanconi anemia proteins function in mitophagy and immunity. Cell 165(4):867–881

Svendsen JM et al (2009) Mammalian BTBD12/SLX4 assembles a Holliday junction resolvase and is required for DNA repair. Cell 138(1):63–77

Tan PL et al (2006) Successful engraftment without radiation after fludarabine-based regimen in Fanconi anemia patients undergoing genotypically identical donor hematopoietic cell transplantation. Pediatr Blood Cancer 46(5):630–636

Taniguchi T et al (2002a) S-phase-specific interaction of the Fanconi anemia protein, FANCD2, with BRCA1 and RAD51. Blood 100(7):2414–2420

Taniguchi T et al (2002b) Convergence of the fanconi anemia and ataxia telangiectasia signaling pathways. Cell 109(4):459–472

Tischkowitz M, Dokal I (2004) Fanconi anaemia and leukaemia - clinical and molecular aspects. Br J Haematol 126(2):176–191

Vaz F et al (2010) Mutation of the RAD51C gene in a Fanconi anemia-like disorder. Nat Genet 42(5):406–409

Velez-Ruelas MA et al (2006) Hematopoietic changes during progression from Fanconi anemia into acute myeloid leukemia: case report and brief review of the literature. Hematology 11(5):331–334

Villamil MA et al (2012) Serine phosphorylation is critical for the activation of ubiquitin-specific protease 1 and its interaction with WD40-repeat protein UAF1. Biochemistry 51(45):9112–9123

Wagner JE et al (2007) Unrelated donor bone marrow transplantation for the treatment of Fanconi anemia. Blood 109(5):2256–2262

Wang M et al (2000) Identification of DNA adducts of acetaldehyde. Chem Res Toxicol 13(11):1149–1157

Wang X, Andreassen PR, D'Andrea AD (2004) Functional interaction of monoubiquitinated FANCD2 and BRCA2/FANCD1 in chromatin. Mol Cell Biol 24(13):5850–5862

Wang X et al (2007) Chk1-mediated phosphorylation of FANCE is required for the Fanconi anemia/BRCA pathway. Mol Cell Biol 27(8):3098–3108

Watters DJ (2003) Oxidative stress in ataxia telangiectasia. Redox Rep 8(1):23–29

Wells PG et al (1997) Oxidative damage in chemical teratogenesis. Mutat Res 396(1–2):65–78

Williams SA et al (2011) Functional and physical interaction between the mismatch repair and FA-BRCA pathways. Hum Mol Genet 20(22):4395–4410

Wilson JB et al (2008) FANCG promotes formation of a newly identified protein complex containing BRCA2, FANCD2 and XRCC3. Oncogene 27(26):3641–3652

Wong AK et al (1997) RAD51 interacts with the evolutionarily conserved BRC motifs in the human breast cancer susceptibility gene brca2. J Biol Chem 272(51):31941–31944

Wu Y, Shin-ya K, Brosh RM Jr (2008) FANCJ helicase defective in Fanconia anemia and breast cancer unwinds G-quadruplex DNA to defend genomic stability. Mol Cell Biol 28(12):4116–4128

Wu-Baer F et al (2003) The BRCA1/BARD1 heterodimer assembles polyubiquitin chains through an unconventional linkage involving lysine residue K6 of ubiquitin. J Biol Chem 278(37):34743–34746

Xia B et al (2006) Control of BRCA2 cellular and clinical functions by a nuclear partner, PALB2. Mol Cell 22(6):719–729
Xia B et al (2007) Fanconi anemia is associated with a defect in the BRCA2 partner PALB2. Nat Genet 39(2):159–161
Yalcin S et al (2008) Foxo3 is essential for the regulation of ataxia telangiectasia mutated and oxidative stress-mediated homeostasis of hematopoietic stem cells. J Biol Chem 283(37):25692–25705
Yamamoto KN et al (2011) Involvement of SLX4 in interstrand cross-link repair is regulated by the Fanconi anemia pathway. Proc Natl Acad Sci U S A 108(16):6492–6496
Yamashita T et al (1998) The Fanconi anemia pathway requires FAA phosphorylation and FAA/FAC nuclear accumulation. Proc Natl Acad Sci U S A 95(22):13085–13090
Yang H et al (2002) BRCA2 function in DNA binding and recombination from a BRCA2-DSS1-ssDNA structure. Science 297(5588):1837–1848
Yang H et al (2005) The BRCA2 homologue Brh2 nucleates RAD51 filament formation at a dsDNA-ssDNA junction. Nature 433(7026):653–657
Yu X et al (2003) The BRCT domain is a phospho-protein binding domain. Science 302(5645):639–642
Zanier R et al (2004) Fanconi anemia C gene product regulates expression of genes involved in differentiation and inflammation. Oncogene 23(29):5004–5013
Zhang QS et al (2008) Tempol protects against oxidative damage and delays epithelial tumor onset in Fanconi anemia mice. Cancer Res 68(5):1601–1608
Zhang QS et al (2010) Fancd2−/− mice have hematopoietic defects that can be partially corrected by resveratrol. Blood 116(24):5140–5148
Zhi G et al (2009) Fanconi anemia complementation group FANCD2 protein serine 331 phosphorylation is important for fanconi anemia pathway function and BRCA2 interaction. Cancer Res 69(22):8775–8783
Zhou W et al (2012) FAN1 mutations cause karyomegalic interstitial nephritis, linking chronic kidney failure to defective DNA damage repair. Nat Genet 44(8):910–915

Ribosomopathies Through a Diamond Lens

5

Anna Aspesi and Steven R. Ellis

Contents

5.1 Introduction

Ribosomopathies are generally thought of as diseases arising from defects in the process of ribosome biogenesis. Initially, the ribosomopathies showed an intriguing bias toward the inherited bone marrow failure syndromes, suggesting an unusual sensitivity of hematopoiesis to failures in the process of making ribosomes (Liu and Ellis 2006). As the field has continued to mature, a growing number of human diseases have been linked to apparent defects in manufacturing ribosomes. Many of these diseases are idiosyncratic in nature involving a single gene with distinct clinical sequelae. Recent reviews have outlined the growing list of ribosomopathies; and we would direct readers to such a review for an updated list (Yelick and Trainor 2015). Our focus here will be on the contributions of defects in ribosome synthesis to a subset of inherited bone marrow failure syndromes, with particular emphasis on Diamond-Blackfan anemia (DBA), the prototypical ribosomopathy. Other ribosomopathies will

A. Aspesi
Department of Health Sciences, University of Eastern Piedmont, Novara, Italy

S. R. Ellis (✉)
Department of Biochemistry and Molecular Genetics, University of Louisville, Louisville, KY, USA
e-mail: srelli01@louisville.edu

G. M. Kupfer et al. (eds.), *Bone Marrow Failure*, Pediatric Oncology,
https://doi.org/10.1007/978-3-319-61421-2_5

be discussed only in the context of how they may contribute to our understanding of the molecular underpinnings of the inherited bone marrow failure syndromes.

Ribosomes are large ribonucleoprotein assemblies engaged in protein synthesis. Many of the fundamental steps involved in peptide bond formation and the process by which the ribosome translocates along an mRNA in synthesizing a nascent polypeptide are thought to reside within the RNA components of the ribosome with the bulk of the ribosomal proteins involved making the process of protein synthesis more accurate and efficient through their interactions with ribosomal RNAs and various factors involved in protein synthesis. The human ribosome is composed of 4 rRNAs and 80 ribosomal proteins distributed between 2 subunits differing in size and shape. The smaller 40S ribosomal subunit is composed of 18S rRNA and 33 ribosomal proteins, whereas the 60S subunit consists of 3 rRNAs, 5S, 5.8S, and 28S, and 47 ribosomal proteins.

5.1.1 Ribosome Biogenesis

The process by which the 84 structural components of the ribosome assemble with one another to form the individual ribosomal subunits is complex and involves several hundred additional proteins and RNAs working together in a temporal fashion from primary rRNA transcripts in the nucleolus to mature functional subunits in the cytoplasm (de la Cruz et al. 2015). Three of the four rRNAs are transcribed together as a polycistronic RNA by RNA polymerase I. In addition to 18S, 5.8S, and 28S rRNAs, this primary transcript includes flanking sequences 5′ and 3′ to the mature rRNAs and two internal transcribed sequences. The mature rRNAs are liberated from this primary transcript through a series of endo and exonucleolytic cleavage reactions. These cleavages occur as substrates are made available as ribosomal proteins bind and fold pre-rRNAs in concert with a multitude of transiently associated factors that participate in subunit maturation. The fourth rRNA, 5S rRNA is transcribed by RNA polymerase III and forms a ribonucleoprotein (RNP) subcomplex with ribosomal proteins Rpl5(uL18) and Rpl11(uL5) facilitated by additional assembly factors. A number of additional factors contribute to the incorporations of the 5S subcomplex into pre-60S particles.

5.1.2 Ribosome Structure

The ribosome itself took shape before the divergence of the three major domains of life, eubacteria, archaebacteria, and eukaryotes. Somewhat surprisingly, in terms of phylogenetic sequence comparisons, the archaebacteria (which tend to live in extreme environments) and eukarya are more closely related to one another than either are to the more familiar eubacteria. The recent proposal for a universal nomenclature for ribosomal proteins is based upon phylogenetic sequence comparisons, classifying ribosomal proteins as universal if family members are found in all three kingdoms and either B or E if family members are restricted to either the eubacterial or archaeal/eukaryal lineages, respectively (Ban et al. 2014).

In terms of structure, Melnikov et al. have described ribosomes as having a conserved core with bacterial- or eukaryotic-specific shells (Melnikov et al. 2012). The universal ribosomal proteins belong to a common structural core of ribosomes necessary for carrying out the basic steps of protein synthesis shared by ribosomes in the three domains of life. Outside of this common core, new ribosomal proteins unique to eubacteria, archaebacteria/eukarya, and eukarya alone have been recruited to work in conjunction with the common core to perform functions more specialized to a particular domain of life. Eukaryotic ribosomes are much larger than their eubacterial and archaebacterial counterparts: including expansion sequences in rRNAs, additional structural elements added to core proteins, new proteins common to archaeal and eukaryal lineages, and several additional proteins unique to the eukaryal lineage (Gamalinda and Woolford Jr. 2014).

The most dramatic differences between bacterial and eukaryotic ribosomes occur on the solvent exposed surfaces of the ribosomal subunits. These distinctive features are presumably necessary for interactions with the myriad of factors involved in assembling ribosomal subunits, transporting nascent subunits from the nucleolus to the cytoplasm, and for aspects of the translational process differing between the different domains of life. Superimposed on these generalized differences between bacterial and eukaryotic ribosomes are novel ribosomal proteins in eukaryotes that have evolved to give ribosomes unique characteristics in a particular tissue or cell type, creating what are now referred to as specialized ribosomes (Kondrashov et al. 2011).

5.2 Diamond-Blackfan Anemia: The Prototypical Ribosomopathy

To date, 18 genes have been linked to Diamond-Blackfan anemia (Danilova and Gazda 2015). The vast majority of the genes encode ribosomal proteins. The ribosomal proteins affected in DBA include proteins of both the 40S and 60S ribosomal subunit. The 40S subunit proteins known to be affected in DBA include Rps19(eS19), Rps26(eS26), Rps10(eS10), Rps24(eS24), Rps17(eS17), Rps7(eS7), Rps27(eS27), Rps28(e28), and Rps29 (uS14). In parenthesis we include the names for the ribosomal proteins using the new universal system of nomenclature (Ban et al. 2014). Looking at the names for these proteins using the new nomenclature reveals that only one of the nine Rps proteins affected in DBA belongs to the common core of the 40S subunit, Rps29(uS14), with the remaining proteins having evolved after the divergence of archaebacteria and eukarya from the eubacteria. As 15 of the 33 proteins of the eukaryotic 40S subunit belong to the common core, this bias is not simply a reflection of the percentage of 40S subunit proteins belonging to common core relative to those recruited later. Whether there is any significance to this bias against proteins of the common core being affected in DBA remains unknown.

The situation is more complicated for proteins of the 60S subunit. The 60S ribosomal proteins known to be affected in DBA include Rpl5(uL18), Rpl11(uL5), Rpl35A(eL33), Rpl15(eL15), Rpl26(uL24), Rpl27(eL27), and Rpl31(eL31). Here the bias toward protein components of the common core seems to fall off with DBA, though it should be noted that Rpl5(uL18) and Rpl11(uL5) are distinct in terms of forming a subcomplex with 5S rRNA prior to being incorporated into the 60S subunit. Moreover, the 5S rRNA subcomplex has been co-opted as a signaling molecule regulating p53 levels in response to ribosome stress (see pathophysiological mechanisms). Intriguingly, the other 60S subunit protein from the common core so far implicated in DBA is Rpl26(uL24), another protein known to play a role in regulating p53 expression (Chen et al. 2012), although through a mechanism distinct from Rpl5(uL18) and Rpl11(uL5).

5.2.1 Pre-rRNA Processing as a Means of Monitoring Ribosomal Protein Function

The ribosomal protein genes affected in DBA harbor heterozygous loss-of-function mutations resulting in haploinsufficiency for the affected ribosomal protein. Ribosomal protein function is routinely monitored through their role in ribosome biogenesis by assessing the effect of mutant alleles on the process by which mature 18S, 5.8S, and 28S rRNAs are generated from the polymerase I primary transcript. Loss-of-function alleles of ribosomal proteins affected in DBA all display characteristic pre-rRNA processing defects, the nature of which are dictated by where these proteins are located in the structural organization of the 40S subunit relative to ends of mature RNAs (Flygare et al. 2007). As noted by O'Donohue et al. (2010), the three most frequently mutated genes in DBA patients that encode proteins of the 40S ribosomal subunit Rps19(25%), Rps26(6.5%), and Rps10(2.5%) are all involved in the maturation of the 3′ end of 18S rRNA. As shown in Fig. 5.1, these proteins are all located in the head region of the 40S subunit, which also contains the 3′ structural domain of 18S rRNA. This led to the hypothesis that processing defects involved in 3′ end maturation may be less severe than those influencing the 5′ end of 18S, thereby resulting in a disease

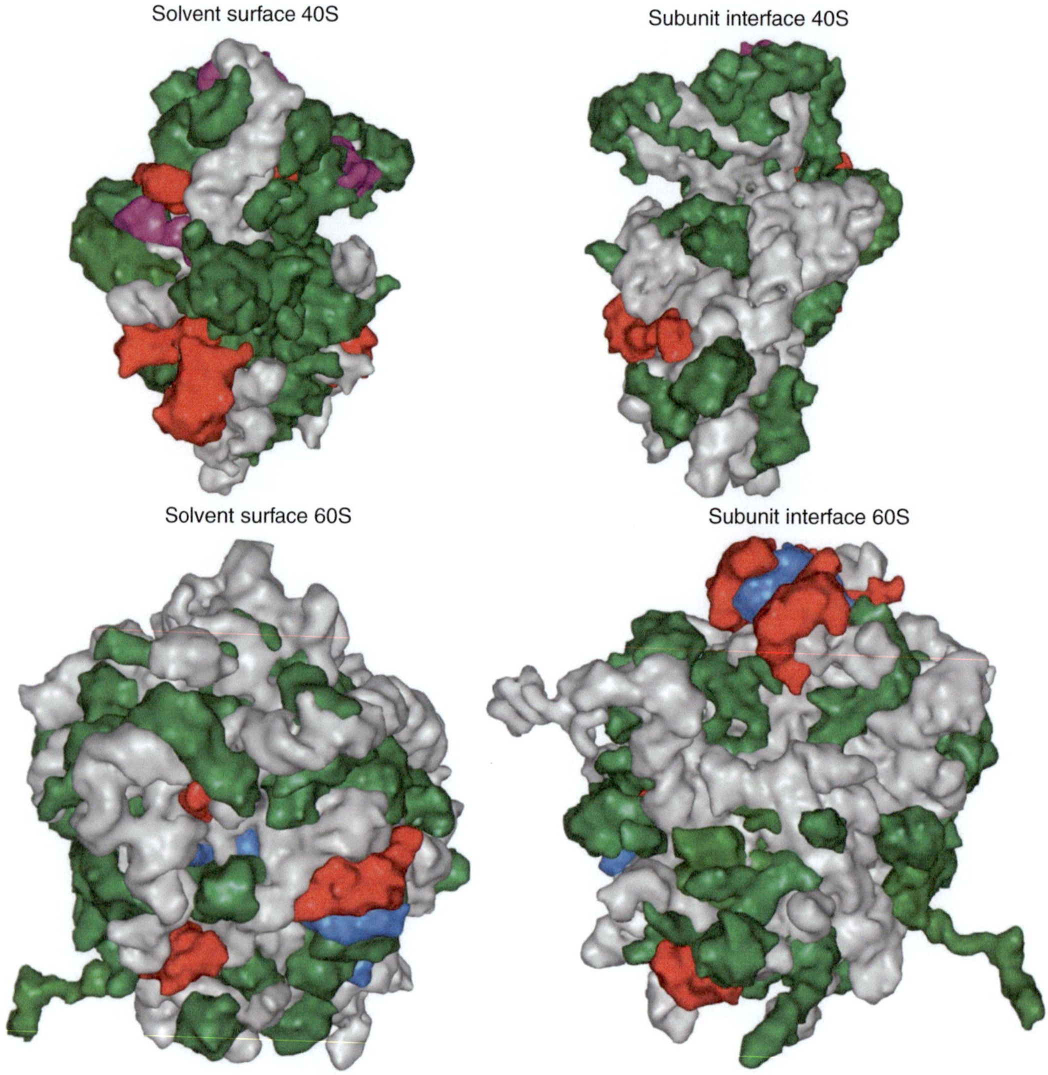

Fig. 5.1 Ribosomal proteins affected in Diamond-Blackfan anemia. The atomic coordinates for the 40S and 60S ribosomal subunits were derived from the work of Khatter et al. (2015) deposited in the protein data bank with the accession code 4UGO. The figure was created using protein workshop software developed by Moreland et al. (2005). Proteins affected in DBA are shown in red with the exception of Rps10, Rps19, and Rps26 of the 40S subunit, which are shown in magenta. Other ribosomal proteins are shown in green. 18S and 28S rRNAs of the 40S and 60S ribosomal subunits, respectively, are shown in gray. 5S and 5.8S rRNAs of the 60S ribosomal subunit are shown in blue

state rather than embryonic lethality (O'Donohue et al. 2010). As can be seen in Fig. 5.1, DBA proteins are also found on base of the 40S structure with the 5′ domain of 18S rRNA, and studies have shown that these proteins influence the 5′ end of 18S rRNA. Therefore, while the frequency of mutations in small subunit proteins is clearly biased toward those in the head domain, being located on the base and influencing 5′end maturation does not preclude a protein from being involved in DBA. In this regard, it is also noteworthy that components of the small subunit processome carrying out many of the earliest steps in the biogenesis of the 40S subunit have been implicated in other ribosomopathies that do not present as bone marrow failure syndromes but nevertheless are not embryonic lethal (Sondalle and Baserga 2014).

Like the proteins of the 40S ribosomal subunit, proteins of the 60S ribosomal subunit also influence pre-rRNA processing. Some of the more dramatic pre-rRNA processing defects observed with 60S subunit ribosomal proteins are evident by capillary electrophoresis without the need for radio-isotopic detection (Farrar et al. 2014). Quarello et al. have suggested that this technique may be amenable to use as a diagnostic aide for DBA (Quarello et al. 2016).

5.2.2 Non-ribosomal Proteins Causing DBA

To date, only two proteins other than ribosomal proteins have been linked to DBA. Both are located on the X chromosome. The first is GATA1, a transcription factor involved in lineage decisions during hematopoiesis, including erythropoiesis. GATA1 thus represents the first gene identified in DBA that provides a clear molecular basis for erythroid phenotype observed in DBA patients (Sankaran et al. 2012). The other protein is Tsr2, which is involved, at least in yeast, in the maturation of 40S ribosomal subunits (Gripp et al. 2014). This is the first factor involved in ribosome biogenesis other than a ribosomal protein that has been implicated in DBA. Factors involved in ribosome biogenesis are only transiently associated with ribosomes and so in contrast to ribosomal proteins may behave catalytically being continuously regenerated after performing their functions in subunit maturation. Consequently such genes may require two loss-of-function alleles to manifest clinically, which may be an exceptionally rare event, unless such a gene is found on the X chromosome.

5.3 Pathophysiologic Mechanisms

Except for GATA1, it is difficult to reconcile the genes affected in DBA with red cell hypoplasia, the sine qua non of Diamond-Blackfan anemia. How a defect in a process as ubiquitous as ribosome biogenesis can cause highly selective disorders affecting a limited number of tissues remains a mystery for DBA and other ribosomopathies. There are two general models for how defects in ribosome synthesis could be involved in the molecular underpinnings of DBA. The first of these is a ribosome stress model where rogue ribosomal proteins failing to assemble into their respective ribosomal subunits have alternative fates including promoting p53 activation and apoptosis (Ellis and Gleizes 2011). The second model evokes changes in translational output arising from reduced amounts of 40S or 60S subunits caused by ribosomal protein haploinsufficiency. Both models have strong experimental support with some caveats, and it seems highly likely that disease phenotypes may involve a combination of the two mechanisms, which are not mutually exclusive. Each will be discussed in turn below.

5.3.1 Ribosome Stress

Pestov et al. were the first to draw attention to the relationship between defects in ribosome synthesis and the activation of p53 via a process they referred to as nucleolar stress (Pestov et al. 2001). We will use the term ribosome stress to reflect the fact that not all stressors that affect ribosome biogenesis may affect nucleolar structure (Nicolas et al. 2016). The importance of p53 activation to DBA pathophysiology became evident with the finding that loss of p53 function rescued phenotypes in a zebra fish and mouse models of DBA (Danilova et al. 2008; Jaako et al. 2015) and cell death in human cellular models of DBA (Dutt et al. 2011). The mechanisms underlying p53 activation in cells with abortive ribosome synthesis began to take shape with studies showing ribosomal proteins were capable of binding to and inhibiting MDM2, a ubiquitin ligase targeting p53 for proteasomal degradation responsible for maintaining low levels of p53 expression in unstressed cells (Marechal et al. 1994). Inhibition of MDM2 via interaction with ribosomal proteins diverted from their normal fate of being assembled into ribosomal subunits to now interacting with MDM2, leads to p53 stabilization and activation. A potentially straightforward model by which a limited number of ribosomal proteins play a role in signaling p53 activation in response to ribosome stress has given way to an embarrassment of riches with an ever-growing list of ribosomal proteins shown to interact with MDM2 (Kim et al. 2014; Xu et al. 2016). Ribosomal proteins known to interact with MDM2 directly leading to p53 activation include Rps3(uS3), Rps7(eS7), Rps14(uS11), Rps15(u19), Rps20(uS10), Rps25(eS25), Rps26(eS26), Rps27(eS27), Rps27a(eS31), Rps27L, Rpl5(uL18), Rpl11(uL5), Rpl23(uL14), Rpl26(uL24), and Rpl37(eL37).

Among these proteins, Rpl5(uL18) and Rpl11(uL5) stand out as being critical among the direct effectors in mediating p53 activation in response to ribosome stress (Donati et al. 2013). With all the other ribosomal proteins potentially involved in ribosome stress signaling, it seems worthwhile to consider whether the signaling mechanism centered on Rpl5/Rpl11 could be rheostatically controlled. In a normal electronic rheostat, resistance is variable controlled through a moving knob or slider, whereas for a ribosome stress model, the moving knob or slider would be the nature, number, and amount of free ribosomal proteins available for interacting with MDM2 and other growth control molecules. Adaptation of a rheostat model to ribosome stress signaling could potentially explain both the surplus of ribosomal protein modulators and the bias toward noncore ribosomal proteins involved in Diamond-Blackfan anemia.

If we assume that Rpl5 and Rpl11 are critical regulators of ribosome stress signaling as part of the 5S RNP subcomplex, one can envision how a defect in 60S subunit biogenesis could lead to the failure of incorporating this subcomplex into nascent 60S particles making it now available for interaction with MDM2 and p53 induction. Less clear was how a defect in 40S subunit biogenesis could signal ribosomal stress through the 5S RNP subcomplex. Fumagalli et al. resolved this issue by showing that the translation of TOP-containing ribosomal protein mRNAs, including Rpl5 and Rpl11, was increased in cells with impaired 40S subunit biogenesis (Fumagalli et al. 2009).

What remains unclear, however, is our knowledge of threshold of ribosome stress signaling required for p53-induced apoptosis, particularly in vivo in different cell types. If the level by which components of the 5S RNP subcomplex were induced by impaired 40S biogenesis were below a particular threshold for p53-induced apoptosis, there could be a role for small subunit ribosomal proteins acting either on their own or in concert with the 5S RNP in inhibiting MDM2 and activating p53.

The nature, number, and amount of small subunit ribosomal proteins available for this rheostatic control of the MDM2-p53 axis could be influenced by which ribosomal protein was limiting for 40S subunit biogenesis under conditions of haploinsufficiency. The elegant studies by Nomura and colleagues in the 1960s revealed that the assembly of ribosomal subunits was a hierarchical process with some primary assembly proteins binding directly to rRNA and other secondary and tertiary binding proteins being more reliant on RNA binding sites created by folding events mediated by the primary binding proteins and protein/protein interactions (Held et al. 1974). The loss of a tertiary binding protein would still allow some degree of assembly of primary and secondary binding proteins and only affect the binding of a limited number of other tertiary binding proteins into the abortive complex. In contrast, the loss of a critical primary binding protein affects the incorporation of a far greater number of proteins into the abortive complex, thus releasing a far greater number of proteins to potentially signal ribosome stress.

While we do not have an assembly map of human 40S subunits comparable to that worked out for the bacterial 30S subunit, viewing human 40S subunit as having a common core with a eukaryotic shell could give us an analogous, if somewhat cruder, perspective. Very little is known regarding the degradation of abortive intermediates that accumulate when ribosomal subunit assembly is compromised, although it does appear that there are cellular quality control mechanisms involved in the degradation of misassembled or nonfunctional ribonucleoprotein complexes (Fujii et al. 2012). Consequently, proteins that get assembled into abortive complexes may be degraded along with rRNA as part of this quality control mechanism. Thus, we would have two general classes of ribosomal proteins during abortive assembly, those that get assembled into the abortive complex and are presumably degraded and those failing to assemble, which could then be free for ribosome stress signaling. Fewer proteins may be available for ribosome stress signaling if assembly were aborted by haploinsufficiency for a protein of the outer shell, whereas the number of proteins released if a protein of the common core were affected may be incompatible with life.

Rps29(uS14) is the current exception to the finding that ribosomal proteins of the 40S subunit affected in DBA belong to the eukaryotic shell. Intriguingly, bacterial S14 is a tertiary binder in the Nomura assembly map (Held et al. 1974) and in eukaryotes Rps29 is incorporated in a late cytoplasmic step in the maturation of 40S subunits (de la Cruz et al. 2015). Thus, the relationship between ribosomal subunit assembly dependencies and the release of ribosomal proteins for various roles in controlling cell cycle progression and apoptosis is clearly more nuanced, allowing certain proteins within the conserved core of the ribosome to be affected in DBA.

As appealing as the ribosome stress model is as an underlying mechanism for the pathogenesis of DBA, there are significant caveats. Foremost among these caveats is that Rpl5(uL18) and Rpl11(uL5), central mediators of ribosome stress signaling, are themselves DBA proteins (Gazda et al. 2008). Thus, there would have to be alternative means of signaling to p53 activation when either of these two proteins is absent, or that p53-independent mechanisms may also contribute to phenotypes in DBA. In a recent tour de force, the Lafontaine laboratory has monitored the effect of reducing the expression of each of the human ribosomal proteins on nucleolar structure and p53 induction (Nicolas et al. 2016). Based on their cutoff criteria for significant induction of p53 (fivefold increase over basal levels), the loss of function of many ribosomal proteins, including virtually all DBA proteins, did not result in what was considered a significant increase in steady-state levels of p53. These rather shocking results, which in some cases differ from previous published reports, may relate to their rather stringent cutoff of significance at fivefold induction, which again points to our lack of knowledge of critical thresholds for p53 activation in physiologically relevant settings. The ever-mounting complexity of factors feeding into models of ribosome stress continues to confound any consensus regarding the role of misassembled ribosomal proteins and p53 activation in DBA pathophysiology.

Before going on to discuss the role of translational alterations in DBA pathophysiology, it is worthwhile discussing other ribosomopathies in the context of ribosome stress. The first of these is the bone marrow failure syndrome Shwachman-Diamond syndrome. Shwachman-Diamond syndrome and Diamond-Blackfan anemia differ in clinical presentation, which is covered elsewhere in this volume. To date, there is a single gene known to be affected in Shwachman-Diamond syndrome given the acronym *SBDS*, for Shwachman-Diamond-Bodian syndrome. SBDS is a conserved protein found in eukaryal and archaeal lineages, which plays a role in the release of eukaryotic initiation factor 6 (eIF6) from nascent 60S subunits exiting the nucleus to the cytoplasm. The presence of bound eIF6 serves as an anti-association factor preventing the joining of 40S and 60S ribosomal subunits until the latter are fully matured (Weis et al. 2015). Thus, the function of SBDS in the release of eIF6 is one of the final steps in 60S subunit maturation before the subunit becomes part of the 60S subunit pool active in translation.

The failure to release eIF6 from nascent 60S subunits in cytoplasm interferes with the recycling of eIF6 to the nucleus where it performs a function in transporting nascent subunits from the nucleus to the cytoplasm. In this manner, the loss of SBDS has a secondary effect on 60S subunit maturation by impeding the transport of 60S subunits from the nucleus to the cytoplasm (Menne et al. 2007). In contrast to DBA where the loss of a ribosomal protein can interfere with the assembly of other ribosomal proteins into nascent subunits leading to the degradation of partially assembled subunits, the 60S subunits that accumulate in the nucleus of cells deficient in SBDS and its yeast ortholog Sdo1 are relatively stable and likely have a relatively full complement of ribosomal proteins, except for those assembling in the cytoplasm (Moore et al. 2010). Importantly, the failure to transport 60S subunits from the nucleus to the cytoplasm does not appear to interfere with the incorporation of the 5S RNP subcomplex into nascent subunits. These fundamental differences in the manner in which ribosomal proteins and SBDS interfere with the maturation of ribosomal subunits likely play a role in the differences in clinical phenotypes between Shwachman-Diamond syndrome and Diamond-Blackfan anemia patients.

Any model for ribosome stress in the pathophysiology of Diamond-Blackfan anemia must deal with the Treacher Collins syndrome conundrum. Treacher Collins is a syndrome characterized by craniofacial anomalies. Importantly for our discussion, patients with Treacher Collins syndrome do not manifest bone marrow failure. This is surprising because the genes affected in TCS interfere with the transcription of rRNAs, and like DBA activation of p53 appears to play a central role in the pathophysiology of TCS. Ribosomal RNA forms the base of any assembly pathway for ribosomal subunits, and reductions in rRNA should interfere with subsequent incorporation of all ribosomal proteins into nascent subunits. Therefore, one might expect that ribosomal proteins failing to assemble as a consequence of reduced transcription of rRNA would play a role in activating p53 similar to that seen in DBA and as such affect erythropoiesis. And yet, there is no evidence for a defect in erythropoiesis in TCS patients.

Transcription of rDNA by RNA polymerase I plays a critical role in defining ribosome levels in cells, and although all three RNA polymerases are thought to be coordinated by various levels of crosstalk during ribosome production, there are likely transient windows when expression of ribosomal RNAs and proteins is uncoupled, leading to imbalances in the ribosome substituents before new steady-state conditions are achieved. Consequently there may be additional levels of control on ribosome stress-mediated signaling when rRNA transcription is affected in a physiological setting, as opposed to the signaling mechanisms involved when there is haploinsufficiency for a ribosomal protein.

5.3.2 Translational Alterations

The Ruggero group has shown that loss of DKC1, the gene affected in X-linked dyskeratosis congenita (DC), can influence the translation of IRES-containing mRNAs and contribute to the pathogenesis of the X-linked form of this bone marrow failure syndrome (Bellodi et al. 2010). While the loss of telomere function is the primary cause of most forms of DC, DKC1 mutations affect a number of additional processes including ribosome synthesis and function (Angrisani et al. 2014). These additional functions of DKC1 presumably contribute to the severity of X-linked forms of the disease (Townsley et al. 2014), and so at least the X-linked form of DC could also be classified as a ribosomopathy.

It seems reasonable to infer that changes in translational output in cells affected by haploinsufficiency for ribosomal proteins could also contribute to the pathogenesis of DBA. Each of the ribosomal proteins affected in DBA has been shown to influence pre-rRNA processing and in many cases has been shown to influence the levels of their respective ribosomal subunit (Flygare et al. 2007; Nicolas et al. 2016; Choesmel et al. 2007). Such losses of ribosomal subunits have been shown to affect global translation in various cellular models of DBA and in some cases have been shown to affect the translation of specific mRNAs encoding proteins involved in hematopoiesis (Horos et al. 2012). One of the more telling examples of an effect on translation that could give rise to the clinical features of DBA were the studies of Ludwig et al. showing that haploinsufficiency for ribosomal proteins affected in DBA could adversely affect the translation of GATA1 mRNA (Ludwig et al. 2014). These studies linked DBA caused by ribosomal protein haploinsufficiency with DBA caused by mutations in GATA1. The mutations in GATA1 found in DBA result in an amino-terminal truncated protein retaining residual activity but lacking a critical domain required for erythropoiesis (Sankaran et al. 2012). Importantly, in cells with normal GATA1 but haploinsufficient for different ribosomal proteins affected in DBA, Ludwig et al. showed that the translation of full-length GATA1 was decreased providing a mechanism whereby reduced levels of ribosomal proteins could selectively affect erythropoiesis.

The exact nature by which ribosomal protein haploinsufficiency affects the translation of GATA1 remains to be identified, but it is worthwhile noting that the effect on GATA1 translation is independent of which subunit is affected. It is difficult to envision a specific translational control mechanism that would give similar effects regardless of which subunit was affected. Thus, it seems possible that a general reduction in protein synthetic capacity could somehow be involved in the pathogenesis of DBA.

Support for a role of general reduction of protein synthesis in the pathogenesis of DBA has recently come from studies from the Abkowitz group. Yang et al. have recently published an elegant study on the timing of heme and globin synthesis in developing erythrocytes (Yang et al. 2016). These studies reveal that cells haploinsufficient for ribosomal proteins affected in DBA exhibit a delay in globin synthesis while heme synthesis continues unabated, leading to heme excess. Heme excess, in turn, leads to increased reactive oxygen species and promotes ferroptosis/apoptosis of erythroid progenitors. Further support for the role of heme toxicity in the pathogenesis of DBA comes from the observation that reducing heme synthesis to parallel globin synthesis or an increase in heme export from cells can rescue phenotypes caused by haploinsufficiency for ribosomal proteins in CD34^{+} cultures induced to differentiate along the erythroid lineage.

Yang et al. also provide a model for how mechanisms of cell death induced by heme toxicity could synergize with ribosome stress signaling to preferentially affect erythropoiesis. In this model, p53 activation in response to ribosome stress could potentially interfere with the synthesis of certain antioxidant defense mechanism sensitizing cells to reactive oxygen species induced by heme excess. Thus, it seems increasingly likely that the two mechanisms implicated in the pathophysiology of DBA interact to preferentially effect erythropoiesis and therefore begin to explain how disrupting a ubiquitous process like ribosome synthesis could engender tissue selectivity in terms of clinical phenotypes.

5.4 Ribosomopathies: A Gateway to Tumorigenesis

The two main models proposed to explain defective erythropoiesis in DBA have also been advocated to account for high incidence of cancer in DBA patients. An increased risk to develop myelodysplastic syndrome (MDS), acute myeloid leukemia (AML), and solid tumors has been observed by studying a large cohort of DBA patients (Vlachos et al. 2012). Shwachman-Diamond syndrome, dyskeratosis congenita, and 5q− syndrome, an acquired condition due to heterozygous loss of the Rps14(uS11) gene (Ebert et al. 2008), located on the long arm of chromosome 5, are all known to be associated with MDS and progression to leukemia. Most recently, next-generation sequencing technologies led to the discovery that somatic mutations in RP genes are rather common in different cancer types. For example, Rpl5(uL18), Rpl10(uL16), and Rpl22(eL22) were found mutated in T-acute lymphoblastic leukemia (De Keersmaecker et al. 2013; Rao et al. 2012), whereas other RPs were mutated in endometrial cancer, colorectal carcinoma, and glioma (Goudarzi and Lindstrom 2016). Heterozygous mutations in several RPs also cause tumors in zebra fish (Amsterdam et al. 2004) and in other animal models including *Drosophila* and mouse (Kazerounian et al. 2016; Stewart and Denell 1993). Therefore, there is rising evidence that ribosome dysfunction can drive malignant transformation.

Tumorigenesis is typically accompanied by stimulation of protein synthesis, which is critical to support unrestrained proliferation in cancer cells. It seems paradoxical that pathologies characterized by hypoproliferative phenotypes may be associated with elevated cancer risk. The causal link between ribosomopathies and cancer might be, once again, the dysregulation of p53-dependent pathways. Persistent activation of p53 in RP depleted cells may provide selective pressure for the expansion of clones with spontaneous mutations that confer proliferative advantage. The acquisition of any compensatory mutation that counterbalances the effects of ribosome stress and prevents apoptosis may contribute to tumorigenesis. Interestingly, a similar mechanism where a clone with growth advantage prevails over the population of cells carrying only the original RP mutation may also be responsible for the spontaneous remission observed in some cases of DBA.

A high cancer risk in cells subjected to ribosome stress may also be the result of alterations in the translation of specific messenger RNAs, particularly oncogenes and tumor suppressors. Other mechanisms have been suggested to explain why RP depletion would increase cancer predisposition. A reduction in the number of ribosomes or qualitative alterations in their composition could impact translational fidelity and lead to cellular transformation (Sulima et al. 2014); moreover, some RPs may have extraribosomal functions relevant for cancer development.

5.5 Concluding Thoughts

There are an increasing number of human diseases caused by mutations in genes encoding either structural components of the ribosome or factors involved in ribosome biogenesis. These diseases collectively known as ribosomopathies continue to provide challenges in terms of underlying pathogenic mechanisms. In some cases it still remains to be seen whether defective ribosome biogenesis plays a major role in disease phenotype, or instead in cases where the factors involved have multiple functions within cells whether defects in ribosome synthesis play a role in modifying disease phenotype. In other diseases, where defects in ribosome synthesis are more clearly defined as having a role in disease pathogenesis, the link between defects in a process as ubiquitous as ribosome biogenesis and seemingly tissue-selective disease phenotypes remains elusive. Many studies have supported a role for p53 activation via ribosome stress in disease pathogenesis, but many questions remain because of the remarkable myriad of factors that have been implicated in ribosome stress signaling. Recent studies on the timing of heme and globin synthesis in erythroid progenitors have also provided fascinating new insights as to how general defects in protein synthesis linked to haploinsufficiency for ribosomal proteins could potentially account for the erythroid selectivity of Diamond-Blackfan anemia. Finally, adding fuel to growing interest in ribosomopathies is the link between many of these diseases and tumorigenesis as evidenced by the cancer predisposition in certain ribosomopathies and the finding of somatic mutations in ribosomal protein genes in tumor genotyping.

References

Amsterdam A et al (2004) Many ribosomal protein genes are cancer genes in zebrafish. PLoS Biol 2(5):E139

Angrisani A et al (2014) Human dyskerin: beyond telomeres. Biol Chem 395(6):593–610

Ban N et al (2014) A new system for naming ribosomal proteins. Curr Opin Struct Biol 24:165–169

Bellodi C et al (2010) Loss of function of the tumor suppressor DKC1 perturbs p27 translation control and contributes to pituitary tumorigenesis. Cancer Res 70(14):6026–6035

Chen J, Guo K, Kastan MB (2012) Interactions of nucleolin and ribosomal protein L26 (RPL26) in translational control of human p53 mRNA. J Biol Chem 287(20):16467–16476

Choesmel V et al (2007) Impaired ribosome biogenesis in Diamond-Blackfan anemia. Blood 109(3):1275–1283

Danilova N, Gazda HT (2015) Ribosomopathies: how a common root can cause a tree of pathologies. Dis Model Mech 8(9):1013–1026

Danilova N, Sakamoto KM, Lin S (2008) Ribosomal protein S19 deficiency in zebrafish leads to developmental abnormalities and defective erythropoiesis through activation of p53 protein family. Blood 112(13):5228–5237

De Keersmaecker K et al (2013) Exome sequencing identifies mutation in CNOT3 and ribosomal genes RPL5 and RPL10 in T-cell acute lymphoblastic leukemia. Nat Genet 45(2):186–190

Donati G et al (2013) 5S ribosomal RNA is an essential component of a nascent ribosomal precursor complex that regulates the Hdm2-p53 checkpoint. Cell Rep 4(1):87–98

Dutt S et al (2011) Haploinsufficiency for ribosomal protein genes causes selective activation of p53 in human erythroid progenitor cells. Blood 117(9):2567–2576

Ebert BL et al (2008) Identification of RPS14 as a 5q- syndrome gene by RNA interference screen. Nature 451(7176):335–339

Ellis SR, Gleizes PE (2011) Diamond Blackfan anemia: ribosomal proteins going rogue. Semin Hematol 48(2):89–96

Farrar JE et al (2014) Exploiting pre-rRNA processing in Diamond Blackfan anemia gene discovery and diagnosis. Am J Hematol 89(10):985–991

Flygare J et al (2007) Human RPS19, the gene mutated in Diamond-Blackfan anemia, encodes a ribosomal protein required for the maturation of 40S ribosomal subunits. Blood 109(3):980–986

Fujii K et al (2012) 40S subunit dissociation and proteasome-dependent RNA degradation in non-functional 25S rRNA decay. EMBO J 31(11):2579–2589

Fumagalli S et al (2009) Absence of nucleolar disruption after impairment of 40S ribosome biogenesis reveals an rpL11-translation-dependent mechanism of p53 induction. Nat Cell Biol 11(4):501–508

Gamalinda M, Woolford JL Jr (2014) Deletion of L4 domains reveals insights into the importance of ribosomal protein extensions in eukaryotic ribosome assembly. RNA 20(11):1725–1731

Gazda HT et al (2008) Ribosomal protein L5 and L11 mutations are associated with cleft palate and abnormal thumbs in Diamond-Blackfan anemia patients. Am J Hum Genet 83(6):769–780

Goudarzi KM, Lindstrom MS (2016) Role of ribosomal protein mutations in tumor development (Review). Int J Oncol 48(4):1313–1324

Gripp KW et al (2014) Diamond-Blackfan anemia with mandibulofacial dystostosis is heterogeneous, including the novel DBA genes TSR2 and RPS28. Am J Med Genet A 164A(9):2240–2249

Held WA et al (1974) Assembly mapping of 30 S ribosomal proteins from Escherichia coli. Further studies. J Biol Chem 249(10):3103–3111

Horos R et al (2012) Ribosomal deficiencies in Diamond-Blackfan anemia impair translation of transcripts essential for differentiation of murine and human erythroblasts. Blood 119(1):262–272

Jaako P et al (2015) Disruption of the 5S RNP-Mdm2 interaction significantly improves the erythroid defect in a mouse model for Diamond-Blackfan anemia. Leukemia 29(11):2221–2229

Kazerounian S et al (2016) Development of Soft Tissue Sarcomas in Ribosomal Proteins L5 and S24 Heterozygous Mice. J Cancer 7(1):32–36

Khatter H et al (2015) Structure of the human 80S ribosome. Nature 520(7549):640–645

Kim TH, Leslie P, Zhang Y (2014) Ribosomal proteins as unrevealed caretakers for cellular stress and genomic instability. Oncotarget 5(4):860–871

Kondrashov N et al (2011) Ribosome-mediated specificity in Hox mRNA translation and vertebrate tissue patterning. Cell 145(3):383–397

de la Cruz J, Karbstein K, Woolford JL Jr (2015) Functions of ribosomal proteins in assembly of eukaryotic ribosomes in vivo. Annu Rev Biochem 84:93–129

Liu JM, Ellis SR (2006) Ribosomes and marrow failure: coincidental association or molecular paradigm? Blood 107(12):4583–4588

Ludwig LS et al (2014) Altered translation of GATA1 in Diamond-Blackfan anemia. Nat Med 20(7):748–753

Marechal V et al (1994) The ribosomal L5 protein is associated with mdm-2 and mdm-2-p53 complexes. Mol Cell Biol 14(11):7414–7420

Melnikov S et al (2012) One core, two shells: bacterial and eukaryotic ribosomes. Nat Struct Mol Biol 19(6):560–567

Menne TF et al (2007) The Shwachman-Bodian-Diamond syndrome protein mediates translational activation of ribosomes in yeast. Nat Genet 39(4):486–495

Moore JBt et al (2010) Distinct ribosome maturation defects in yeast models of Diamond-Blackfan anemia and Shwachman-Diamond syndrome. Haematologica 95(1):57–64

Moreland JL et al (2005) The Molecular Biology Toolkit (MBT): a modular platform for developing molecular visualization applications. BMC Bioinformatics 6:21

Nicolas E et al (2016) Involvement of human ribosomal proteins in nucleolar structure and p53-dependent nucleolar stress. Nat Commun 7:11390

O'Donohue MF et al (2010) Functional dichotomy of ribosomal proteins during the synthesis of mammalian 40S ribosomal subunits. J Cell Biol 190(5):853–866

Pestov DG, Strezoska Z, Lau LF (2001) Evidence of p53-dependent cross-talk between ribosome biogenesis and the cell cycle: effects of nucleolar protein Bop1 on G(1)/S transition. Mol Cell Biol 21(13):4246–4255

Quarello P et al (2016) Ribosomal RNA analysis in the diagnosis of Diamond-Blackfan Anaemia. Br J Haematol 172(5):782–785

Rao S et al (2012) Inactivation of ribosomal protein L22 promotes transformation by induction of the stemness factor, Lin28B. Blood 120(18):3764–3773

Sankaran VG et al (2012) Exome sequencing identifies GATA1 mutations resulting in Diamond-Blackfan anemia. J Clin Invest 122(7):2439–2443

Sondalle SB, Baserga SJ (2014) Human diseases of the SSU processome. Biochim Biophys Acta 1842(6):758–764

Stewart MJ, Denell R (1993) Mutations in the Drosophila gene encoding ribosomal protein S6 cause tissue overgrowth. Mol Cell Biol 13(4):2524–2535

Sulima SO et al (2014) Bypass of the pre-60S ribosomal quality control as a pathway to oncogenesis. Proc Natl Acad Sci U S A 111(15):5640–5645

Townsley DM, Dumitriu B, Young NS (2014) Bone marrow failure and the telomeropathies. Blood 124(18):2775–2783

Vlachos A et al (2012) Incidence of neoplasia in Diamond Blackfan anemia: a report from the Diamond Blackfan Anemia Registry. Blood 119(16):3815–3819

Weis F et al (2015) Mechanism of eIF6 release from the nascent 60S ribosomal subunit. Nat Struct Mol Biol 22(11):914–919

Xu X, Xiong X, Sun Y (2016) The role of ribosomal proteins in the regulation of cell proliferation, tumorigenesis, and genomic integrity. Sci China Life Sci 59(7):656–672

Yang Z et al (2016) Delayed globin synthesis leads to excess heme and the macrocytic anemia of Diamond Blackfan anemia and del(5q) myelodysplastic syndrome. Sci Transl Med 8(338):338ra67

Yelick PC, Trainor PA (2015) Ribosomopathies: global process, tissue specific defects. Rare Dis 3(1):e1025185

Dyskeratosis Congenita and the Telomere Biology Disorders

6

Lois Dodson and Alison A. Bertuch

Contents

L. Dodson · A. A. Bertuch (✉)
Department of Pediatrics, Section of Hematology/Oncology, Baylor College of Medicine and Texas Children's Hospital, Houston, TX, USA

Department of Molecular and Human Genetics, Baylor College of Medicine, Houston, TX, USA
e-mail: abertuch@bcm.edu

6.1 Introduction

Historically, a diagnosis of dyskeratosis congenita (DC) was given to patients manifesting a mucocutaneous triad of reticulated skin pigmentation, dysplastic nails, and oral leukoplakia (Fig. 6.1). While these findings are highly penetrant, DC also encompasses many more clinical features and spares few organ systems (Table 6.1). Among the numerous findings, bone marrow failure (BMF), pulmonary fibrosis, hepatic cirrhosis, and cancer contribute significantly to morbidity and early

G. M. Kupfer et al. (eds.), *Bone Marrow Failure*, Pediatric Oncology,
https://doi.org/10.1007/978-3-319-61421-2_6

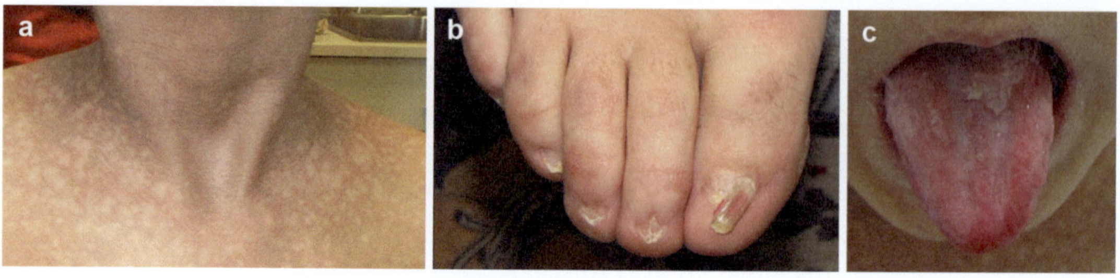

Fig. 6.1 The DC mucocutaneous triad. (**a**) Reticulated skin pigmentation, (**b**) nail dystrophy, and (**c**) oral leukoplakia in an adolescent female. Each of these features was absent at the time of her presentation with BMF in early childhood

Table 6.1 Potential manifestations of DC and the TBDs

Prenatal growth	Intrauterine growth restriction, low birth weight
Postnatal growth	Short stature (in very severely affected patients)
CNS	Microcephaly, cerebellar hypoplasia (defining feature of HHS), cerebral calcifications, and cysts (distinctive pattern seen in CP)
Eyes	Epiphora, lacrimal duct stenosis Blepharitis, sparse eyelashes, trichiasis, entropion, ectropion Conjunctivitis, corneal ulceration, cataracts Retinal vascular changes including exudative retinopathy (defining feature of RS and CP) Optic nerve atrophy
Dental	Caries, missing teeth, periodontitis, decreased crown/root ratio, taurodontism
Gastrointestinal	Oral leukoplakia Esophageal stricture Peptic ulceration Noninfectious enteropathy, intractable diarrhea, enterocolitis Gastrointestinal telangiectasias with tendency for bleeding (prominent feature of CP)
Hepatic	Abnormal liver function tests Nodular regenerative hyperplasia Noncirrhotic portal hypertension Hepatic fibrosis, cirrhosis
Pulmonary	Abnormal pulmonary function tests with restrictive pattern and decreased DL_{CO} Fibrosis, usual interstitial pneumonia Emphysema Arteriovenous malformations with or without shunting Hepatopulmonary syndrome
Skeletal	Osteopenia, osteoporosis with tendency to fracture (prominent feature of CP), avascular necrosis of hips and shoulders
Genitourinary—females	Labial adhesions and leukoplakia, hymenal stricture, urethral stricture
Genitourinary—males	Urethral stricture, meatal stenosis, meatal leukoplakia, small testes, undescended testes, phimosis, hypospadias
Skin/nails/hair	Reticular pigmentation, especially neck and thorax Hyperkeratosis Hyperhidrosis Dystrophic nails; may progress to absence Early graying, alopecia
Hematologic	Anemia, and/or thrombocytopenia, and/or neutropenia Elevated MCV for age, elevated hemoglobin F for age Hypocellular bone marrow

Table 6.1 (continued)

Immunologic	Lymphopenia, decreased B- and NK-cell counts Decreased IgG, IgM, IgA Reduced T cell response to specific antigens and mitogens Severe combined immunodeficiency (feature of HHS)
Oncologic	Squamous cell carcinoma, particularly of the head/neck region and tongue Myelodysplastic syndrome Acute myeloid leukemia Hepatocellular carcinoma
Neurodevelopmental	Learning disability, developmental delay, intellectual disability, depression, anxiety

mortality. Defects in telomere length maintenance underlie the clinical manifestations of DC. Advances in genetic and telomere length testing have revealed a spectrum of related disorders, based on shared genetic causes and telomere defects, collectively known as the telomere biology disorders (TBDs), syndromes of telomere shortening, short telomere syndromes (or disorders), and telomeropathies. This chapter highlights the importance of telomere length maintenance and summarizes the diagnosis, clinical manifestations, and treatment challenges of DC. The molecular defects conferred by pathogenic variants in the 14 genes currently associated with DC and the TBDs are comprehensively reviewed. Overlapping clinical considerations with the severe variants, Hoyeraal-Hreidarsson syndrome (HHS), Revesz syndrome (RS), and Coats plus (CP), and familial pulmonary fibrosis are also discussed.

6.2 Telomere Length Maintenance and DC

The natural ends of chromosomes, referred to as telomeres, are distinguished from other chromosomal regions by the presence of tandem repeats of simple G-rich DNA sequence (TTAGGG in humans) in association with a cadre of telomere-specific proteins (Moyzis et al. 1988; Palm and de Lange 2008). The function of this specialized nucleoprotein structure is to prevent natural chromosome termini from being recognized as double-stranded DNA breaks and acted upon as such, which can result in telomere-telomere fusions and genomic instability. Whereas the bulk of chromosomal DNA is faithfully replicated by the semiconservative DNA replication machinery, chromosome termini are replicated incompletely due to the so-called end replication problem (Watson 1972; Olovnikov 1973). In the absence of a mechanism to replenish lost terminal telomeric repeats, telomeres shorten with each cell division cycle (Harley et al. 1990). Eventually a threshold is reached, triggering a DNA damage checkpoint response and cellular senescence (Allsopp and Harley 1995). This signal to stop proliferation occurs prior to the loss of the telomere's protective properties and normally occurs in somatic cells. When such checkpoints are abrogated, however, further telomere shortening results in loss of the telomere's end protection function and, ultimately, genomic instability instigated by telomere-telomere fusions (Counter et al. 1992).

One approach used to measure telomere length in blood cells, and which is available clinically, combines fluorescence in situ hybridization (FISH) using a telomeric DNA-specific probe with flow cytometry to distinguish various leukocyte subsets (Baerlocher et al. 2006; Baerlocher and Lansdorp 2003). This method is often referred to as telomere flow FISH. When applied to cohort of several hundred individuals from infancy to the ninth decade of life, telomere flow FISH revealed that telomere lengths progressively shorten in granulocytes and lymphocytes as humans age, with the greatest decline in several cell types occurring in the first 20 years of life (Aubert et al. 2012). In addition, at any given age, telomere

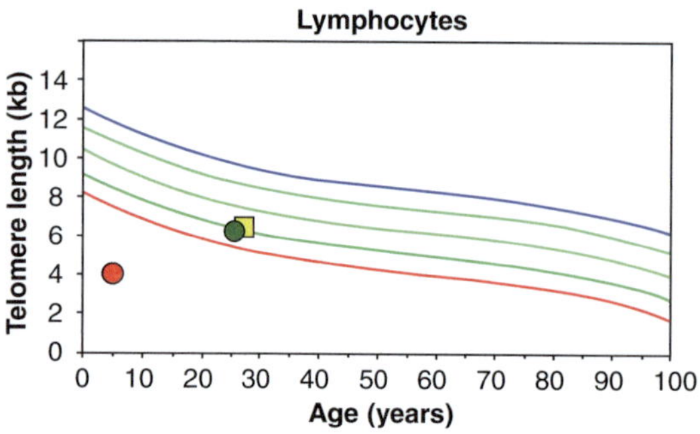

Fig. 6.2 Very short telomeres revealed by telomere flow FISH analysis. The curves from bottom to top represent the 1st, 10th, 50th, 90th, and 99th percentiles. Telomere length below the 1st percentile line is considered very short and is highly sensitive and specific for DC. Shown here are the results of telomere length testing obtained on the lymphocytes of a 4-year-old boy with BMF (red circle) and his parents (green circle and yellow square). The results prompted analysis of TBD-associated genes, which revealed a de novo pathogenic variant in *TINF2*

lengths within the 1st to 99th percentiles vary substantially (Fig. 6.2). For example, at birth, telomeres in the pan-lymphocyte population measure 8–13 kilobases within this normal range. Thus, telomere lengths must be interpreted with respect to a patient's age in order to determine whether they fall outside the normal range.

Not all cells undergo progressive telomere shortening with cell division. Certain cell types, such as germ cells, stem cells, and highly proliferative cells, are able to maintain telomere length via the action of telomerase, a specialized reverse transcriptase that catalyzes the de novo addition of telomeric repeat sequences onto the chromosome termini using sequences within an integral RNA subunit as the template (Greider and Blackburn 1987). However, telomerase expression is limiting, and, consequently, loss of a single functional copy of a telomerase constituent gene, as observed in the TBD spectrum, results in haploinsufficiency and abnormally short telomeres (Marrone et al. 2004; Armanios et al. 2005; Goldman et al. 2005).

In addition to telomerase, additional factors are required for normal telomere length maintenance and function. These include a telomere-specific protein complex known as shelterin (Palm and de Lange 2008). Collectively, the six shelterin members serve several functions including promoting the formation of a specialized conformation of the telomere, known as the t-loop, inhibiting the DNA damage response, recruiting telomerase, facilitating semiconservative replication of the telomeric tracts, and promoting cohesion of sister chromatid telomeres until anaphase.

Dyskeratosis congenita is the prototype for a TBD and is molecularly characterized by the presence of very short telomeres, defined as lengths less than the 1st percentile for age (Alter et al. 2007, 2012). In particular, very short telomere length across lymphocyte subsets (naive T cells, memory T cells, B cells, and NK/NKT cells) as measured by automated telomere flow FISH is both highly sensitive and specific for a diagnosis of DC (Fig. 6.2). While granulocyte telomere length is also very short in patients with DC, this finding alone is nonspecific as it may be observed in variety of conditions associated with BMF (Alter et al. 2007, 2012, 2015).

The initial clue that DC was the result of defective telomere maintenance came from the observations that the protein dyskerin, which is encoded by the X-linked DC-associated gene, *DKC1*, was in complex with telomerase (Mitchell et al. 1999a). It was further shown that cells with *DKC1* mutations had a reduction in the telomerase RNA subunit, hTR, reduced telomerase activity, and short telomeres. Subsequently, mutations in 13 additional genes have been found in patients with DC and related TBDs (to be discussed further below) (Armanios et al. 2005; Vulliamy et al. 2001, 2005, 2008; Walne et al. 2007; Savage et al. 2008; Zhong et al. 2011; Stanley et al. 2016; Kocak et al. 2014; Guo et al. 2014; Ballew et al. 2013a; Simon et al. 2016; Anderson et al. 2012; Takai et al. 2016). While some of the proteins encoded by these genes also have non-telomeric roles, the common thread is a role in telomere maintenance and function (Fig. 6.3). The genes encode telomerase core components (*TERT* and *TERC*), factors required for telomerase biogenesis (*DKC1*, *NHP2*, *NOP2*, *NAF1*, and *PARN*), telomerase trafficking (*WRAP53*), telomerase recruitment (*ACD*), telomere replication and end structure (*RTEL1*, *CTC1*, *STN1*, and *POT1*), and multiple aspects of telomere biology (*TINF2*). Pathogenic variants in one of these genes will be

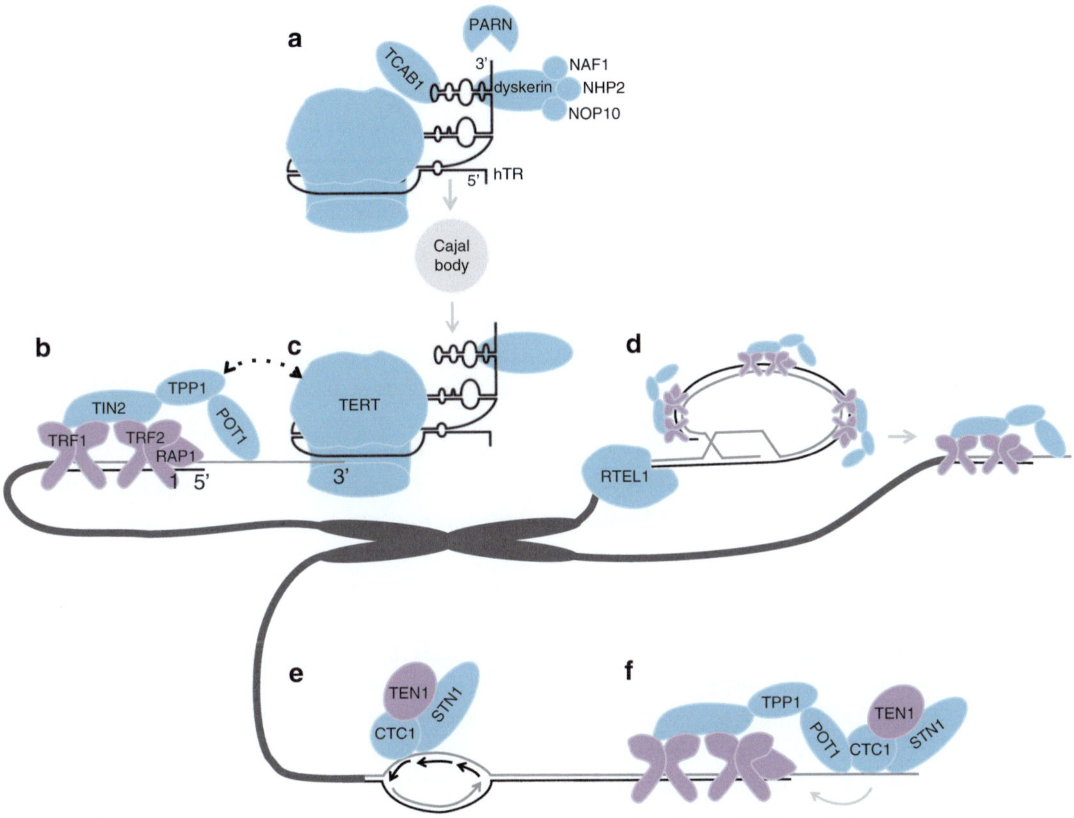

Fig. 6.3 Normal function of the products of genes implicated in TBDs. (**a**) Stability of hTR requires dyskerin, NHP2, NOP10, NAF1, and PARN. TCAB1 delivers hTR to Cajal bodies, where it localizes until S phase. (**b**) Telomere-associated TPP1 recruits telomerase to telomeres via interaction of its TEL patch with the TEN domain of TERT. The TPP1/POT1 heterodimer stimulates telomerase processivity. TPP1/POT1 localization to telomeres requires TPP1 interaction with TIN2. (**c**) TERT, the enzymatic component of telomerase, extends the G-overhang of telomeres by adding telomeric repeat DNA. hTR, the RNA component of telomerase, provides the template for TERT. (**d**) Shelterin facilitates the formation of t-loops. t-loops and members of shelterin protect the G-overhang from aberrant DNA damage signaling. RTEL1 is a helicase that resolves the t-loop during replication. (**e**) CTC1 and STN1 are members of the CST complex. The CST complex facilitates replication of double-stranded telomeric DNA. (**f**) CST is recruited to the G-overhang by POT1. The CST complex and POT1 facilitate C-strand fill-in after post-replicative nucleolytic processing, thereby maintaining the G-overhang. CST and POT1 inhibit telomerase elongation of telomeres (not pictured)

identified in only ~60–70% of patients, and, therefore, the absence of a detectable variant does not rule out the diagnosis of DC or a related TBD.

6.3 Diagnosis and Clinical Features of DC and Related TBDs

The incidence of DC has been estimated to be 1/1,000,000 (Walne et al. 2005). The Canadian Inherited Marrow Failure Study, which includes centers that care for >95% of eligible pediatric patients diagnosed with an inherited BMF syndrome (IBMFS) in Canada, reported a diagnosis of DC in 3.9% of a cohort of 274 pediatric IBMFS patients enrolled between 2001 and 2010 (Tsangaris et al. 2011). The increasing availability and use of telomere flow FISH and comprehensive genetic testing is likely to result in greater numbers, with fewer patients diagnosed with unclassifiable IBMFS or idiopathic aplastic anemia (Ghemlas et al. 2015; Keel et al. 2016).

Diagnostic criteria for DC vary. Some reserve the term for patients with the mucocutaneous triad (classical DC) (Fig. 6.1) or who have at least two of the major features (reticulated skin pigmentation, dysplastic nails, leukoplakia, and BMF) and two or more of the other somatic features known to occur in DC (Table 6.1) (Dokal 2011). Others will render the diagnosis if a pathogenic variant in a gene associated with DC is identified along with BMF, myelodysplastic syndrome, or pulmonary fibrosis, or if telomere lengths fall below the 1st percentile and two or more features of DC are present (Dokal et al. 2015). Apparently healthy individuals with very short telomeres and a pathogenic variant in a DC-associated gene may be identified by family studies, prior to the development of any clinical features of DC. This latter category of at-risk patients is important to recognize as they may benefit from genetic counseling, disease surveillance, anticipatory guidance, and preventive care.

Most significantly, the clinical features of DC can vary over time in any given patient and may vary among affected family members. The time course of onset of manifestations is also variable. For example, a young child may present with BMF prior to the development of features of the mucocutaneous triad, or a middle-aged adult may present with liver disease and pulmonary fibrosis without overt BMF. Awareness of the array of clinical features of DC is important to timely diagnosis and provision of care, avoiding unnecessary diagnostic studies or ineffective therapies (e.g., the utilization of immunosuppressive therapy for BMF). Table 6.1 outlines the various clinical features that have been recognized from detailed studies on large cohorts as well as in small case series and case reports. Several of the most clinically significant manifestations are discussed below.

Bone marrow failure is highly penetrant in DC with estimates of up to 80% of patients developing BMF by the age of 30 years (Alter et al. 2009; Kirwan and Dokal 2008). This may manifest from mild unilineage cytopenia to marked pancytopenia with severe neutropenia and red blood cell and platelet transfusion dependence in the context of a hypocellular bone marrow. Thrombocytopenia is frequently the first blood cell count abnormality. While macrocytosis and elevation in hemoglobin F may be present, absence of these findings does not exclude an underlying TBD. There are no pathognomonic features in the bone marrow that allow the diagnosis of a TBD based on histopathology alone. Mild dysplasia in erythroid or myeloid precursors or megakaryocytes may be present and stable over time. Progressive dysplasia involving two or three lineages with or without the appearance of a cytogenetic clone may herald the development of myelodysplastic syndrome or acute myeloid leukemia.

Lung disease may also be responsible for significant morbidity and mortality in patients with DC (Giri et al. 2011). In most cases, interstitial lung disease, specifically pulmonary fibrosis, is diagnosed in the years following hematopoietic stem cell transplantation (HSCT) (Giri et al. 2011). However, HSCT is not a prerequisite for the development of pulmonary fibrosis in patients with DC (Giri et al. 2011) nor is preceding BMF (Parry et al. 2011a). Symptoms associated with pulmonary fibrosis include chronic cough and exertional dyspnea. Inspiratory rales and digital clubbing may be present. Pulmonary function tests reveal a restrictive pattern with a decreased forced vital capacity and decreased diffusion capacity for carbon monoxide (DL_{co}). The radiographic appearance is most often described as usual interstitial pneumonia.

Notably, adult-onset idiopathic pulmonary fibrosis is the most common manifestation of a TBD based on the prevalence and the percent of cases associated with pathogenic variants in *TERT* and *TERC* (Armanios 2009). In these cases, diagnosis is made in the fourth to sixth decades of life. The patients may have concurrently varying degrees of hematologic abnormalities (macrocytosis, anemia, thrombocytopenia in ~25%) and liver disease and rarely a mucocutaneous feature of DC (Borie et al. 2016; Newton et al. 2016). Notably, co-occurrence of aplastic anemia not only in a patient with IPF but also in one of their family members is highly predictive of an underlying telomerase gene mutation (Parry et al. 2011b). In addition to *TERT* and

TERC, heterozygous mutations in *RTEL1* and *PARN* and more rarely in *NAF1*, *TINF2*, and *DKC1* (hemizygous) have been found to be causal risk factors for these adult-onset cases (Stanley et al. 2016; Parry et al. 2011a; Armanios et al. 2007; Alder et al. 2015; Tsakiri et al. 2007; Diaz de Leon et al. 2010; Kropski et al. 2014; Cogan et al. 2015).

Telomere defects also result in gastrointestinal and hepatic manifestations. Approximately 20% of the Johns Hopkins Telomere Syndrome Registry cohort reported significant gastrointestinal disease (Jonassaint et al. 2013). In that same study, a systematic review of the literature identified over 40 cases of patients with DC or HHS with gastrointestinal features. The most common findings were esophageal stenosis, enteropathy, and enterocolitis. Notably, over half of the 23 reported cases with lower tract disease (including chronic diarrhea, severe enteropathy, and enterocolitis) occurred in infants 18 months of age or younger, all of whom carried a diagnosis of HHS. However, these features were also found in older children and young adults with classical DC. This indicates that lower tract disease is associated with early onset disease.

Liver disease manifestations can range from asymptomatic elevation of liver transaminases to cirrhotic end-stage liver disease. As with pulmonary fibrosis, kinships with a predominant liver disease phenotype with occurrences of hematologic abnormalities among family members have been described and attributed to *TERT* and *TERC* variants (Calado et al. 2009a). Noncirrhotic portal hypertension and hepatopulmonary syndrome (HPS) have also been reported in patients with DC, with earlier onset than pulmonary fibrosis (median age 25 years) (Gorgy et al. 2015; Abramowsky et al. 2003; Brown et al. 1993).

DC is also a cancer predisposition syndrome, likely due to the genomic instability that can arise in the context of very short, deprotected telomeres. A study from the National Cancer Institute calculated an actuarial risk of 40% by age 50 years (Alter et al. 2009, 2010). Cancers most commonly reported in patients with DC include squamous cell carcinoma of the head and neck, anogenital region, and skin, myelodysplastic syndrome, acute myeloid leukemia, and Hodgkin and non-Hodgkin lymphoma. Of these, squamous cell carcinoma of the head and neck region had the highest incidence and with a predilection for the tongue rather than the oropharynx (Alter et al. 2010). Most cancers emerge after the second decade of life. As HSCT outcomes improve, the incidence and prevalence of cancer in DC cohorts may observe an increase. No case series or prospective studies have been reported on specific cancer treatment outcomes in DC; however, patients with DC are known to have increased sensitivity to chemotherapeutics and radiation therapy.

6.4 Severe DC/TBD Variants

Hoyeraal-Hreidarsson syndrome (HHS) and Revesz syndrome (RS) are severe variants of DC. Patients diagnosed with these syndromes manifest clinical features of DC but also have additional syndrome-defining features. HHS is typically diagnosed in the first few years of life and is defined by the presence of cerebellar hypoplasia (Hoyeraal et al. 1970; Hreidarsson et al. 1988; Aalfs et al. 1995; Berthet et al. 1994; Ohga et al. 1997). BMF develops at a very young age. Additional features often include intrauterine growth restriction, neurodevelopmental delay, microcephaly, ataxia, and immunodeficiency (Berthet et al. 1995; Yaghmai et al. 2000). In some cases, severe combined immunodeficiency of the T+, B−, and NK− type is present, and death due to viral infection has been reported in many cases (Ballew et al. 2013b; Lamm et al. 2009; Touzot et al. 2012). Infants also may present to gastroenterologists with bloody, noninfectious enterocolitis (Sznajer et al. 2003). Variants in a subset of the genes associated with the other TBDs have been found in patients with HHS. This may reflect the greater extent to which pathogenic variants in these genes affect telomere length. These include monoallelic variants in *TINF2*, *DKC1*, and *RTEL1* and biallelic variants in *TERT*, *ACD*, *RTEL1*, and *PARN* (Kocak et al. 2014; Ballew et al. 2013a, b; Walne et al. 2008, 2013; Knight et al. 1999a; Marrone et al. 2007; Deng et al. 2013; Le Guen et al. 2013; Gramatges et al. 2013; Burris et al. 2016; Tummala et al. 2015). As with classical DC and other TBDs, some patients with HHS will remain genetically uncharacterized. However, very short telomeres are nearly uniformly present, which provides diagnostic support.

RS is another severe variant of DC and has the defining feature of bilateral exudative retinopathy, also known as Coats' disease (Savage et al. 2008; Walne et al. 2008; Scheinfeld et al. 2007; Riyaz et al. 2007; McElnea et al. 2013; Sasa et al. 2012; Revesz et al. 1992; Kajtar and Mehes 1994; Gleeson et al. 2012; Duprey and Steger 1988). Additional features that may be present include features of DC, including BMF and the mucocutaneous triad, intrauterine growth restriction, microcephaly, cerebellar hypoplasia, intracranial calcification, and sparse hair. As with HHS, RS is typically diagnosed during the first few years of life. While ophthalmologic findings are present in approximately 30% of patients with DC, exudative retinopathy is rare (Tsilou et al. 2010). Therefore, bilateral exudative retinopathy appears to be associated only with severe, early onset disease. Nearly all cases of RS with a genetic diagnosis are due to pathogenic variants in *TINF2* and are associated with very short telomeres (Savage et al. 2008; Walne et al. 2008). Siblings with a novel *TERT* missense variant were reported; however, they lacked other central nervous system findings (Sharma et al. 2014). Thus, initial targeted sequencing of *TINF2* is likely to be sufficient to establish a genetic diagnosis in patients with RS.

Coats plus (CP) is also within the TBD spectrum. Similar to RS, patients with CP have bilateral exudative retinopathy and intracranial calcification (Crow et al. 2004). However, in CP, the pattern of calcification is characteristic, with asymmetric involvement of the thalamus, basal ganglia, dentate, and deep cortex and with associated leukoencephalopathy and brain cysts. Additional features include osteopenia with tendency to fracture and poor bone healing; recurrent gastrointestinal bleeding due to vascular ectasias in the stomach, small intestines, and liver; intrauterine growth restriction; failure to thrive; the mucocutaneous triad of DC; and cytopenias, although not typically progressing to severe BMF (Crow et al. 2004; Linnankivi et al. 2006; Briggs et al. 2008). The gastrointestinal vascular ectasias may result in significant morbidity and fatal hemorrhage (Simon et al. 2016; Takai et al. 2016; Linnankivi et al. 2006; Briggs et al. 2008; Polvi et al. 2012).

Three genes have been implicated in CP to date, *CTC1*, which accounts for the majority of reported cases with an ascertained genetic cause, *STN1*, and *POT1* (Simon et al. 2016; Anderson et al. 2012; Takai et al. 2016; Polvi et al. 2012). Importantly, unlike DC, HHS, and RS, CP is not uniformly associated with very short telomeres. In one study, two of three individuals with *CTC1* pathogenic variants had telomere lengths less than the 1st percentile in both pan-lymphocyte and granulocyte populations as analyzed by telomere flow FISH; the third individual had lengths at the 1st percentile (Anderson et al. 2012). Two other studies, however, found no significant differences in the relative telomere length in a total of 13 patients with *CTC1* pathogenic variants as compared to controls as measured by quantitative PCR (qPCR) (Polvi et al. 2012; Walne et al. 2012). Similarly, of the two patients with CP due to pathogenic variants in *STN1*, only one exhibited significantly shorter than expected telomere lengths, as measured by telomere restriction fragment analysis (Simon et al. 2016). Whether these differences reflect differences in methodology remains unclear. At this time, however, telomere lengths within the range of normal do not rule out a diagnosis of CP due to a defect in one of these genes.

6.5 Treatment for Severe Complications of DC and the TBDs

As outlined above, DC and the TBDs affect multiple organ systems. Treatments for the disease manifestations are limited and directed toward specific organ system involvement. Periodic monitoring of peripheral blood counts and bone marrow, pulmonary, and liver function tests is recommended to allow for early detection of disease development and progression. This may allow for the timely offering of supportive care and potentially greater options for treatment intervention. Treatments focused on life-threatening complications of BMF, pulmonary fibrosis, and liver disease in DC and the TBDs are described below.

6.5.1 Hematopoietic Stem Cell Transplantation

Allogeneic HSCT is the only curative treatment for BMF in patients with DC. Historically, HSCT with myeloablative conditioning regimens has been associated with marked risks of transplant-related morbidity and mortality, especially the long-term risks of pulmonary fibrosis and liver cirrhosis (de la Fuente and Dokal 2007). Defective telomere maintenance and poor repair of DNA damage localized to telomeres are thought to underlie the sensitivity of patients with DC to myeloablative conditioning regimens. A systematic review of 109 patients reported in the literature revealed generally poor outcomes with 5- and 10-year survival estimates of 57% and 23%, respectively (Barbaro and Vedi 2016). The 5-year survival for those transplanted after 2000 (n = 47), since when approaches to transplantation for DC-related BMF have evolved to favor lower doses or elimination of alkylating agents and radiation, was significantly higher at 70%. However, the 10-year survival was still dismal at 28%. While 5-year survival was greater for those receiving reduced intensity conditioning regimens (RIC), the increase lost significance in multivariate analysis, which identified age >20 years at HSCT and alternative donor source as poor prognostic indicators. As fewer patients underwent RIC, most deaths after RIC occurred early, and the median follow-up was much shorter than for myeloablative regimens, an improvement in long-term outcome with RIC that may be revealed ultimately with larger RIC cohorts and longer follow-up. Regardless, until therapies are developed that can attenuate the development of non-hematopoietic pathologies that are inherent to DC itself, the long-term impact of HSCT on survival for DC will be limited.

6.5.2 Androgen Therapy

Androgens, such as oxymetholone and danazol, have been used to treat BMF in patients with DC and the TBDs. Retrospective reports from the National Cancer Institute inherited BMF study and the Dyskeratosis Congenita Registry in the United Kingdom demonstrated responses in some but not all patients (Khincha et al. 2014; Islam et al. 2013). The most frequent response was improvement in anemia, with some patients demonstrating improved platelet counts and, less commonly, neutrophil counts. The duration of response was variable, from a few months to several years. The most common adverse effects in these retrospective case series were lipid changes with increases in triglyceride and decreases in high-density lipoprotein levels.

The mechanism of action of androgens is poorly understood. Investigators at the National Institutes of Health demonstrated an increase in *TERT* expression and telomerase activity in hematopoietic cells cultured in the presence of androgens (Calado et al. 2009b). This suggested that androgens might slow the rate of telomere loss. They then tested this question in a prospective study on the use of danazol for patients within the TBD spectrum (Townsley et al. 2016). Eligible patients had an adjusted peripheral blood leukocyte telomere length at or below the 1st percentile [as measured by qPCR], a mutation in a TBD gene, or both and at least one blood count below moderately low thresholds, pulmonary fibrosis, or both. Twenty-one of the 27 patient cohorts had a variant in *TERT*, *TERC*, *DKC1*, or *RTEL1*. The median age was 41 years, with the youngest subject 17 years of age. Danazol was administered orally at a dose of 800 mg/day. The primary and secondary efficacy end points of the study were a 20% reduction in the annual rate of telomere shortening estimated for patients with telomerase gene mutations measured at 24 months and hematologic response to treatment at various time points, respectively. Each of the first 12 patients treated for 24 months was found to have met the primary end point, with 11 of the 12 demonstrating a gain in telomere length over the 24-month interval. Thus, there was sufficient evidence for rejection of the null hypothesis and early study closure. Hematologic responses were observed in ~80% of patients at 3 months (19 of 24) and 24 months (10 of 12). While these results were encouraging, it is important to note that ten subjects withdrew from the study due to adverse effects, three prior to 3 months and an additional six prior to 12 months. Thus, at 12 months, only ~51% remained on study and were demonstrating a hematologic response. Lymphocyte telomere length was measured by both qPCR and telomere flow FISH in seven subjects. Although similar trends were generally observed, the measurements varied substantially. Future studies using telomere flow FISH and designed to assess the impact on other clinical parameters such as pulmonary fibrosis are warranted.

Potential adverse effects of androgen therapy are liver enzyme elevations, lipid abnormalities, and masculinization, which were observed in the above retrospective and prospective studies (Khincha et al. 2014; Townsley et al. 2016). Peliosis (blood-filled cysts) of the liver and spleen and formation of hepatic tumors are potential life-threatening complications (Pavlatos et al. 2001). Peliosis can occur after a period of months or years of therapy. Splenic peliosis and rupture have been reported in two patients with a TBD who were simultaneously on G-CSF and oxymetholone (Giri et al. 2007). This led to a recommendation to avoid the concurrent use of androgens and cytokines in patients with DC. It is important to note, however, that androgens alone predispose to peliosis (Pavlatos et al. 2001). Therefore, any patient on androgen therapy should be monitored periodically for the development of hepatic and splenic peliosis.

6.5.3 Lung and Liver Transplantation

Two antifibrotic agents, nintedanib and pirfenidone, are currently approved to treat idiopathic pulmonary fibrosis in the United States, each shown in clinical trials to slow the progression of the disease. However, it is unknown whether these agents are effective in pulmonary fibrosis due to an underlying TBD. Lung transplantation is the only curative therapy for pulmonary fibrosis in DC and related TBDs. Three case series of adults who underwent lung transplantation for telomere-mediated pulmonary fibrosis have been reported (Silhan et al. 2014; Borie et al. 2015; Tokman et al. 2015). A total of 31 adults received transplants (ages 35–64 years), nearly all with *TERT* or *TERC* pathogenic variants, except for two who met criteria for a TBD but lacked a genetic etiology. The combined case series revealed that these patients are at high risk of severe cytopenias in association with immunosuppressive agents, secondary infectious complications, acute renal failure, and calcineurin inhibitor-induced chronic renal insufficiency. These studies indicate that lung transplantation is feasible in adults with telomere-mediated pulmonary fibrosis; however, specialized approaches are needed, particularly with respect to posttransplantation immunosuppressive regimens.

Whether similar outcomes will be observed in younger patients with DC, particularly those who have received HSCT, remains to be determined. One adolescent with known diagnosis of DC at the time of lung transplantation has been reported (Giri et al. 2011). Unlike the adults in the case series described above, the patient had undergone HSCT 9 years prior. Details of the posttransplantation course were limited, except that 18 months after lung transplant, he had mild leukopenia and neutropenia, which prevented the use of mycophenolate mofetil, and 21 months posttransplant, the patient was alive and doing well, with resolution of his respiratory symptoms. While this case report is encouraging, coexisting liver disease or other serious comorbidities in many patients with DC may present barriers to lung transplantation.

Far fewer cases of liver transplantation have been reported in patients with DC and related TBDs (Gorgy et al. 2015; Mahansaria et al. 2015; Singh et al. 2015). Details of successful liver transplantation of a 34-year-old patient with cirrhosis and a known diagnosis of DC were recently reported. The patient also had severe hepatopulmonary syndrome, interstitial lung disease, and a past history of bone marrow transplantation for BMF. The case illustrated the critical consideration prior to liver transplantation of whether the pulmonary morbidity of a TBD patient is primarily due to hepatopulmonary syndrome, and, thus, reversible with liver transplantation, or due to restrictive lung disease.

6.6 Genetics of DC and the TBDs

As stated above, DC and the TBDs are genetically heterogeneous with 14 genes associated with these disorders to date (Table 6.2). Autosomal dominant, autosomal recessive, and X-linked recessive patterns of inheritance are observed. Adding further complexity, kinships have been described in which there is increasing severity and earlier onset of disease in successive generations, a phenomenon referred to as disease anticipation (Armanios et al. 2005; Vulliamy et al. 2004). Genetic counseling is crucial as the parents and siblings of an affected child may be at risk of disease manifestations even if the child has disease associated with biallelic mutations. Each of the genes is discussed below as well as the impact of gene dosage on the clinical phenotype.

6.6.1 Telomerase Core Subunits

Not surprisingly, pathogenic variants in the genes encoding the core subunits of telomerase are associated with DC and the TBDs. These are *TERC*, which encodes the telomerase RNA component, hTR, and *TERT*, which encodes the reverse transcriptase, TERT (Nakamura et al. 1997; Meyerson et al. 1997). hTR provides the template for TERT reverse transcription of telomeric repeats onto the chromosome end (Feng et al. 1995). It also contributes to other aspects

Table 6.2 DC-associated genes

Gene (product)	Inheritance	Disease association	Effect of disease-associated variants
TERT (TERT)	AD AR	IPF, LD, AA, MDS, AL, DC DC, HHS	Reduce telomerase activity, processivity, or recruitment
TERC (hTR)	AD	IPF, LD, AA, MDS, AL, DC	Reduce telomerase activity
DKC1 (dyskerin)	XLR, inherited or de novo	DC, HHS	Reduce hTR stability and telomerase activity
NHP2 (NHP2)	AR	DC	Reduce hTR stability and telomerase activity
NOP10 (NOP10)	AR	DC	Reduce hTR stability and telomerase activity
NAF1 (NAF1)	AD	DC, IPF, LD, MDS	Reduce hTR stability and telomerase activity
PARN (PARN)	AD AR	IPF DC, HHS	Reduce hTR stability and telomerase activity
WRAP53 (TCAB1)	AR	DC	Impair telomerase trafficking
ACD (TPP1)	AD AR	AA HHS	Reduce telomerase recruitment to telomeres
RTEL1 (RTEL1)	AD AR	IPF HHS	Impair telomere replication
CTC1 (CTC1)	AR	CP, DC	Impair telomere replication, impair C-strand fill-in
STN1 (STN1)	AR	CP	Impair telomere replication, impair C-strand fill-in
POT1 (POT1)	AR	CP	Impair C-strand fill-in, impair inhibition of telomerase
TINF2 (TIN2)	AD, mostly de novo	DC, HHS, RS, IPF	Reduce telomerase recruitment to telomeres, telomerase-independent telomere shortening, impair sister telomere cohesion

AD autosomal dominant, *AR* autosomal recessive, *XLR* X-linked recessive, *DC* dyskeratosis congenita, *HHS* Hoyeraal-Hreidarsson syndrome, *CP* Coats plus, *RS* Revesz syndrome, *AA* aplastic anemia, *AL* acute leukemia, *IPF* idiopathic pulmonary fibrosis, *LD* liver disease, *MDS* myelodysplastic syndrome of TERT enzymology and provides a scaffold for factors such as TCAB1 and dyskerin (Egan and Collins 2012). There is a spectrum of presentations associated with mutations in these genes. Heterozygous pathogenic *TERT* and *TERC* variants are most often associated with adult-onset pulmonary fibrosis (Armanios et al. 2007; Tsakiri et al. 2007), accounting for 18% of familial cases (Borie et al. 2016). In addition, autosomal dominant transmission of *TERT* and *TERC* variants has been associated with adult-onset cases of aplastic anemia, myelodysplastic syndrome, liver disease, and classical DC presenting in the first two decades of life (Armanios et al. 2005; Vulliamy et al. 2001, 2004; Calado et al. 2009a; Yamaguchi et al. 2003, 2005). Rare cases of inheritance of biallelic pathogenic *TERT* variants have been reported in children with DC and HHS (Marrone et al. 2007; Gramatges et al. 2013).

More than 75 unique variants in *TERT* and approximately 60 in *TERC* have been found in cases within the TBD spectrum, and most of these variants are private (Podlevsky et al. 2008; Bertuch 2016). Accordingly, careful functional evaluation of *TERT* and *TERC* variants is required to determine pathogenicity, which converges on a reduction of telomerase activity at the chromosome end. Pathogenicity can occur by reducing TERT or hTR level, enzymatic activity, or processivity (the ability to add multiple repeats with a single binding event) (Alder et al. 2011; Gramatges et al. 2013). Notably, several variants in *TERT* that were previously reported to be TBD-associated exhibited normal activity and processivity in in vitro assays (Robart and Collins 2010; Zaug et al. 2013). Normal in vitro telomerase activity and processivity, however, do not rule out pathogenicity as the variant allele may impact the ability to maintain telomere length in cells. Indeed, variants have been identified which retain normal in vitro telomerase activity but when overexpressed in cells impart failure to maintain telomeres because of defective telomerase association with telomeres, impaired processivity, or lower ability of telomerase to utilize dGTP (Chu et al. 2016).

6.6.2 Telomerase Assembly and Stability

Several factors are required for the assembly of telomerase in vivo, and pathogenic variants in these, too, have been found in TBD patients (Fig. 6.3a). Variants in *DKC1* are the most common cause of DC and the predominant cause of X-linked DC. *DKC1* cases are often sporadic due to de novo mutations (Knight et al. 1999b) and present as classical DC or HHS with onset in the first decade of life (Heiss et al. 1998). Decreased hTR and, consequently, decreased telomerase activity and telomere shortening are present in these patients (Mitchell et al. 1999a; Wong et al. 2004).

Dyskerin is a constituent of the telomerase holoenzyme, linked to the complex via its interaction with the H/ACA box region of hTR (Mitchell et al. 1999a, b). Nascent H/ACA RNA transcripts, like hTR, assemble into a pre-ribonucleoprotein (pre-RNP) complex with a dyskerin-NOP10-NHP2-NAF1 tetramer. This H/ACA-RNP complex translocates from the site of transcription to the nucleolus, where GAR1 replaces NAF1 and maturation of the RNP occurs (Darzacq et al. 2006; Wang and Meier 2004; Richard et al. 2006). Variants in *DKC1* were suggested to disrupt binding of dyskerin to its cognate RNAs, including hTR, based on the crystal structure of the archaeal protein (Rashid et al. 2006). However, biochemical assays with in vitro translated dyskerin from DC alleles showed that pathogenic variants do not affect tetramer formation (Trahan et al. 2010) or RNP formation with an hTR construct. Therefore, it is possible that hTR-dyskerin interaction is intact in *DKC1* variant cells and another defect causes the reduction in hTR level. For example, it has been proposed that dyskerin normally inhibits hTR degradation by the exosome and that pathogenic variants in *DKC1* disrupt this function, leading to a reduction in the level of hTR (Tseng et al. 2015; Shukla et al. 2016).

In addition to its role in telomere biology, dyskerin is a pseudouridine synthase. The RNA component of H/ACA-RNP complexes shares snoRNA or scaRNA sequence complementarity with target ribosomal or spliceosomal RNA, respectively. Through this sequence-specific targeting, dyskerin pseudouridylates RNA (Angrisani et al. 2014). This modification is part of ribosome and spliceosome biogenesis. A mouse model of *DKC1*-associated DC showed deficiencies in pseudouridylation of ribosomal RNA, suggesting that human *DKC1*-associated DC may be a ribosomopathy (Mochizuki et al. 2004; Ruggero et al. 2003). However, in one study, cells derived from patients harboring *DKC1* pathogenic variants were not found to have defects in rRNA pseudouridylation or processing (Wong and Collins 2006), In another, using patient-derived cells with *DKC1* variants and corrected for telomerase deficiency, minor deficiencies in rRNA pseudouridylation were present, but were not associated with rRNA stability or reduction in protein synthesis (Thumati et al. 2013). Thus, while it has long been speculated that ribosomal defects play a role in DC (Heiss et al. 1998), experimental evidence has yet to delineate this contribution.

As *DKC1* variants were known to cause DC, variants in *NOP10*, *NHP2*, and *NAF1*, which encode additional components of the dyskerin-NOP10-NHP2-NAF1 tetramer, were anticipated in cohorts of patients with genetically uncharacterized DC. In one such cohort of 171 patients from unrelated families, variants in *NOP10* were found in association with disease in one family (Walne et al. 2007). Three affected members of the family were homozygous for a *NOP10* missense variant and had short telomeres. This alteration did not affect dyskerin-NOP10-NHP2-NAF1 tetramer formation but did impede pre-RNP assembly with hTR and a subset of other H/ACA RNAs in vitro (Trahan et al. 2010). To date, no additional patients with *NOP10* variants have been reported in the literature.

In the same cohort (reduced to 117 genetically uncharacterized patients), mutations in *NHP2* were found in two families (Vulliamy et al. 2008). One case had a homozygous missense variant in *NHP2* and a DC phenotype along with the additional clinical features of testicular atrophy, opportunistic infections, intellectual disability, intracranial calcification, and liver cirrhosis. The other case had compound heterozygous missense variants in *NHP2* and classical DC. Both patients had very short telomeres and reduced hTR level. Further supporting the pathogenic nature of these variants, they were found to prevent NHP2 inclusion in the tetramer and impaired the formation of pre-RNP with all tested H/ACA RNAs, including hTR (Trahan et al. 2010). As with *NOP10*, no additional patients with *NHP2* variants have been reported in the literature to date.

Variants in *NAF1* have also been associated with TBDs. In 25 kindreds with genetically uncharacterized familial pulmonary fibrosis, heterozygous *NAF1* variants were identified in two families (Stanley et al. 2016). In the first family, three heterozygous individuals were affected with disease. One was 56 years old with a diagnosis of DC, although clinical details were not available. Another had pulmonary fibrosis-emphysema, liver disease, and myelodysplasia. The last individual had emphysema. The person in the second family had pulmonary fibrosis and BMF. Telomeres were very short in the affected individuals. hTR level was reduced in patient cells, and expression of the *NAF1* variants in cancer cells recapitulated the effect on hTR. Finally, haploinsufficiency was established in a heterozygous knockout mouse model. Although the levels of snoRNAs were reduced, there were no significant differences in ribosomal RNA pseudouridinylation. Thus, as with dyskerin, the primary defect of loss of NAF1 function in patient cells is mediated through telomerase deficiency.

Although GAR1 replaces NAF1 in H/ACA RNPs, its absence does not appear to impact telomerase. Whereas knockdown of NAF1, NOP10, or NHP2 reduces hTR level, knockdown of GAR1 does not (Vulliamy et al. 2008). Consistent with a lack of an effect on telomerase, pathogenic variants in *GAR1* have not been found in association with the TBDs to date, including in the 171 proband DC cohort that yielded patients with variants in *NOP10* and *NHP2* (Walne et al. 2007; Vulliamy et al. 2008).

Variants in *NAF1*, *NHP2*, and *NOP10* segregated with disease in the above kindreds, and patient-derived cells had decreased hTR levels. However, the scarcity of patients identified with variants in *NOP10*, *NHP2*, and *NAF1* is notable. It is possible that a narrow window exists for these proteins to have both partial loss-of-function and be compatible with life. In this scenario, more deleterious mutations would cause loss of viability before diagnosis, and less deleterious mutations would be tolerated. Then, these few cases would represent pathogenic variants causing protein function to land within the narrow window.

PARN is one of the recent additions to the list of genes implicated in DC and the TBDs. Monoallelic pathogenic variants in *PARN* were first reported in several kindreds with autosomal dominant pulmonary fibrosis (Stuart et al. 2015). Subsequently, biallelic *PARN* variants were found to cause autosomal recessive DC and HHS (Burris et al. 2016; Tummala et al. 2015; Dhanraj et al. 2015; Moon et al. 2015). Incomplete penetrance has been observed in several of the autosomal dominant pulmonary fibrosis kindreds with *PARN* mutations. All probands had telomere length below the 50th percentile; however several variant carriers were unaffected and had normal telomere length as measured by qPCR (Stuart et al. 2015). Therefore, carrier parents of children with DC or HHS caused by *PARN* variants are at risk for pulmonary fibrosis, but the degree of risk is uncertain.

PARN (poly(A)-specific ribonuclease) is a 3′ deadenylase that removes posttranscriptionally added adenosines from the 3′ end of RNA. PARN was first described in mRNA metabolism but more recently was found to act on H/ACA RNAs (Berndt et al. 2012). As hTR has an H/ACA domain, this suggested that a failure to deadenylate hTR is the basis for *PARN* pathogenic variants causing TBD phenotypes (Stuart et al. 2015; Moon et al. 2015). Consistent with this, cells with deficiency in PARN activity exhibited increased polyadenylated hTR. In a current model, the overall level of hTR is reduced because polyadenylated hTR is targeted to the exosome and degraded (Tseng et al. 2015; Shukla et al. 2016; Nguyen et al. 2015).

PAPD5 (a noncanonical poly(A) polymerase) posttranscriptionally adds adenosines to the 3′ end of hTR. Depleting PAPD5 or reducing exosome activity can restore hTR level in PARN-deficient cells (Tseng et al. 2015; Shukla et al. 2016; Nguyen et al. 2015). Importantly, these findings have provided a conceptual framework for potential targeted therapy for not only PARN-deficient patients but also patients with variants in other genes impacting hTR levels, such as *DKC1* (Tseng et al. 2015; Shukla et al. 2016).

PARN processes other transcripts in addition to hTR. Its processing of snoRNA and scaRNA implicates PARN in the biogenesis of ribosomal and spliceosomal RNAs, respectively. Support of this has come from the finding of an aberrant ribosome fractionation profile in an HHS patient with *PARN* variants, indicating ribosome biogenesis was altered (Dhanraj et al. 2015). However, it remains to be determined whether alterations in the ribosome profile or splicing contribute to the cellular or clinical phenotype of patients with *PARN* variants.

6.6.3 Telomerase Trafficking and Recruitment to Telomeres

As noted above, telomerase activity is tightly regulated with limiting amounts expressed in restricted populations. Its restricted association and action at telomeres in the S phase of the cell cycle impose another level of regulation. TCAB1 (encoded by *WRAP53*) binds hTR's CAB box motif (Jady et al. 2004) and recruits hTR from the nucleolus to Cajal bodies (Venteicher et al. 2009; Lee et al. 2014), sites of RNP modification and assembly (Fig. 6.3a). The telomerase RNP accumulates in Cajal bodies until S phase, when it moves to telomeres (Zhu et al. 2004; Tomlinson et al. 2006, 2008; Cristofari et al. 2007).

Compound heterozygous variants in *WRAP53* were found to cause classical DC in two of nine unrelated patients with previously genetically uncharacterized DC (Zhong et al. 2011). As expected, the patients had very short telomeres. In patient-derived cells, TCAB1 mislocalized to the cytoplasm instead of the Cajal bodies. Dyskerin and hTR in these cells also mislocalized, residing in nucleoli instead of Cajal bodies (Zhong et al. 2011; Batista et al. 2011). In vitro telomerase activity was maintained, yet telomeres shortened over time (Batista et al. 2011). Together, these results demonstrated that mislocalization of telomerase is a mechanism which can compromise telomere maintenance in vivo.

The shelterin complex member TPP1 is another important player for in vivo telomerase action, and its disruption is also implicated in the TBDs (Fig. 6.3b, c). TPP1 forms a heterodimer with POT1. POT1 binds and protects the terminal single-stranded 3′ extension of telomeric DNA (referred to as the G-overhang) (Palm and de Lange 2008), which is the substrate of telomerase. TPP1 recruits telomerase to telomeres via its TEL patch and stimulates telomerase processivity (Nandakumar et al. 2012; Zhong et al. 2012; Wang et al. 2007; Xin et al. 2007; Latrick and Cech 2010).

A variant in *ACD*, which encodes TPP1, was found to segregate with short telomeres in one family (Kocak et al. 2014). This variant, which resulted in the deletion of a single amino acid in the TEL patch, was carried by identical twins, one who had IUGR and died at 4 months because of complications of pertussis and the other who also had IUGR and was diagnosed with HHS during the first year of life. This patient had telomere length below the 1st percentile and underwent HSCT for BMF at 3 years of age. These affected twins carried an additional missense variant. Functional studies showed that the deletion allele significantly reduced telomerase recruitment and processivity via disruption of the TEL patch, while the missense allele only slightly reduced the interaction between TIN2 and TPP1, with no detectable downstream effect (Kocak et al. 2014; Bisht et al. 2016). Gene editing showed that the deletion allele alone was sufficient to cause telomere shortening and eventual senescence in cancer cell lines (Bisht et al. 2016). Still, family members heterozygous for the deletion allele had short telomeres but were healthy (Kocak et al. 2014). Thus, it is possible that the missense allele or another modifier contributed to the development of severe disease in the twins. Another unrelated family was reported in which the same deletion allele was identified and segregated with short telomeres (Guo et al. 2014). Disease anticipation was observed in this family, with individuals heterozygous for the deletion allele having earlier onset of aplastic anemia or other blood disorders and cancer in each of three generations. TPP1 from the deletion allele localized to telomeres but failed to recruit telomerase (Guo et al. 2014), consistent with the finding that this is a partial loss-of-function allele with a specific deficit in TPP1-telomerase interaction (Bisht et al. 2016).

6.6.4 Replication of Telomeres and Establishment of Telomere End Structure

While telomerase is important for the replenishment of terminal repeats lost as a result of the end replication problem, additional factors are crucial for telomere length maintenance and function. These include those required for replication of telomeric DNA, which spans up to 14 kilobase pairs in length along the chromosome end, as well as those required for the regulation of telomere end structure, known as the t-loop. Correspondingly, variants in genes encoding these key factors have been observed in DC and the related TBDs.

RTEL1, a DNA helicase, is one such factor. To date, 18 patients with biallelic *RTEL1* variants from 13 families have been reported. All but one of these patients had a diagnosis of HHS, and most had severe B- and NK-cell deficiency among other disease manifestations presenting in early childhood (Ballew et al. 2013a, b; Deng et al. 2013; Le Guen et al. 2013; Walne et al. 2013). The one patient without a diagnosis of HHS had IUGR, microcephaly, marked short stature, and severe immunodeficiency and died in infancy (Ballew et al. 2013b). Thus, no patient with classical DC and biallelic *RTEL1* variants has been reported, underscoring the severe impact of biallelic mutations in *RTEL1* on human health. Indeed, monoallelic *RTEL1* variants are also associated with disease, with several pulmonary fibrosis kinships and few cases of DC (Ballew et al. 2013a; Stuart et al. 2015; Kannengiesser et al. 2015).

RTEL1 facilitates the replication of telomeric DNA, which is rich in G and C nucleotides and forms complex secondary structures (Vannier et al. 2013). It has also been proposed to play a crucial role in unwinding the t-loop in the S phase of the cell cycle (Fig. 6.3d) (Vannier et al. 2012; Sarek et al. 2015). Marked problems with telomere structure in cells with mutations in *RTEL1* were demonstrated by an increase in the formation of t-circles, which are thought to reflect aberrant t-loop excision; an increase in signal-free ends and sister telomere loss, indicating a loss of telomeric DNA sequence; fragile telomeres, indicative of collapsed replication forks; and telomere fusions (Cogan et al. 2015; Ballew et al. 2013b; Deng et al. 2013; Le Guen et al. 2013; Walne et al. 2013).

Aside from telomere dysfunction, cells derived from patients with pathogenic variants in *RTEL1* display genome instability. This was shown by decreased ability to repair cross-links (Ballew et al. 2013b), increased 53BP1 foci, and increased anaphase bridges (Le Guen et al. 2013). It has been suggested that the severe immunodeficiency seen in these patients may be due to the extra-telomeric defect in DNA repair caused by pathogenic variants in *RTEL1* (Ballew et al. 2013b). Additionally, patient cells with pathogenic variants in *RTEL1* had impaired nuclear export of the spliceosomal pre-U2 RNP and defective splicing (Schertzer et al. 2015). The effect of this remains to be explored but could account for some of the disease characteristics of patients.

As described above, pathogenic variants in *CTC1*, *STN1*, or *POT1* cause autosomal recessive CP. Patients with CP often have one truncating and one missense *CTC1* variant (Anderson et al. 2012; Polvi et al. 2012; Walne et al. 2012). To date, 36 patients with CP caused by variants in *CTC1* have been reported (Anderson et al. 2012; Polvi et al. 2012; Walne et al. 2012; Keller et al. 2012; Bisserbe et al. 2015; Netravathi et al. 2015). However, patients with *CTC1* pathogenic variants can have a phenotype that deviates from CP, as demonstrated by a patient who presented with classical DC and by patients who lacked retinopathy or brain abnormalities (Walne et al. 2012; Keller et al. 2012).

Several steps are required for the replication of telomeric DNA, which consists of thousands of base pairs of G-rich sequence on the 5′ to 3′ strand and the G-overhang. The first step is semiconservative replication of the telomeric tract by the replisome. Next, there is exonucleolytic processing of the C-rich strand, resulting in G-overhangs on both daughters of semiconservative replication. In cells that express telomerase, the G-overhang is then extended by telomerase. Lastly, DNA polymerase alpha (polα)/primase coverts the extended G-overhang to an appropriate size by a process known as C-strand fill-in. The CST complex plays a role in several of these steps; it stimulates polα-/primase-mediated repair of single-stranded gaps that are formed during replication of double-stranded telomeric DNA tracts (Fig. 6.3e), negatively regulates telomerase, and stimulates polα-/primase-mediated C-strand fill-in (Fig. 6.3f) (Rice and Skordalakes 2016; Chen and Lingner 2013). POT1 also negatively regulates telomerase and is required for regeneration of the G-overhang after telomere replication (Palm and de Lange 2008). As noted above, telomeres are variably short in patients with *CTC1*, *STN1*, and *POT1* pathogenic variants. Telomere defects, however, have been detected in cells from such patients including telomere dysfunction-induced damage foci, excessive G-overhangs, and telomere signal-free ends (Simon et al. 2016; Takai et al. 2016). These defects are thought to arise from deregulation of telomerase coupled with a defect in C-strand fill-in. As a result, the G-overhangs are excessively long, and, after the second round of replication, the product of replication of the telomeric C strand is abruptly short (Takai et al. 2016). Therefore, pathogenic variants in these proteins may cause proliferative defects via telomere dysfunction and/or stochastic truncations rather than progressive telomere shortening as observed in DC or the other TBDs with defects in telomerase or its action.

6.6.5 Multifactorial

Pathogenic variants in *TINF2*, which encodes TIN2, were the first to implicate the shelterin complex in DC (Savage et al. 2008). Registry data indicate *TINF2* variants account for approximately 11% of DC-spectrum disorders, including HHS and RS (Walne et al. 2008). Interestingly, variants in *TINF2* are the most frequent genetic cause of RS to date. Most patients with *TINF2* variants develop aplastic anemia before the age of 10 years. In contrast to other DC-associated genes in which variants distribute throughout the encoded protein and are frequently inherited, *TINF2* variants cluster to a 34 amino acid long region in exon 6 (i.e., the DC cluster) and are most often de novo (Walne et al. 2008; Frank et al. 2015). The de novo nature of *TINF2* variants is notable as telomere lengths in affected individuals are markedly short in a single generation (Walne et al. 2008) in contrast to the progressive shortening that may be observed over successive generations in families with heterozygous *TERT* or *TERC* variants (Armanios et al. 2005; Vulliamy et al. 2004).

Telomere length maintenance requires both telomeric repeat addition by telomerase and the prevention of telomere loss by nucleolytic processing. As TIN2 is a member of the shelterin complex (Fig. 6.3b), which impacts both of these activities, groups have investigated the role of *TINF2* variants in regulating both. Expression of variant TIN2 in human cancer cell lines resulted in telomere shortening, abrogated TIN2 interaction with telomerase, and impaired telomerase recruitment to telomeres (Frank et al. 2015; Yang et al. 2011). Therefore, it was proposed that failure of telomerase recruitment to telomeres underlies the telomere shortening. However, mice with a variant in *TINF2* identical to one observed in patients exhibited telomere dysfunction and failure of length maintenance independent of telomerase (Frescas and de Lange 2014). This suggests that TIN2 pathogenic variants cause a failure of telomere maintenance via telomere dysfunction in addition to causing a decrease in telomerase action on telomeres. Lastly, TIN2 interacts with heterochromatin protein 1γ (HP1γ) via a binding site within the DC cluster, and this interaction is required for sister telomere cohesion in cancer cell lines (Canudas et al. 2011). Some *TINF2* DC variants cause reduction of TIN2 binding to HP1γ, and deficient sister telomere cohesion is observed in some patient-derived cells. Thus, disruption in sister telomere cohesion may be a third mechanism for telomere shortening or simply underlie the defect in telomerase recruitment and telomere protection.

6.7 Closing Thoughts

The therapeutic challenges with DC and the TBDs are significant. Treatment modalities that can reduce rates of telomere shortening or, better, restore telomere length are needed, and these must impact the critical tissues affected by these disorders (e.g., bone marrow, lung, liver, and gastrointestinal tract). While abnormally short telomeres characterize DC and the TBDs, the molecular mechanisms underlying the shortening are diverse and may not be equally amenable to any given approach (e.g., upregulation of telomerase activity). Expansion of the clinical phenotypes of DC and the TBDs is likely to continue with the activities of several registries in the USA and abroad as well as with the reporting of small case series and case reports, which often provoke larger cohort studies. Examples of this are the recent reports of hepatopulmonary syndrome and pulmonary arteriovenous malformations without apparent liver disease as significant causes of pulmonary morbidity in patients with DC (Gorgy et al. 2015; Khincha et al. 2017). Efforts to uncover the genetic etiology in the 30–40% of patients with DC who lack pathogenic variants in any of the known genes is a continued need, which will not only aid families and clinicians but also increase our understanding of the fundamentals of telomere biology.

References

Aalfs CM, van den Berg H, Barth PG, Hennekam RC (1995) The Hoyeraal-Hreidarsson syndrome: the fourth case of a separate entity with prenatal growth retardation, progressive pancytopenia and cerebellar hypoplasia. Eur J Pediatr 154(4):304–308

Abramowsky C, Romero R, Heffron T (2003) Pathology of noncirrhotic portal hypertension: clinicopathologic study in pediatric patients. Pediatr Dev Pathol 6(5):421–426. https://doi.org/10.1007/s10024-003-1002-8

Alder JK, Cogan JD, Brown AF, Anderson CJ, Lawson WE, Lansdorp PM, Phillips JA, Loyd JE, Chen JJ-L, Armanios M, Artandi SE (2011) Ancestral mutation in telomerase causes defects in repeat addition processivity and manifests as familial pulmonary fibrosis. PLoS Genet 7(3):e1001352

Alder JK, Stanley SE, Wagner CL, Hamilton M, Hanumanthu VS, Armanios M (2015) Exome sequencing identifies mutant TINF2 in a family with pulmonary fibrosis. Chest 147(5):1361–1368. https://doi.org/10.1378/chest.14-1947

Allsopp RC, Harley CB (1995) Evidence for a critical telomere length in senescent human fibroblasts. Exp Cell Res 219(1):130–136. https://doi.org/10.1006/excr.1995.1213

Alter BP, Baerlocher GM, Savage SA, Chanock SJ, Weksler BB, Willner JP, Peters JA, Giri N, Lansdorp PM (2007) Very short telomere length by flow fluorescence in situ hybridization identifies patients with dyskeratosis congenita. Blood 110(5): 1439–1447

Alter BP, Giri N, Savage SA, Rosenberg PS (2009) Cancer in dyskeratosis congenita. Blood 113(26):6549–6557. https://doi.org/10.1182/blood-2008-12-192880 blood-2008-12-192880 [pii]

Alter BP, Giri N, Savage SA, Peters JA, Loud JT, Leathwood L, Carr AG, Greene MH, Rosenberg PS (2010) Malignancies and survival patterns in the National Cancer Institute inherited bone marrow failure syndromes cohort study. Br J Haematol 150(2):179–188. https://doi.org/10.1111/j.1365-2141.2010.08212.x

Alter BP, Rosenberg PS, Giri N, Baerlocher GM, Lansdorp PM, Savage SA (2012) Telomere length is associated with disease severity and declines with age in dyskeratosis congenita. Haematologica 97(3):353–359. https://doi.org/10.3324/haematol.2011.055269

Alter BP, Giri N, Savage SA, Rosenberg PS (2015) Telomere length in inherited bone marrow failure syndromes. Haematologica 100(1):49–54. https://doi.org/10.3324/haematol.2014.114389

Anderson BH, Kasher PR, Mayer J, Szynkiewicz M, Jenkinson EM, Bhaskar SS, Urquhart JE, Daly SB, Dickerson JE, O'Sullivan J, Leibundgut EO, Muter J, Abdel-Salem GM, Babul-Hirji R, Baxter P, Berger A, Bonafe L, Brunstom-Hernandez JE, Buckard JA, Chitayat D, Chong WK, Cordelli DM, Ferreira P, Fluss J, Forrest EH, Franzoni E, Garone C, Hammans SR, Houge G, Hughes I, Jacquemont S, Jeannet PY, Jefferson RJ, Kumar R, Kutschke G, Lundberg S, Lourenco CM, Mehta R, Naidu S, Nischal KK, Nunes L, Ounap K, Philippart M, Prabhakar P, Risen SR, Schiffmann R, Soh C, Stephenson JB, Stewart H, Stone J, Tolmie JL, van der Knaap MS, Vieira JP, Vilain CN, Wakeling EL, Wermenbol V, Whitney A, Lovell SC, Meyer S, Livingston JH, Baerlocher GM, Black GC, Rice GI, Crow YJ (2012) Mutations in CTC1, encoding conserved telomere maintenance component 1, cause Coats plus. Nat Genet 44(3):338–342. https://doi.org/10.1038/ng.1084

Angrisani A, Vicidomini R, Turano M, Furia M (2014) Human dyskerin: beyond telomeres. Biol Chem 395(6):593–610. https://doi.org/10.1515/hsz-2013-0287

Armanios M (2009) Syndromes of telomere shortening. Annu Rev Genomics Hum Genet 10:45–61. https://doi.org/10.1146/annurev-genom-082908-150046

Armanios M, Chen JL, Chang YP, Brodsky RA, Hawkins A, Griffin CA, Eshleman JR, Cohen AR, Chakravarti A, Hamosh A, Greider CW (2005) Haploinsufficiency of telomerase reverse transcriptase leads to anticipation in autosomal dominant dyskeratosis congenita. Proc Natl Acad Sci U S A 102(44):15960–15964

Armanios MY, Chen JJ, Cogan JD, Alder JK, Ingersoll RG, Markin C, Lawson WE, Xie M, Vulto I, Phillips JA III, Lansdorp PM, Greider CW, Loyd JE (2007) Telomerase mutations in families with idiopathic pulmonary fibrosis. N Engl J Med 356(13):1317–1326

Aubert G, Baerlocher GM, Vulto I, Poon SS, Lansdorp PM (2012) Collapse of telomere homeostasis in hematopoietic cells caused by heterozygous mutations in telomerase genes. PLoS Genet 8(5):e1002696. https://doi.org/10.1371/journal.pgen.1002696

Baerlocher GM, Lansdorp PM (2003) Telomere length measurements in leukocyte subsets by automated multicolor flow-FISH. Cytometry A 55(1):1–6. https://doi.org/10.1002/cyto.a.10064

Baerlocher GM, Vulto I, de Jong G, Lansdorp PM (2006) Flow cytometry and FISH to measure the average length of telomeres (flow FISH). Nat Protoc 1(5):2365–2376

Ballew BJ, Yeager M, Jacobs K, Giri N, Boland J, Burdett L, Alter BP, Savage SA (2013a) Germline mutations of regulator of telomere elongation helicase 1, RTEL1, in Dyskeratosis congenita. Hum Genet 132(4):473–480. https://doi.org/10.1007/s00439-013-1265-8

Ballew BJ, Joseph V, De S, Sarek G, Vannier JB, Stracker T, Schrader KA, Small TN, O'Reilly R, Manschreck C, Harlan Fleischut MM, Zhang L, Sullivan J, Stratton K, Yeager M, Jacobs K, Giri N, Alter BP, Boland J, Burdett L, Offit K, Boulton SJ, Savage SA, Petrini JH (2013b) A recessive founder mutation in regulator of telomere elongation helicase 1, RTEL1, underlies severe immunodeficiency and features of Hoyeraal Hreidarsson syndrome. PLoS Genet 9(8):e1003695. https://doi.org/10.1371/journal.pgen.1003695

Barbaro P, Vedi A (2016) Survival after hematopoietic stem cell transplant in patients with dyskeratosis congenita: systematic review of the literature. Biol Blood Marrow Transplant 22(7):1152–1158. https://doi.org/10.1016/j.bbmt.2016.03.001

Batista LF, Pech MF, Zhong FL, Nguyen HN, Xie KT, Zaug AJ, Crary SM, Choi J, Sebastiano V, Cherry A, Giri N, Wernig M, Alter BP, Cech TR, Savage SA, Reijo Pera RA, Artandi SE (2011) Telomere shortening and loss of self-renewal in dyskeratosis congenita induced pluripotent stem cells. Nature 474(7351):399–402. https://doi.org/10.1038/nature10084

Berndt H, Harnisch C, Rammelt C, Stohr N, Zirkel A, Dohm JC, Himmelbauer H, Tavanez JP, Huttelmaier

S, Wahle E (2012) Maturation of mammalian H/ACA box snoRNAs: PAPD5-dependent adenylation and PARN-dependent trimming. RNA 18(5):958–972. https://doi.org/10.1261/rna.032292.112

Berthet F, Caduff R, Schaad UB, Roten H, Tuchschmid P, Boltshauser E, Seger RA (1994) A syndrome of primary combined immunodeficiency with microcephaly, cerebellar hypoplasia, growth failure and progressive pancytopenia. Eur J Pediatr 153(5):333–338

Berthet F, Tuchschmid P, Boltshauser E, Seger RA (1995) The Hoyeraal-Hreidarsson syndrome: don't forget the associated immunodeficiency. Eur J Pediatr 154(12):998

Bertuch AA (2016) The molecular genetics of the telomere biology disorders. RNA Biol 13(8):696–706. https://doi.org/10.1080/15476286.2015.1094596

Bisht K, Smith EM, Tesmer VM, Nandakumar J (2016) Structural and functional consequences of a disease mutation in the telomere protein TPP1. Proc Natl Acad Sci U S A 113(46):13021–13026. https://doi.org/10.1073/pnas.1605685113

Bisserbe A, Tertian G, Buffet C, Turhan A, Lambotte O, Nasser G, Alvin P, Tardieu M, Riant F, Bergametti F, Tournier-Lasserve E, Denier C (2015) Cerebro-retinal microangiopathy with calcifications and cysts due to recessive mutations in the CTC1 gene. Rev Neurol (Paris) 171(5):445–449. https://doi.org/10.1016/j.neurol.2015.01.566

Borie R, Kannengiesser C, Hirschi S, Le Pavec J, Mal H, Bergot E, Jouneau S, Naccache JM, Revy P, Boutboul D, Peffault de la Tour R, Wemeau-Stervinou L, Philit F, Cordier JF, Thabut G, Crestani B, Cottin V (2015) Severe hematologic complications after lung transplantation in patients with telomerase complex mutations. J Heart Lung Transplant 34(4):538–546. https://doi.org/10.1016/j.healun.2014.11.010

Borie R, Tabeze L, Thabut G, Nunes H, Cottin V, Marchand-Adam S, Prevot G, Tazi A, Cadranel J, Mal H, Wemeau-Stervinou L, Bergeron Lafaurie A, Israel-Biet D, Picard C, Reynaud Gaubert M, Jouneau S, Naccache JM, Mankikian J, Menard C, Cordier JF, Valeyre D, Reocreux M, Grandchamp B, Revy P, Kannengiesser C, Crestani B (2016) Prevalence and characteristics of TERT and TERC mutations in suspected genetic pulmonary fibrosis. Eur Respir J 48(6):1721–1731. https://doi.org/10.1183/13993003.02115-2015

Briggs TA, Abdel-Salam GM, Balicki M, Baxter P, Bertini E, Bishop N, Browne BH, Chitayat D, Chong WK, Eid MM, Halliday W, Hughes I, Klusmann-Koy A, Kurian M, Nischal KK, Rice GI, Stephenson JB, Surtees R, Talbot JF, Tehrani NN, Tolmie JL, Toomes C, van der Knaap MS, Crow YJ (2008) Cerebroretinal microangiopathy with calcifications and cysts (CRMCC). Am J Med Genet A 146A(2):182–190. https://doi.org/10.1002/ajmg.a.32080

Brown KE, Kelly TE, Myers BM (1993) Gastrointestinal involvement in a woman with dyskeratosis congenita. Dig Dis Sci 38(1):181–184

Burris AM, Ballew BJ, Kentosh JB, Turner CE, Norton SA, NCI DCEG Cancer Genomics Research Laboratory, NCI DCEG Cancer Sequencing Working Group, Giri N, Alter BP, Nellan A, Gamper C, Hartman KR, Savage SA (2016) Hoyeraal-Hreidarsson syndrome due to PARN mutations: fourteen years of follow-up. Pediatr Neurol 56:62–68 e61. https://doi.org/10.1016/j.pediatrneurol.2015.12.005

Calado RT, Regal JA, Kleiner DE, Schrump DS, Peterson NR, Pons V, Chanock SJ, Lansdorp PM, Young NS (2009a) A spectrum of severe familial liver disorders associate with telomerase mutations. PLoS One 4(11):e7926. https://doi.org/10.1371/journal.pone.0007926

Calado RT, Yewdell WT, Wilkerson KL, Regal JA, Kajigaya S, Stratakis CA, Young NS (2009b) Sex hormones, acting on the TERT gene, increase telomerase activity in human primary hematopoietic cells. Blood 114(11):2236–2243. https://doi.org/10.1182/blood-2008-09-178871 blood-2008-09-178871 [pii]

Canudas S, Houghtaling BR, Bhanot M, Sasa G, Savage SA, Bertuch AA, Smith S (2011) A role for heterochromatin protein 1γ at human telomeres. Genes Dev 25(17):1807–1819. https://doi.org/10.1101/gad.17325211

Chen LY, Lingner J (2013) CST for the grand finale of telomere replication. Nucleus 4(4):277–282. https://doi.org/10.4161/nucl.25701

Chu TW, MacNeil DE, Autexier C (2016) Multiple mechanisms contribute to the cell growth defects imparted by human telomerase insertion in fingers domain mutations associated with premature aging diseases. J Biol Chem 291(16):8374–8386. https://doi.org/10.1074/jbc.M116.714782

Cogan JD, Kropski JA, Zhao M, Mitchell DB, Rives L, Markin C, Garnett ET, Montgomery KH, Mason WR, McKean DF, Powers J, Murphy E, Olson LM, Choi L, Cheng DS, Blue EM, Young LR, Lancaster LH, Steele MP, Brown KK, Schwarz MI, Fingerlin TE, Schwartz DA, Lawson WE, Loyd JE, Zhao Z, Phillips JA III, Blackwell TS (2015) Rare variants in RTEL1 are associated with familial interstitial pneumonia. Am J Respir Crit Care Med 191(6):646–655. https://doi.org/10.1164/rccm.201408-1510OC

Counter CM, Avilion AA, LeFeuvre CE, Stewart NG, Greider CW, Harley CB, Bacchetti S (1992) Telomere shortening associated with chromosome instability is arrested in immortal cells which express telomerase activity. EMBO J 11(5):1921–1929

Cristofari G, Adolf E, Reichenbach P, Sikora K, Terns RM, Terns MP, Lingner J (2007) Human telomerase RNA accumulation in Cajal bodies facilitates telomerase recruitment to telomeres and telomere elongation. Mol Cell 27(6):882–889. https://doi.org/10.1016/j.molcel.2007.07.020

Crow YJ, McMenamin J, Haenggeli CA, Hadley DM, Tirupathi S, Treacy EP, Zuberi SM, Browne BH, Tolmie JL, Stephenson JB (2004) Coats' plus: a progressive familial syndrome of bilateral Coats' disease, characteristic cerebral calcification, leukoencephalopathy, slow pre- and post-natal linear growth and defects of bone marrow and integument. Neuropediatrics 35(1):10–19. https://doi.org/10.1055/s-2003-43552

Darzacq X, Kittur N, Roy S, Shav-Tal Y, Singer RH, Meier UT (2006) Stepwise RNP assembly at the site of H/ACA RNA transcription in human cells. J Cell Biol 173(2):207–218. https://doi.org/10.1083/jcb.200601105

de la Fuente J, Dokal I (2007) Dyskeratosis congenita: advances in the understanding of the telomerase defect and the role of stem cell transplantation. Pediatr Transplant 11(6):584–594. https://doi.org/10.1111/j.1399-3046.2007.00721.x

Deng Z, Glousker G, Molczan A, Fox AJ, Lamm N, Dheekollu J, Weizman OE, Schertzer M, Wang Z, Vladimirova O, Schug J, Aker M, Londono-Vallejo A, Kaestner KH, Lieberman PM, Tzfati Y (2013) Inherited mutations in the helicase RTEL1 cause telomere dysfunction and Hoyeraal-Hreidarsson syndrome. Proc Natl Acad Sci U S A 110(36):E3408–E3416. https://doi.org/10.1073/pnas.1300600110

Dhanraj S, Gunja SM, Deveau AP, Nissbeck M, Boonyawat B, Coombs AJ, Renieri A, Mucciolo M, Marozza A, Buoni S, Turner L, Li H, Jarrar A, Sabanayagam M, Kirby M, Shago M, Pinto D, Berman JN, Scherer SW, Virtanen A, Dror Y (2015) Bone marrow failure and developmental delay caused by mutations in poly(A)-specific ribonuclease (PARN). J Med Genet 52(11):738–748. https://doi.org/10.1136/jmedgenet-2015-103292

Diaz de Leon A, Cronkhite JT, Katzenstein AL, Godwin JD, Raghu G, Glazer CS, Rosenblatt RL, Girod CE, Garrity ER, Xing C, Garcia CK (2010) Telomere lengths, pulmonary fibrosis and telomerase (TERT) mutations. PLoS One 5(5):e10680. https://doi.org/10.1371/journal.pone.0010680

Dokal I (2011) Dyskeratosis congenita. Hematology Am Soc Hematol Educ Program 2011:480–486. https://doi.org/10.1182/asheducation-2011.1.480

Dokal I, Vulliamy T, Mason P, Bessler M (2015) Clinical utility gene card for: dyskeratosis congenita - update 2015. Eur J Hum Genet 23(4). https://doi.org/10.1038/ejhg.2014.170

Duprey PA, Steger JW (1988) An unusual case of dyskeratosis congenita with intracranial calcifications. J Am Acad Dermatol 19(4):760–762

Egan ED, Collins K (2012) Biogenesis of telomerase ribonucleoproteins. RNA 18(10):1747–1759. https://doi.org/10.1261/rna.034629.112

Feng J, Funk WD, Wang SS, Weinrich SL, Avilion AA, Chiu CP, Adams RR, Chang E, Allsopp RC, Yu J et al (1995) The RNA component of human telomerase. Science 269(5228):1236–1241

Frank AK, Tran DC, Qu RW, Stohr BA, Segal DJ, Xu L (2015) The Shelterin TIN2 subunit mediates recruitment of telomerase to telomeres. PLoS Genet 11(7):e1005410. https://doi.org/10.1371/journal.pgen.1005410

Frescas D, de Lange T (2014) A TIN2 dyskeratosis congenita mutation causes telomerase-independent telomere shortening in mice. Genes Dev 28(2):153–166. https://doi.org/10.1101/gad.233395.113

Ghemlas I, Li H, Zlateska B, Klaassen R, Fernandez CV, Yanofsky RA, Wu J, Pastore Y, Silva M, Lipton JH, Brossard J, Michon B, Abish S, Steele M, Sinha R, Belletrutti M, Breakey VR, Jardine L, Goodyear L, Sung L, Dhanraj S, Reble E, Wagner A, Beyene J, Ray P, Meyn S, Cada M, Dror Y (2015) Improving diagnostic precision, care and syndrome definitions using comprehensive next-generation sequencing for the inherited bone marrow failure syndromes. J Med Genet 52(9):575–584. https://doi.org/10.1136/jmedgenet-2015-103270

Giri N, Pitel PA, Green D, Alter BP (2007) Splenic peliosis and rupture in patients with dyskeratosis congenita on androgens and granulocyte colony-stimulating factor. Br J Haematol 138(6):815–817. https://doi.org/10.1111/j.1365-2141.2007.06718.x BJH6718 [pii]

Giri N, Lee R, Faro A, Huddleston CB, White FV, Alter BP, Savage SA (2011) Lung transplantation for pulmonary fibrosis in dyskeratosis congenita: case report and systematic literature review. BMC Blood Disord 11:3. https://doi.org/10.1186/1471-2326-11-3

Gleeson M, O'Marcaigh A, Cotter M, Brosnahan D, Vulliamy T, Smith OP (2012) Retinal vasculopathy in autosomal dominant dyskeratosis congenita due to TINF2 mutation. Br J Haematol 159(5):498. https://doi.org/10.1111/bjh.12088

Goldman F, Bouarich R, Kulkarni S, Freeman S, Du HY, Harrington L, Mason PJ, Londono-Vallejo A, Bessler M (2005) The effect of TERC haploinsufficiency on the inheritance of telomere length. Proc Natl Acad Sci U S A 102(47):17119–17124. https://doi.org/10.1073/pnas.0505318102 0505318102 [pii]

Gorgy AI, Jonassaint NL, Stanley SE, Koteish A, DeZern AE, Walter JE, Sopha SC, Hamilton JP, Hoover-Fong J, Chen AR, Anders RA, Kamel IR, Armanios M (2015) Hepatopulmonary syndrome is a frequent cause of dyspnea in the short telomere disorders. Chest 148(4):1019–1026. https://doi.org/10.1378/chest.15-0825

Gramatges MM, Qi X, Sasa GS, Chen JJ, Bertuch AA (2013) A homozygous telomerase T-motif variant resulting in markedly reduced repeat addition processivity in siblings with Hoyeraal Hreidarsson syndrome. Blood 121(18):3586–3593. https://doi.org/10.1182/blood-2012-08-447755

Greider CW, Blackburn EH (1987) The telomere terminal transferase of Tetrahymena is a ribonucleoprotein enzyme with two kinds of primer specificity. Cell 51(6):887–898

Guo Y, Kartawinata M, Li J, Pickett HA, Teo J, Kilo T, Barbaro PM, Keating B, Chen Y, Tian L, Al-Odaib A, Reddel RR, Christodoulou J, Xu X, Hakonarson H, Bryan TM (2014) Inherited bone marrow failure associated with germline mutation of ACD, the gene encoding telomere protein TPP1. Blood 124(18):2767–2774. https://doi.org/10.1182/blood-2014-08-596445

Harley CB, Futcher AB, Greider CW (1990) Telomeres shorten during ageing of human fibroblasts. Nature 345(6274):458–460. https://doi.org/10.1038/345458a0

Heiss NS, Knight SW, Vulliamy TJ, Klauck SM, Wiemann S, Mason PJ, Poustka A, Dokal I (1998) X-linked dyskeratosis congenita is caused by mutations in a highly conserved gene with putative nucleolar functions. Nat Genet 19(1):32–38. https://doi.org/10.1038/ng0598-32

Hoyeraal HM, Lamvik J, Moe PJ (1970) Congenital hypoplastic thrombocytopenia and cerebral malformations in two brothers. Acta Paediatr Scand 59(2): 185–191

Hreidarsson S, Kristjansson K, Johannesson G, Johannsson JH (1988) A syndrome of progressive pancytopenia with microcephaly, cerebellar hypoplasia and growth failure. Acta Paediatr Scand 77(5):773–775

Islam A, Rafiq S, Kirwan M, Walne A, Cavenagh J, Vulliamy T, Dokal I (2013) Haematological recovery in dyskeratosis congenita patients treated with danazol. Br J Haematol 162(6):854–856. https://doi.org/10.1111/bjh.12432

Jady BE, Bertrand E, Kiss T (2004) Human telomerase RNA and box H/ACA scaRNAs share a common Cajal body-specific localization signal. J Cell Biol 164(5):647–652. https://doi.org/10.1083/jcb.200310138 jcb.200310138 [pii]

Jonassaint NL, Guo N, Califano JA, Montgomery EA, Armanios M (2013) The gastrointestinal manifestations of telomere-mediated disease. Aging Cell 12(2):319–323. https://doi.org/10.1111/acel.12041

Kajtar P, Mehes K (1994) Bilateral coats retinopathy associated with aplastic anaemia and mild dyskeratotic signs. Am J Med Genet 49(4):374–377. https://doi.org/10.1002/ajmg.1320490404

Kannengiesser C, Borie R, Menard C, Reocreux M, Nitschke P, Gazal S, Mal H, Taille C, Cadranel J, Nunes H, Valeyre D, Cordier JF, Callebaut I, Boileau C, Cottin V, Grandchamp B, Revy P, Crestani B (2015) Heterozygous RTEL1 mutations are associated with familial pulmonary fibrosis. Eur Respir J 46:474. https://doi.org/10.1183/09031936.00040115

Keel SB, Scott A, Sanchez-Bonilla M, Ho PA, Gulsuner S, Pritchard CC, Abkowitz JL, King MC, Walsh T, Shimamura A (2016) Genetic features of myelodysplastic syndrome and aplastic anemia in pediatric and young adult patients. Haematologica 101(11):1343–1350. https://doi.org/10.3324/haematol.2016.149476

Keller RB, Gagne KE, Usmani GN, Asdourian GK, Williams DA, Hofmann I, Agarwal S (2012) CTC1 mutations in a patient with dyskeratosis congenita. Pediatr Blood Cancer 59(2):311–314. https://doi.org/10.1002/pbc.24193

Khincha PP, Wentzensen IM, Giri N, Alter BP, Savage SA (2014) Response to androgen therapy in patients with dyskeratosis congenita. Br J Haematol 165(3):349–357. https://doi.org/10.1111/bjh.12748

Khincha PP, Bertuch AA, Agarwal S, Townsley DM, Young NS, Keel S, Shimamura A, Boulad F, Simoneau T, Justino H, Kuo C, Artandi S, McCaslin C, Cox DW, Chaffee S, Collins BF, Giri N, Alter BP, Raghu G, Savage SA (2017) Pulmonary arteriovenous malformations: an uncharacterised phenotype of dyskeratosis congenita and related telomere biology disorders. Eur Respir J 49(1):1601640. https://doi.org/10.1183/13993003.01640-2016

Kirwan M, Dokal I (2008) Dyskeratosis congenita: a genetic disorder of many faces. Clin Genet 73(2):103–112

Knight SW, Heiss NS, Vulliamy TJ, Aalfs CM, McMahon C, Richmond P, Jones A, Hennekam RC, Poustka A, Mason PJ, Dokal I (1999a) Unexplained aplastic anaemia, immunodeficiency, and cerebellar hypoplasia (Hoyeraal-Hreidarsson syndrome) due to mutations in the dyskeratosis congenita gene, DKC1. Br J Haematol 107(2):335–339 bjh1690 [pii]

Knight SW, Heiss NS, Vulliamy TJ, Greschner S, Stavrides G, Pai GS, Lestringant G, Varma N, Mason PJ, Dokal I, Poustka A (1999b) X-linked dyskeratosis congenita is predominantly caused by missense mutations in the DKC1 gene. Am J Hum Genet 65(1):50–58. https://doi.org/10.1086/302446 S0002-9297(07)63727-6 [pii]

Kocak H, Ballew BJ, Bisht K, Eggebeen R, Hicks BD, Suman S, O'Neil A, Giri N, NCI DCEG Cancer Genomics Research Laboratory, NCI DCEG Cancer Sequencing Working Group, Maillard I, Alter BP, Keegan CE, Nandakumar J, Savage SA (2014) Hoyeraal-Hreidarsson syndrome caused by a germline mutation in the TEL patch of the telomere protein TPP1. Genes Dev 28(19):2090–2102. https://doi.org/10.1101/gad.248567.114

Kropski JA, Mitchell DB, Markin C, Polosukhin VV, Choi L, Johnson JE, Lawson WE, Phillips JA, Cogan JD, Blackwell TS, Loyd JE (2014) A novel dyskerin (DKC1) mutation is associated with familial interstitial pneumonia. Chest 146(1):e1–e7. https://doi.org/10.1378/chest.13-2224

Lamm N, Ordan E, Shponkin R, Richler C, Aker M, Tzfati Y (2009) Diminished telomeric 3′ overhangs are associated with telomere dysfunction in Hoyeraal-Hreidarsson syndrome. PLoS One 4(5):e5666. https://doi.org/10.1371/journal.pone.0005666

Latrick CM, Cech TR (2010) POT1-TPP1 enhances telomerase processivity by slowing primer dissociation and aiding translocation. EMBO J 29(5):924–933. https://doi.org/10.1038/emboj.2009.409

Le Guen T, Jullien L, Touzot F, Schertzer M, Gaillard L, Perderiset M, Carpentier W, Nitschke P, Picard C, Couillault G, Soulier J, Fischer A, Callebaut I, Jabado N, Londono-Vallejo A, de Villartay JP, Revy P (2013) Human RTEL1 deficiency causes Hoyeraal-Hreidarsson syndrome with short telomeres and genome instability. Hum Mol Genet 22(16):3239–3249. https://doi.org/10.1093/hmg/ddt178

Lee JH, Lee YS, Jeong SA, Khadka P, Roth J, Chung IK (2014) Catalytically active telomerase holoenzyme is assembled in the dense fibrillar component of the nucleolus during S phase. Histochem Cell Biol 141(2):137–152. https://doi.org/10.1007/s00418-013-1166-x

Linnankivi T, Valanne L, Paetau A, Alafuzoff I, Hakumaki JM, Kivela T, Lonnqvist T, Makitie O, Paakkonen L,

Vainionpaa L, Vanninen R, Herva R, Pihko H (2006) Cerebroretinal microangiopathy with calcifications and cysts. Neurology 67(8):1437–1443. https://doi.org/10.1212/01.wnl.0000236999.63933.b0

Mahansaria SS, Kumar S, Bharathy KG, Kumar S, Pamecha V (2015) Liver transplantation after bone marrow transplantation for end stage liver disease with severe hepatopulmonary syndrome in dyskeratosis congenita: a literature first. J Clin Exp Hepatol 5(4):344–347. https://doi.org/10.1016/j.jceh.2015.10.003

Marrone A, Stevens D, Vulliamy T, Dokal I, Mason PJ (2004) Heterozygous telomerase RNA mutations found in dyskeratosis congenita and aplastic anemia reduce telomerase activity via haploinsufficiency. Blood 104(13):3936–3942

Marrone A, Walne A, Tamary H, Masunari Y, Kirwan M, Beswick R, Vulliamy T, Dokal I (2007) Telomerase reverse transcriptase homozygous mutations in autosomal recessive dyskeratosis congenita and Hoyeraal-Hreidarsson syndrome. Blood 110:4198

McElnea EM, van der Spek N, Smith O, Fitzsimon S, Patel CK, O'Marcaigh A (2013) Revesz syndrome masquerading as bilateral cicatricial retinopathy of prematurity. J AAPOS 17(6):634–636. https://doi.org/10.1016/j.jaapos.2013.07.016

Meyerson M, Counter CM, Eaton EN, Ellisen LW, Steiner P, Caddle SD, Ziaugra L, Beijersbergen RL, Davidoff MJ, Liu Q, Bacchetti S, Haber DA, Weinberg RA (1997) hEST2, the putative human telomerase catalytic subunit gene, is up-regulated in tumor cells and during immortalization. Cell 90(4):785–795

Mitchell JR, Wood E, Collins K (1999a) A telomerase component is defective in the human disease dyskeratosis congenita. Nature 402(6761):551–555

Mitchell JR, Cheng J, Collins K (1999b) A box H/ACA small nucleolar RNA-like domain at the human telomerase RNA 3′ end. Mol Cell Biol 19(1):567–576

Mochizuki Y, He J, Kulkarni S, Bessler M, Mason PJ (2004) Mouse dyskerin mutations affect accumulation of telomerase RNA and small nucleolar RNA, telomerase activity, and ribosomal RNA processing. Proc Natl Acad Sci U S A 101(29):10756–10761. https://doi.org/10.1073/pnas.0402560101 0402560101 [pii]

Moon DH, Segal M, Boyraz B, Guinan E, Hofmann I, Cahan P, Tai AK, Agarwal S (2015) Poly(A)-specific ribonuclease (PARN) mediates 3′-end maturation of the telomerase RNA component. Nat Genet 47(12):1482–1488. https://doi.org/10.1038/ng.3423

Moyzis RK, Buckingham JM, Cram LS, Dani M, Deaven LL, Jones MD, Meyne J, Ratliff RL, Ratliff RL, Wu JR (1988) A highly conserved repetitive DNA sequence, (TTAGGG)n, present at the telomeres of human chromosomes. Proc Natl Acad Sci U S A 85(18):6622–6626

Nakamura TM, Morin GB, Chapman KB, Weinrich SL, Andrews WH, Lingner J, Harley CB, Cech TR (1997) Telomerase catalytic subunit homologs from fission yeast and human. Science 277(5328):955–959

Nandakumar J, Bell CF, Weidenfeld I, Zaug AJ, Leinwand LA, Cech TR (2012) The TEL patch of telomere protein TPP1 mediates telomerase recruitment and processivity. Nature 492(7428):285–289. https://doi.org/10.1038/nature11648

Netravathi M, Kumari R, Kapoor S, Dakle P, Dwivedi MK, Roy SD, Pandey P, Saini J, Ramakrishna A, Navalli D, Satishchandra P, Pal PK, Kumar A, Faruq M (2015) Whole exome sequencing in an Indian family links Coats plus syndrome and dextrocardia with a homozygous novel CTC1 and a rare HES7 variation. BMC Med Genet 16:5. https://doi.org/10.1186/s12881-015-0151-8

Newton CA, Batra K, Torrealba J, Kozlitina J, Glazer CS, Aravena C, Meyer K, Raghu G, Collard HR, Garcia CK (2016) Telomere-related lung fibrosis is diagnostically heterogeneous but uniformly progressive. Eur Respir J 48(6):1710–1720. https://doi.org/10.1183/13993003.00308-2016

Nguyen D, Grenier St-Sauveur V, Bergeron D, Dupuis-Sandoval F, Scott MS, Bachand F (2015) A polyadenylation-dependent 3′ end maturation pathway is required for the synthesis of the human telomerase RNA. Cell Rep 13(10):2244–2257. https://doi.org/10.1016/j.celrep.2015.11.003

Ohga S, Kai T, Honda K, Nakayama H, Inamitsu T, Ueda K (1997) What are the essential symptoms in the Hoyeraal-Hreidarsson syndrome? Eur J Pediatr 156(1):80–81

Olovnikov A (1973) A theory of marginotomy: the incomplete copying of template margin in enzymatic synthesis of polynucleotides and biological significance of the phenomenon. J Theor Biol 41:181–190

Palm W, de Lange T (2008) How shelterin protects mammalian telomeres. Annu Rev Genet 42:301–334

Parry EM, Alder JK, Lee SS, Phillips JA III, Loyd JE, Duggal P, Armanios M (2011a) Decreased dyskerin levels as a mechanism of telomere shortening in X-linked dyskeratosis congenita. J Med Genet 48(5):327–333. https://doi.org/10.1136/jmg.2010.085100

Parry EM, Alder JK, Qi X, Chen JJ, Armanios M (2011b) Syndrome complex of bone marrow failure and pulmonary fibrosis predicts germline defects in telomerase. Blood 117(21):5607–5611. https://doi.org/10.1182/blood-2010-11-322149

Pavlatos AM, Fultz O, Monberg MJ, Vootkur A (2001) Review of oxymetholone: a 17alpha-alkylated anabolic-androgenic steroid. Clin Ther 23(6):789–801; discussion 771

Podlevsky JD, Bley CJ, Omana RV, Qi X, Chen JJ (2008) The telomerase database. Nucleic Acids Res 36(Database issue):D339–D343. https://doi.org/10.1093/nar/gkm700

Polvi A, Linnankivi T, Kivela T, Herva R, Keating JP, Makitie O, Pareyson D, Vainionpaa L, Lahtinen J, Hovatta I, Pihko H, Lehesjoki AE (2012) Mutations in CTC1, encoding the CTS telomere maintenance complex component 1, cause cerebroretinal microangiopathy with calcifications and cysts. Am J Hum Genet 90(3):540–549. https://doi.org/10.1016/j.ajhg.2012.02.002

Rashid R, Liang B, Baker DL, Youssef OA, He Y, Phipps K, Terns RM, Terns MP, Li H (2006) Crystal structure of a Cbf5-Nop10-Gar1 complex and implications in RNA-guided pseudouridylation and dyskeratosis congenita. Mol Cell 21(2):249–260. https://doi.org/10.1016/j.molcel.2005.11.017

Revesz T, Fletcher S, al-Gazali LI, DeBuse P (1992) Bilateral retinopathy, aplastic anaemia, and central nervous system abnormalities: a new syndrome? J Med Genet 29(9):673–675

Rice C, Skordalakes E (2016) Structure and function of the telomeric CST complex. Comput Struct Biotechnol J 14:161–167. https://doi.org/10.1016/j.csbj.2016.04.002

Richard P, Kiss AM, Darzacq X, Kiss T (2006) Cotranscriptional recognition of human intronic box H/ACA snoRNAs occurs in a splicing-independent manner. Mol Cell Biol 26(7):2540–2549. https://doi.org/10.1128/MCB.26.7.2540-2549.2006

Riyaz A, Riyaz N, Jayakrishnan MP, Mohamed Shiras PT, Ajith Kumar VT, Ajith BS (2007) Revesz syndrome. Indian J Pediatr 74(9):862–863

Robart AR, Collins K (2010) Investigation of human telomerase holoenzyme assembly, activity, and processivity using disease-linked subunit variants. J Biol Chem 285(7):4375–4386. https://doi.org/10.1074/jbc.M109.088575 M109.088575 [pii]

Ruggero D, Grisendi S, Piazza F, Rego E, Mari F, Rao PH, Cordon-Cardo C, Pandolfi PP (2003) Dyskeratosis congenita and cancer in mice deficient in ribosomal RNA modification. Science 299(5604): 259–262

Sarek G, Vannier JB, Panier S, Petrini JH, Boulton SJ (2015) TRF2 recruits RTEL1 to telomeres in S phase to promote t-loop unwinding. Mol Cell 57(4):622–635. https://doi.org/10.1016/j.molcel.2014.12.024

Sasa GS, Ribes-Zamora A, Nelson ND, Bertuch AA (2012) Three novel truncating TINF2 mutations causing severe dyskeratosis congenita in early childhood. Clin Genet 81(5):470–478. https://doi.org/10.1111/j.1399-0004.2011.01658.x

Savage SA, Giri N, Baerlocher GM, Orr N, Lansdorp PM, Alter BP (2008) TINF2, a component of the shelterin telomere protection complex, is mutated in dyskeratosis congenita. Am J Hum Genet 82(2):501–509

Scheinfeld MH, Lui YW, Kolb EA, Engel HM, Gomes WA, Weidenheim KM, Bello JA (2007) The neuroradiological findings in a case of Revesz syndrome. Pediatr Radiol 37(11):1166–1170. https://doi.org/10.1007/s00247-007-0592-0

Schertzer M, Jouravleva K, Perderiset M, Dingli F, Loew D, Le Guen T, Bardoni B, de Villartay JP, Revy P, Londono-Vallejo A (2015) Human regulator of telomere elongation helicase 1 (RTEL1) is required for the nuclear and cytoplasmic trafficking of pre-U2 RNA. Nucleic Acids Res 43(3):1834–1847. https://doi.org/10.1093/nar/gku1402

Sharma A, Myers K, Ye Z, D'Orazio J (2014) Dyskeratosis congenita caused by a novel TERT point mutation in siblings with pancytopenia and exudative retinopathy. Pediatr Blood Cancer 61:2302. https://doi.org/10.1002/pbc.25161

Shukla S, Schmidt JC, Goldfarb KC, Cech TR, Parker R (2016) Inhibition of telomerase RNA decay rescues telomerase deficiency caused by dyskerin or PARN defects. Nat Struct Mol Biol 23(4):286–292. https://doi.org/10.1038/nsmb.3184

Silhan LL, Shah PD, Chambers DC, Snyder LD, Riise GC, Wagner CL, Hellstrom-Lindberg E, Orens JB, Mewton JF, Danoff SK, Arcasoy MO, Armanios M (2014) Lung transplantation in telomerase mutation carriers with pulmonary fibrosis. Eur Respir J 44(1):178–187. https://doi.org/10.1183/09031936.00060014

Simon AJ, Lev A, Zhang Y, Weiss B, Rylova A, Eyal E, Kol N, Barel O, Cesarkas K, Soudack M, Greenberg-Kushnir N, Rhodes M, Wiest DL, Schiby G, Barshack I, Katz S, Pras E, Poran H, Reznik-Wolf H, Ribakovsky E, Simon C, Hazou W, Sidi Y, Lahad A, Katzir H, Sagie S, Aqeilan HA, Glousker G, Amariglio N, Tzfati Y, Selig S, Rechavi G, Somech R (2016) Mutations in STN1 cause Coats plus syndrome and are associated with genomic and telomere defects. J Exp Med 213(8):1429–1440. https://doi.org/10.1084/jem.20151618

Singh A, Pandey VK, Tandon M, Pandey CK (2015) Dyskeratosis congenita induced cirrhosis for liver transplantation-perioperative management. Indian J Anaesth 59(5):312–314. https://doi.org/10.4103/0019-5049.156888

Stanley SE, Gable DL, Wagner CL, Carlile TM, Hanumanthu VS, Podlevsky JD, Khalil SE, DeZern AE, Rojas-Duran MF, Applegate CD, Alder JK, Parry EM, Gilbert WV, Armanios M (2016) Loss-of-function mutations in the RNA biogenesis factor NAF1 predispose to pulmonary fibrosis-emphysema. Sci Transl Med 8(351):351ra107. https://doi.org/10.1126/scitranslmed.aaf7837

Stuart BD, Choi J, Zaidi S, Xing C, Holohan B, Chen R, Choi M, Dharwadkar P, Torres F, Girod CE, Weissler J, Fitzgerald J, Kershaw C, Klesney-Tait J, Mageto Y, Shay JW, Ji W, Bilguvar K, Mane S, Lifton RP, Garcia CK (2015) Exome sequencing links mutations in PARN and RTEL1 with familial pulmonary fibrosis and telomere shortening. Nat Genet 47(5):512–517. https://doi.org/10.1038/ng.3278

Sznajer Y, Baumann C, David A, Journel H, Lacombe D, Perel Y, Blouin P, Segura JF, Cezard JP, Peuchmaur M, Vulliamy T, Dokal I, Verloes A (2003) Further delineation of the congenital form of X-linked dyskeratosis congenita (Hoyeraal-Hreidarsson syndrome). Eur J Pediatr 162(12):863–867. https://doi.org/10.1007/s00431-003-1317-5

Takai H, Jenkinson E, Kabir S, Babul-Hirji R, Najm-Tehrani N, Chitayat DA, Crow YJ, de Lange T (2016) A POT1 mutation implicates defective telomere end fill-in and telomere truncations in Coats plus. Genes Dev 30(7):812–826. https://doi.org/10.1101/gad.276873.115

Thumati NR, Zeng XL, Au HH, Jang CJ, Jan E, Wong JM (2013) Severity of X-linked dyskeratosis congenita

(DKCX) cellular defects is not directly related to dyskerin (DKC1) activity in ribosomal RNA biogenesis or mRNA translation. Hum Mutat 34(12):1698–1707. https://doi.org/10.1002/humu.22447

Tokman S, Singer JP, Devine MS, Westall GP, Aubert JD, Tamm M, Snell GI, Lee JS, Goldberg HJ, Kukreja J, Golden JA, Leard LE, Garcia CK, Hays SR (2015) Clinical outcomes of lung transplant recipients with telomerase mutations. J Heart Lung Transplant 34(10):1318–1324. https://doi.org/10.1016/j.healun.2015.05.002

Tomlinson RL, Ziegler TD, Supakorndej T, Terns RM, Terns MP (2006) Cell cycle-regulated trafficking of human telomerase to telomeres. Mol Biol Cell 17(2):955–965. https://doi.org/10.1091/mbc.E05-09-0903 E05-09-0903 [pii]

Tomlinson RL, Abreu EB, Ziegler T, Ly H, Counter CM, Terns RM, Terns MP (2008) Telomerase reverse transcriptase is required for the localization of telomerase RNA to cajal bodies and telomeres in human cancer cells. Mol Biol Cell 19(9):3793–3800. https://doi.org/10.1091/mbc.E08-02-0184

Touzot F, Gaillard L, Vasquez N, Le Guen T, Bertrand Y, Bourhis J, Leblanc T, Fischer A, Soulier J, de Villartay JP, Revy P (2012) Heterogeneous telomere defects in patients with severe forms of dyskeratosis congenita. J Allergy Clin Immunol 129(2):473–482, 482 e471–473. https://doi.org/10.1016/j.jaci.2011.09.043

Townsley DM, Dumitriu B, Liu D, Biancotto A, Weinstein B, Chen C, Hardy N, Mihalek AD, Lingala S, Kim YJ, Yao J, Jones E, Gochuico BR, Heller T, Wu CO, Calado RT, Scheinberg P, Young NS (2016) Danazol treatment for telomere diseases. N Engl J Med 374(20):1922–1931. https://doi.org/10.1056/NEJMoa1515319

Trahan C, Martel C, Dragon F (2010) Effects of dyskeratosis congenita mutations in dyskerin, NHP2 and NOP10 on assembly of H/ACA pre-RNPs. Hum Mol Genet 19(5):825–836. https://doi.org/10.1093/hmg/ddp551 ddp551 [pii]

Tsakiri KD, Cronkhite JT, Kuan PJ, Xing C, Raghu G, Weissler JC, Rosenblatt RL, Shay JW, Garcia CK (2007) Adult-onset pulmonary fibrosis caused by mutations in telomerase. Proc Natl Acad Sci U S A 104(18):7552–7557

Tsangaris E, Klaassen R, Fernandez CV, Yanofsky R, Shereck E, Champagne J, Silva M, Lipton JH, Brossard J, Michon B, Abish S, Steele M, Ali K, Dower N, Athale U, Jardine L, Hand JP, Odame I, Canning P, Allen C, Carcao M, Beyene J, Roifman CM, Dror Y (2011) Genetic analysis of inherited bone marrow failure syndromes from one prospective, comprehensive and population-based cohort and identification of novel mutations. J Med Genet 48(9):618–628. https://doi.org/10.1136/jmg.2011.089821

Tseng CK, Wang HF, Burns AM, Schroeder MR, Gaspari M, Baumann P (2015) Human telomerase RNA processing and quality control. Cell Rep 13(10):2232–2243. https://doi.org/10.1016/j.celrep.2015.10.075

Tsilou ET, Giri N, Weinstein S, Mueller C, Savage SA, Alter BP (2010) Ocular and orbital manifestations of the inherited bone marrow failure syndromes: Fanconi anemia and dyskeratosis congenita. Ophthalmology 117(3):615–622. https://doi.org/10.1016/j.ophtha.2009.08.023

Tummala H, Walne A, Collopy L, Cardoso S, de la Fuente J, Lawson S, Powell J, Cooper N, Foster A, Mohammed S, Plagnol V, Vulliamy T, Dokal I (2015) Poly(A)-specific ribonuclease deficiency impacts telomere biology and causes dyskeratosis congenita. J Clin Invest 125(5):2151–2160. https://doi.org/10.1172/JCI78963

Vannier JB, Pavicic-Kaltenbrunner V, Petalcorin MI, Ding H, Boulton SJ (2012) RTEL1 dismantles T loops and counteracts telomeric G4-DNA to maintain telomere integrity. Cell 149(4):795–806. https://doi.org/10.1016/j.cell.2012.03.030

Vannier JB, Sandhu S, Petalcorin MI, Wu X, Nabi Z, Ding H, Boulton SJ (2013) RTEL1 is a replisome-associated helicase that promotes telomere and genome-wide replication. Science 342(6155):239–242. https://doi.org/10.1126/science.1241779

Venteicher AS, Abreu EB, Meng Z, McCann KE, Terns RM, Veenstra TD, Terns MP, Artandi SE (2009) A human telomerase holoenzyme protein required for Cajal body localization and telomere synthesis. Science 323(5914):644–648. https://doi.org/10.1126/science.1165357.323/5914/644

Vulliamy T, Marrone A, Goldman F, Dearlove A, Bessler M, Mason PJ, Dokal I (2001) The RNA component of telomerase is mutated in autosomal dominant dyskeratosis congenita. Nature 413(6854):432–435

Vulliamy T, Marrone A, Szydlo R, Walne A, Mason PJ, Dokal I (2004) Disease anticipation is associated with progressive telomere shortening in families with dyskeratosis congenita due to mutations in TERC. Nat Genet 36(5):447–449

Vulliamy TJ, Walne A, Baskaradas A, Mason PJ, Marrone A, Dokal I (2005) Mutations in the reverse transcriptase component of telomerase (TERT) in patients with bone marrow failure. Blood Cells Mol Dis 34(3):257–263. https://doi.org/10.1016/j.bcmd.2004.12.008 S1079-9796(05)00030-6 [pii]

Vulliamy T, Beswick R, Kirwan M, Marrone A, Digweed M, Walne A, Dokal I (2008) Mutations in the telomerase component NHP2 cause the premature ageing syndrome dyskeratosis congenita. Proc Natl Acad Sci U S A 105(23):8073–8078

Walne AJ, Marrone A, Dokal I (2005) Dyskeratosis congenita: a disorder of defective telomere maintenance? Int J Hematol 82(3):184–189. https://doi.org/10.1532/IJH97.05067

Walne AJ, Vulliamy T, Marrone A, Beswick R, Kirwan M, Masunari Y, Al-Qurashi FH, Aljurf M, Dokal I (2007) Genetic heterogeneity in autosomal recessive dyskeratosis congenita with one subtype due to mutations in the telomerase-associated protein NOP10. Hum Mol Genet 16(13):1619–1629

Walne AJ, Vulliamy T, Beswick R, Kirwan M, Dokal I (2008) TINF2 mutations result in very short telomeres:

analysis of a large cohort of patients with dyskeratosis congenita and related bone marrow failure syndromes. Blood 112(9):3594–3600

Walne A, Bhagat T, Kirwan M, Gitaux C, Desguerre I, Leonard N, Nogales E, Vulliamy T, Dokal I (2012) Mutations in the telomere capping complex in bone marrow failure and related syndromes. Haematologica 98:334. https://doi.org/10.3324/haematol.2012.071068

Walne AJ, Vulliamy T, Kirwan M, Plagnol V, Dokal I (2013) Constitutional mutations in RTEL1 cause severe dyskeratosis congenita. Am J Hum Genet 92(3):448–453. https://doi.org/10.1016/j.ajhg.2013.02.001

Wang C, Meier UT (2004) Architecture and assembly of mammalian H/ACA small nucleolar and telomerase ribonucleoproteins. EMBO J 23(8):1857–1867. https://doi.org/10.1038/sj.emboj.7600181

Wang F, Podell ER, Zaug AJ, Yang Y, Baciu P, Cech TR, Lei M (2007) The POT1-TPP1 telomere complex is a telomerase processivity factor. Nature 445(7127):506–510

Watson JD (1972) Origin of concatemeric T7 DNA. Nat New Biol 239:197–201

Wong JM, Collins K (2006) Telomerase RNA level limits telomere maintenance in X-linked dyskeratosis congenita. Genes Dev 20(20):2848–2858

Wong JM, Kyasa MJ, Hutchins L, Collins K (2004) Telomerase RNA deficiency in peripheral blood mononuclear cells in X-linked dyskeratosis congenita. Hum Genet 115(5):448–455. https://doi.org/10.1007/s00439-004-1178-7

Xin H, Liu D, Wan M, Safari A, Kim H, Sun W, O'Connor MS, Songyang Z (2007) TPP1 is a homologue of ciliate TEBP-beta and interacts with POT1 to recruit telomerase. Nature 445(7127):559–562. https://doi.org/10.1038/nature05469

Yaghmai R, Kimyai-Asadi A, Rostamiani K, Heiss NS, Poustka A, Eyaid W, Bodurtha J, Nousari HC, Hamosh A, Metzenberg A (2000) Overlap of dyskeratosis congenita with the Hoyeraal-Hreidarsson syndrome. J Pediatr 136(3):390–393. https://doi.org/10.1067/mpd.2000.104295 S0022-3476(00)09009-0 [pii]

Yamaguchi H, Baerlocher GM, Lansdorp PM, Chanock SJ, Nunez O, Sloand E, Young NS (2003) Mutations of the human telomerase RNA gene (TERC) in aplastic anemia and myelodysplastic syndrome. Blood 102(3):916–918. https://doi.org/10.1182/blood-2003-01-0335 2003-01-0335 [pii]

Yamaguchi H, Calado RT, Ly H, Kajigaya S, Baerlocher GM, Chanock SJ, Lansdorp PM, Young NS (2005) Mutations in TERT, the gene for telomerase reverse transcriptase, in aplastic anemia. N Engl J Med 352(14):1413–1424. https://doi.org/10.1056/NEJMoa042980.352/14/1413

Yang D, He Q, Kim H, Ma W, Songyang Z (2011) TIN2 protein dyskeratosis congenita missense mutants are defective in association with telomerase. J Biol Chem 286(26):23022–23030. https://doi.org/10.1074/jbc.M111.225870

Zaug AJ, Crary SM, Jesse Fioravanti M, Campbell K, Cech TR (2013) Many disease-associated variants of hTERT retain high telomerase enzymatic activity. Nucleic Acids Res 41(19):8969–8978. https://doi.org/10.1093/nar/gkt653

Zhong F, Savage SA, Shkreli M, Giri N, Jessop L, Myers T, Chen R, Alter BP, Artandi SE (2011) Disruption of telomerase trafficking by TCAB1 mutation causes dyskeratosis congenita. Genes Dev 25(1):11–16. https://doi.org/10.1101/gad.2006411.25/1/11

Zhong FL, Batista LF, Freund A, Pech MF, Venteicher AS, Artandi SE (2012) TPP1 OB-fold domain controls telomere maintenance by recruiting telomerase to chromosome ends. Cell 150(3):481–494. https://doi.org/10.1016/j.cell.2012.07.012

Zhu Y, Tomlinson RL, Lukowiak AA, Terns RM, Terns MP (2004) Telomerase RNA accumulates in Cajal bodies in human cancer cells. Mol Biol Cell 15(1):81–90. https://doi.org/10.1091/mbc.E03-07-0525

Diamond-Blackfan Anemia

7

Shilpa M. Hattangadi and Jeffrey M. Lipton

Contents

7.1 Introduction

Diamond-Blackfan anemia (DBA) is a rare inherited hypoplastic anemia that usually presents in early infancy. It was first reported by Josephs (1936) and defined as a distinct clinical entity by Diamond and Blackfan (1938). DBA is characterized by a severe macrocytic anemia, reticulocytopenia, and a normocellular bone marrow with a paucity of erythroid precursors.

Clinically, DBA is primarily defined by the failure of terminal erythroid differentiation, but patients also frequently display numerous physical anomalies including short stature and a predisposition to malignancy. DBA has an incidence of approximately 5–10 cases per million live births with no ethnic or gender preference (except for very rare instances of X-linked recessive inheritance) (Vlachos et al. 2008, 2014). Because it is so rare, most of our understand-

S. M. Hattangadi (✉)
Yale Cooperative Center for Excellence in Molecular Hematology, Yale University School of Medicine, New Haven, CT, USA

Pediatric Hematology-Oncology, Yale University School of Medicine, New Haven, CT, USA
e-mail: Shilpa.hattangadi@yale.edu

J. M. Lipton
Division of Hematology/Oncology and Stem Cell Transplantation, Cohen Children's Medical Center of New York, New Hyde Park, NY, USA

The Feinstein Institute for Medical Research, Manhasset, NY, USA

Hofstra North Shore-LIJ School of Medicine, Hempstead, NY, USA
e-mail: jlipton@northwell.edu

G. M. Kupfer et al. (eds.), *Bone Marrow Failure*, Pediatric Oncology,
https://doi.org/10.1007/978-3-319-61421-2_7

ing of the disease thus far has come from patient registries from North America, France, England, and Italy (reviewed in (Shimamura and Alter 2010)). Classically, patients present in the first year of life (median age of diagnosis is 8 weeks of life) with a profound red cell aplasia, macrocytic anemia with reticulocytopenia, and absent or reduced erythroid precursors on bone marrow examination. Rarely the anemia can present in utero, and, since the identification of causative genes and an improved awareness of the disorder, cases are more frequently being identified in adulthood (Vlachos et al. 2014; Lipton et al. 2006).

Although red cell aplasia is the hallmark of DBA, the misappellation Diamond-Blackfan **anemia** would preferably be described as Diamond-Blackfan **syndrome**, because in addition to the hematologic abnormalities, birth defects and growth retardation are frequent features of the disorder. About half of patients with DBA have one congenital anomaly and 25% have two or more (Clinton and Gazda 1993). In fact, in a significant minority of instances, the physical anomaly is the presenting manifestation of the disorder while the anemia is mild or develops later or not at all (also called "non-classic" DBA). The most common physical abnormalities in DBA are craniofacial, thumb, and cardiac or genitourinary defects (Table 7.1, compiled from (Vlachos et al. 2008; Shimamura and Alter 2010; Lipton et al. 2006; Bagby et al. 2004; Vlachos and Muir 2010)). Short stature is also a constitutional feature of the disease that can be exacerbated by early and/or excessive glucocorticoid (GC) therapy, iron overload, and chronic anemia. Intrauterine growth retardation (IUGR) is also found in about 25% of patients, and there is minimal catch-up growth after birth (Vlachos et al. 2008). The major diagnostic criteria of DBA are anemia (often severe), macrocytosis, reticulocytopenia, and absent or decreased mature erythroid precursors in the bone marrow (Table 7.2, from Vlachos et al. (2008)). Elevated erythrocyte adenosine deaminase (eADA) activity is characteristic of DBA erythropoiesis and is found in around 85% of patients. Macrocytosis can be masked by concomitant iron deficiency or thalassemia trait.

Table 7.1 Prevalence and range of congenital anomalies found in DBA (compiled from Vlachos et al. (2008), Shimamura and Alter (2010), Lipton et al. (2006), Bagby et al. (2004), Vlachos and Muir (2010))

Craniofacial	4–50%	Cleft palate
		Cleft lip (0.2%)
		Hypertelorism
		Broad flat nasal bridge
		Microcephaly
		Micrognathia
		Hydrocephalus
		Microtia
		Low-set ears
		Low hairline
Abnormal thumbs	8–38%	Triphalangeal
		Duplex or bifid
		Hypoplastic
		Flat thenar muscles
		Subluxed
		Absent radial artery
Growth retardation	13–30%	Short stature
		Low birth weight (5–25%)
Genitourinary	3–19%	Absent kidney
		Horseshoe kidney
		Hypospadias
		Ectopic kidney/ureters
		Undescended testes
		Inguinal hernia
Cardiac	3–15%	Ventricular septal defect
		Atrial septal defect
		Tetralogy of Fallot
		Pulmonary stenosis
Ophthalmological	5%	Small epicanthal folds
		Hypotelorism
		Strabismus
		Congenital cataract
		Congenital glaucoma
Neck	2%	Short neck
		Webbed neck
		Sprengel deformity
		Klippel-Feil deformity
Central nervous system	2%	Developmental delay
		Hypopituitary
		Chiari malformation
		Myelomeningocele

Table 7.2 Diagnostic criteria of DBA (from Vlachos et al. (2008))

Diagnostic criteria
Age <1 year
Macrocytic anemia with no other cytopenias present
Reticulocytopenia
Normal bone marrow cellularity with paucity of erythroid precursors
Supporting criteria
Major
Gene mutation in literature associated with "classical" DBA
Positive family history
Congenital anomalies associated with "classical" DBA
Minor
Elevated erythrocyte adenosine deaminase activity
Elevated Hgb F level
No evidence of another inherited bone marrow failure syndrome

Moreover, macrocytosis, fetal hemoglobin levels, and elevated eADA activity are obscured in DBA patients undergoing red cell transfusion for severe anemia prior to hematologic evaluation.

An important observation is that patients with DBA who share the same allelic *RP* gene mutation may have very discordant hematologic and non-hematologic manifestations of DBA. Furthermore incomplete penetrance and variable expression in multiplex families is characteristic of the disorder. Parents and siblings of an affected patient who carry the pathogenic mutation may have elevated eADA activity, with or without macrocytosis in the absence of anemia ("non-classic" DBA). In some family members, the anemia may be transient while elevated eADA activity and macrocytosis persist long after the anemia resolves. In addition, it is reported that approximately 20% of all DBA patients undergo remission from either steroid or transfusion dependence even after years of steroid or transfusion dependence. These remissions are long-lived though about 15% of these patients "relapse." Neutrophil counts are generally normal, but there are instances of concomitant neutropenia and thrombocytopenia in patients with mutations in *RPL35a* and *GATA1*, respectively, and occasionally in other genotypes. Rarely DBA can progress to frank aplastic anemia with involvement of all three lineages. And while bone marrow examination generally reveals normal cellularity with a paucity of erythroid precursors and normal myeloid precursors and megakaryocytes, bone marrow cellularity decreases disproportionately with age compared to normal individuals (Giri et al. 2000). Erythroid colony size, number, and maturation obtained from bone marrow precursors are impaired (Lipton et al. 1986). The rate of apoptosis in erythroid progenitor cell cultures from patients with DBA is increased and accentuated after erythropoietin (Epo) deprivation (Perdahl et al. 1994), and although somewhat debatable as to degree, accelerated apoptosis is a salient feature of the DBA erythron (Lipton and Ellis 2009).

7.2 Pathophysiology and Genetics

DBA is most often inherited in an autosomal dominant manner with incomplete penetrance, but there are also more rare X-linked forms of the disorder. A majority of sporadic cases are new dominant variants. Pathogenic mutations in 18 genes have thus far been confirmed in about 65–70% of patients with DBA (Vlachos et al. 2014; Clinton and Gazda 1993): 16 genes encoding ribosomal proteins and 2 non-ribosomal genes, *GATA1* (Sankaran et al. 2012) and *TSR2* (Mercurio et al. 2016). Study of the pathogenesis of DBA has since helped to define a class of inherited bone marrow failure syndromes (IBMFS) referred to as "ribosomopathies" (Chap. 5). Understanding DBA as a disorder of ribosome biogenesis and function still begs the question of how defects in such a fundamental and ubiquitous process as translation cause a fairly limited distribution of distinctly tissue-specific phenotypes, specifically red cell aplasia, developmental abnormalities, and cancer predisposition.

The first gene encoding a ribosomal protein to be implicated in DBA, the *RPS19* gene at 19q13.2, identified through a serendipitous translocation (Draptchinskaia et al. 1999), is coincidentally the most common with a quarter of patients with DBA having abnormalities in *RPS19*. Since that discovery, with the advent of newer single nucleotide polymorphism (SNP)-based or quantitative polymerase chain (qPCR)-based copy number variation assays as well as whole exome sequencing (WES) techniques, pathogenic variants have been identified in 16 ribosomal genes encoding either the small 40S subunit ribosomal proteins RPS7, RPS10, RPS17, RPS19, RPS24, RPS26, RPS27, RPS28, or RPS29 or the large 60S subunit ribosomal proteins RPL5, RPL11, RPL15, RPL26, RPL27, RPL31, or RPL35A, and in *GATA1* and *TSR2* (reviewed in Clinton and Gazda (1993)). Others are being reported and need to be confirmed. Most are missense or nonsense mutations but deletions are also reported. Haploinsufficiency of any of the ribosomal subunit-associated proteins in mammalian cells interferes with normal ribosome assembly (O'Donohue et al. 2010). Excess free ribosomal proteins redirected to the nucleus lead to nucleolar stress, which in turn lead to p53 activation and programmed demise of the erythron. But this is likely not the entire story.

Mutations in genes encoding ribosomal proteins in DBA are always heterozygous (homozygosity likely being incompatible with life), supporting that haploinsufficiency of these proteins is sufficient to cause the phenotype, but phenotypes do vary depending upon the particular gene involved. Thus the phenotype of affected patients with varied mutations may share the aregenerative macrocytic anemia, the short stature, and the increased risk of malignancy, but particular physical anomalies are associated with specific genes. For example, orofacial anomalies such as cleft palate were more common in patients with *RPL5* and *RPS26* and other rare mutations than those with pathogenic variants in *RPL11* and *RPS19* (Gazda et al. 2008; Quarello et al. 2010; Cmejla et al. 2009; Gripp et al. 2014). Pathogenic variants in *RPL11* were predominantly associated with isolated thumb abnormalities (Clinton and Gazda 1993; Gazda et al. 2008). In vitro studies have only made the genotype-phenotype correlation appear more complex; recent work by Moniz and colleagues found that even the extent of apoptosis and cell cycle arrest in erythroid progenitors from patients with either RPL11 or RPS19 haploinsufficiency was distinct. Murine studies support these data showing discrete cell cycle abnormalities in rpl5 ± embryonic stem (ES) cells absent in rps19 ± ES cells (Singh et al. 2014). In addition patients with RPL35a haploinsufficiency tend to be neutropenic as well as anemic (Farrar et al. 2008). And while there is quite variable expression and penetrance of *RP* genes associated with DBA and there are some clear genotype-phenotype correlations, these are remarkably rare with no apparent correlations with important phenotypes such as steroid responsiveness, remission, and cancer predisposition (Vlachos et al. 2012).

The association of RP haploinsufficiency and red cell failure is not restricted to patients with DBA-associated germline mutations. Patients with a subtype of myelodysplastic syndrome (MDS) called del(5q) syndrome have a single cytogenetic abnormality in the form of deletion of the long arm of chromosome 5 and present with a syndrome resembling "acquired" DBA with severe macrocytic anemia, thrombocytosis, and a lower rate of progression to acute myeloid leukemia (AML) than other subtypes of MDS. Interestingly, an RNA interference screen targeting each gene in the deleted 5q region revealed that knockdown of RPS14 recapitulates the erythroid defect characterizing del(5q) syndrome (Ebert et al. 2008a). And although patients with del(5q) MD generally present in late adulthood and have no physical anomalies, cases presenting in childhood and adolescence that mimic non-classical DBA have also been described (Vlachos et al. 2013).

Most recently, pathogenic mutations were discovered in two non-ribosomal genes with distinct DBA phenotypes. In two unrelated families with mandibulofacial dysostosis (MFD) suggestive of Treacher-Collins syndrome (TCS) and a macrocytic anemia diagnostic of DBA (Gripp et al. 2014), an X-linked mutation was found in TSR2, a direct binding partner of the ribosomal protein RPS26. Two male siblings with DBA without physical defects were discovered to have an X-linked mutation at a splicing site in *GATA1*, a master erythroid transcription factor (Sankaran et al. 2012). While these subtle phenotypic differences along with lack of ribosomal protein gene mutations with autosomal dominant inheritance may place these patients in a category outside "classical" DBA, they are typical of non-classical presentations in patients with RP haploinsufficiency. A better understanding of the phenotype-genotype correlation may help us develop more precise categories for DBA patients that can guide improved diagnostic and treatment strategies in the future as well.

Our understanding of the molecular pathophysiology of DBA was hindered for a long time by the lack of animal models for the disease. Although mouse and fish models do not fully recapitulate the clinical syndrome, advances in mouse and zebrafish models have shed light on the complexities differentiating the intrinsic cellular defects causing erythroid progenitor apoptosis from that causing physical anomalies. While the homozygous *Rps19* knockout mouse was embryonic lethal (Matsson et al. 2004), a novel mouse model where *Rps19* is downregulated using the inducible transgenic expression of *Rps19* shRNA resulted in a DBA-like phenotype with macrocytic anemia culminating in bone marrow failure. The hematopoietic defect was rescued by both expression of *Rps19* and inactivation of p53 (Jaako et al. 2011). A murine model of the del(5q) syndrome was recapitulated by conditionally deleting a DNA region similar to the 5q region of humans (including Rps14) from hematopoietic stem cells (Barlow et al. 2010). Heterozygous loss of this region resulted in the macrocytic anemia and erythroid and megakaryocytic dysplasia indicative of the disease in humans. Mice with defects in *Rps19*, *Rps20*, *Rps24*, and *Rpl38* also have growth defects in addition to the hematopoietic phenotypes (Raiser et al. 2014).

Zebrafish have also proven to be a useful tool in the understanding of the pathophysiology of DBA. Specifically, zebrafish models of DBA lacking Rpl11 or Rps19 show developmental defects and failed terminal erythropoiesis (Jaako et al. 2011; Chakraborty et al. 2009). Rps14 loss in zebrafish resulted in animals with a profound anemia and developmental defects like short body length, defective bronchial arch development, and brain and cardiac edema (Payne et al. 2012), and notably the anemia was alleviated with L-leucine treatment (an activator of mRNA translation). While p53-depletion rescues the physical defects in these fish, supporting that p53 stabilization is central to the proapoptotic phenotype induced by nucleosomal stress, the erythropoietic defects appear to be p53 independent (Torihara et al. 2011; Yadav et al. 2014). On the other hand, both the physical and erythroid defects in Rpl35-deficient zebrafish are ameliorated after stimulating the mTOR pathway with leucine or arginine treatments, suggesting that improved protein translation even with reduced numbers of functional ribosomes by activating the mTOR pathway may be crucial and offering a potential new treatment strategy as well. A human trial of L-leucine in DBA is ongoing.

This leads to two main hypotheses as to the mechanisms underlying the apoptosis of erythroid progenitors. The first mechanism is the paradigm above, namely, defective ribosome assembly results in free ribosomal proteins, which return to the nucleosome and lead to nucleolar stress, which then induces p53-*dependent* apoptosis. The principle mechanism linking nucleolar disruption with p53 activation and subsequent cell cycle arrest is through human double minute 2 (HDM2, MDM2 in mice), the ubiquitous E3 ligase that negatively regulates p53 by targeting it for degradation (James et al. 2014). Free ribosomal proteins and ribosome assembly factors like can bind to MDM2 and prevent its binding to p53 (Fig. 7.1). The second mechanism is that insufficient ribosomes resulting from ribosome protein haploinsufficiency could prevent the normal translation of erythroid-important proteins. Insufficient globin protein, for example, would disrupt the tight heme-globin balance necessary during the vast production of hemoglobin, as its disruption results in excess free heme, normally bound in complex with globins. Free heme is known to induce oxidative stress, which can then lead to 53-*independent* apoptosis. Both mechanisms assume that erythroid progenitors (or progenitors from those tissues showing developmental defects in DBA) are more sensitive to loss of functional ribosomes than those in other organs. This may be true for erythroid cells, given that erythroblasts have a rapid proliferation rate and an especially high demand for protein translation for coordinated hemoglobin production (Lajtha and Oliver 1961).

Scientific evidence supports the second hypothesis as well. Free excess heme can lead to apoptosis in erythroid precursors, and the heme exporter FLVCR1 was found to export cytoplasmic heme from these cells (Quigley et al. 2004). Conditional loss of the FLVCR exporter in neonates resulted in a macrocytic anemia in mice similar to that seen in human ribosomopathies. The FLVCR-null mice died in mid-gestation but displayed craniofacial and limb abnormali-

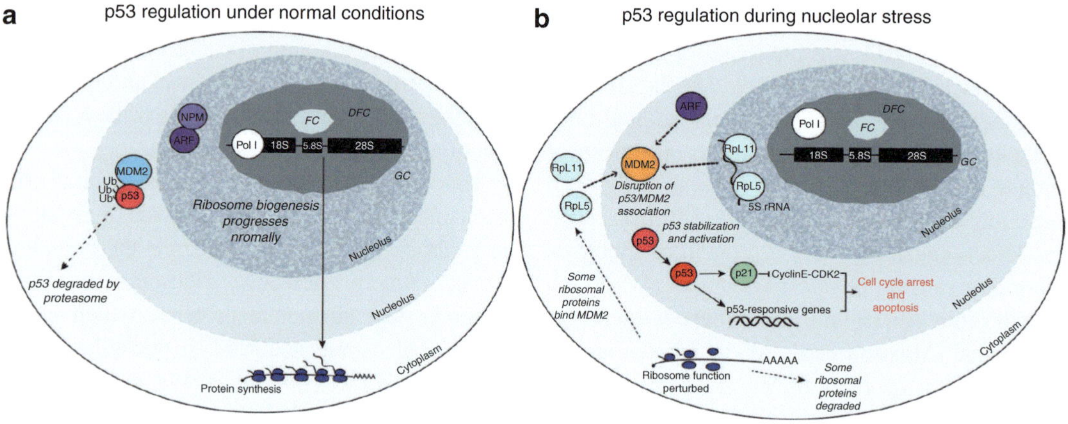

Fig. 7.1 Regulation of p53 during nucleolar stress conditions (adapted from James et al. (2014)). (**a**) During normal, non-stressed conditions, the E3 ubiquitin ligase MDM2 associates with p53, promoting p53's degradation (Brooks and Gu 2006). (**b**) During nucleolar stress, normal ribosome biogenesis and function are perturbed. The normal association between MDM2 and p53 is disrupted; additional proteins such as ribosomal proteins (RpL5, RpL11) with the 5S rRNA (Sloan et al. 2013; Donati et al. 2013) and Arf can associate with MDM2 (Llanos et al. 2001). p53 is stabilized and activates the cell cycle inhibitor p21 and other p53-responsive genes. These events lead to cell cycle arrest and apoptosis

ties similar to DBA as well (Keel et al. 2008). Interestingly, late erythroid cells from DBA patients showed alternatively spliced isoforms of FLVCR1 transcript and protein levels and function were disrupted (Rey et al. 2008). More recently, the Abkowitz group uncovered that a slow rate of globin synthesis relative to heme production occurs in cells from patients with DBA or del(5q) syndrome and that erythropoiesis fails when heme exceeds globin (Yang et al. 2016). Interestingly, the Sankaran group found that ribosomal protein haploinsufficiency resulted in decreased full-length *GATA1* mRNA translation in vitro and that GATA1 protein was globally decreased in primary hematopoietic cells from patients with mutations in RPS19 (Ludwig et al. 2014). Others (Parrella et al. 2014) confirmed that mutations in GATA1 in progenitors from DBA patients resulted in a shortened isoform of the protein, GATA-1s, indicating that the activity of GATA1 is decreased in patients with DBA and that the "defective translation" hypothesis may apply to more erythroid-important proteins than just the globins. Adding to the complexity are the observations that ribosome structure favoring some RPs over others in assembly may be tissue specific (Xue and Barna 2012) and that the translation of certain proteins by canonical cap-mediated translation is favored over IRES-mediated translation disproportionately affecting the erythron (Horos et al. 2012).

7.3 Cancer Predisposition

Patients with DBA show much variability in clinical presentation, disease severity, and response to therapy, but similar to the other inherited bone marrow failure syndromes (IBMFS) Fanconi anemia (FA) and dyskeratosis congenita (DC), DBA is also a cancer predisposition syndrome. Cancer risks appear lower in DBA than FA or DC however. In the literature, over 30 cases of cancer have been reported in close to 1000 patients with DBA (reviewed in Vlachos et al. (2008), Shimamura and Alter (2010), Lipton and Ellis (2010), Yaris et al. (2006), Alter et al. (2003)), comprised of roughly half acute myeloid leukemia (AML) or myelodysplastic syndrome (MDS) and half solid tumors including osteosarcoma. The reported proportion of approximately 4% is higher than the expected <1% for a cohort <30 years of age. The median age for cancer in these reports was 15 years (range 1–43 years), much younger than the median of 68 years in the general population (Ries et al. 2004). The majority of cancer cases were charac-

Table 7.3 Observed to expected ratios of cancers in DBA patients (from Vlachos et al. (2012a))

Cancer type	No. of observed cancers[a]	O/E ratio	95% CI
Events with significant O/E ratios			
All cancers	18[a]	5.4	3.2–8.6
Colon (adenocarcinoma)	3	36.2	7.5–105.8
Bones (osteogenic)	2	32.6	4.0–117.7
Female genital[b]	3	12.0	2.5–35.1
AML[c]	2	27.9	3.4–100.9
MDS[c]	4	287.0	77.2–734.7
Events with nonsignificant O/E ratios			
Oral cavity	1	15.9	0.4–88.3
Soft tissue sarcoma	1	9.8	0.3–54.8
Lung	1	8.3	0.2–46.4
Testis	1	8.3	0.2–46.1
Non-Hodgkin lymphoma	1	5.7	0.1–31.7
Melanoma	1	4.5	0.1–25.3
Breast	2	4.1	0.5–14.9

[a]Eighteen cancers in 17 individuals. On person had breast cancer, colon cancer, and MDS at ages 43, 49, and 51 years
[b]Female genital included cervix, uterus, and vaginal cancers
[c]MDS is not included in the other cancers. One patient had MDS followed by AML so was counted in both groups

terized by poor outcomes. Longitudinal follow-up of cohorts of DBA patients revealed that these statistics weren't so far off. The crude frequency reported from Boston Children's Hospital was 6.6% (Janov et al. 1996), a French cohort 3.8% (Willig et al. 1999), the Italian registry 0/96 (unpublished), and the National Cancer Institute's IBMFS cohort 5% (unpublished). The most recent examination of the comprehensive Diamond-Blackfan Anemia Registry of North America (DBAR) confirmed that the cancer incidence in DBA is significantly elevated (Table 7.3, from Vlachos et al. (2012)). Among 608 patients with up to 20 years of follow-up, 15 solid tumors, 2 cases of AML, and 2 cases of MDS were diagnosed at a median age of 41 years in patients who had not received a bone marrow transplant. The observed-to-expected ratio for all cancers (excluding MDS) combined was 5.4 ($p < 0.05$); significant observed-to-expected ratios were 287 for myelodysplastic syndrome, 36 for colon carcinoma, 33 for osteosarcoma, 28 for acute myeloid leukemia, and 12 for female genital cancers. The median survival was 56 years, and the cumulative incidence of cancer in DBA was approximately 20% by age 46 years. This data confirms that DBA is also a cancer predisposition syndrome and that the incidence of MDS and leukemia, in contrast to the literature, is shifted to older patients not necessarily recognized prior to the development of unbiased patient registries. Surveillance strategies must be developed even in the absence of identifiable DBA "cancer genotypes."

The mechanism of leukemogenesis in Fanconi anemia is thought to be that ongoing apoptotic hematopoiesis puts selective pressure on the myeloid lineage. Malignant clones then emerge, harboring mutations that allow them to evade cell cycle regulation and apoptosis, creating MDS and leukemia (Lensch et al. 1999). A similar mechanism could exist for malignant transformation in DBA. Previous data on the molecular pathogenesis of DBA suggests that nucleolar stress induces p53-dependent apoptosis or cell cycle arrest. Mutations in p53 or HDM2, a negative regulator of p53, could then confer a selective proliferative advantage to particular clones, favoring leukemic transformation (Lipton and Ellis 2009). Haploinsufficient ribosomal protein genes in zebrafish have been found to result in fish prone to peripheral nerve sheath tumors with marked local reduction in p53 protein expression (Amsterdam et al. 2004), suggesting that loss of p53 is essential for tumor development in ribosomopathies.

Alternative mechanisms include a more direct link between abortive ribosome biogenesis and leukemogenesis than p53-dependent regulation.

Analogous to the mechanism proposed for the erythroid specificity of DBA, aberrant ribosome biogenesis may contribute to the disrupted translation of specific transcripts and the use of alternative translation initiation sites leading to altered translation of oncogenes and tumor suppressors. In this way, the proteome of cells, with certain types of ribosome dysfunction, may promote malignant transformation (Raiser et al. 2014). With the advent of whole exome sequencing in current cancer therapy, mutations in numerous ribosomal protein genes have been found in many cancer types (Goudarzi and

Lindström 2016), suggesting that some of these may function directly as tumor suppressors. For example, mutations in ribosomal protein genes have been found in endometrial cancer (RPL22), T-cell acute lymphoblastic leukemia (RPL10, RPL5, and RPL11), chronic lymphocytic leukemia (RPS15), colorectal cancer (RPS20), and glioma (RPL5). Intriguingly, maturation of the 60S subunit was found to be a quality control (QC) checkpoint in the regulation of normal proliferation in yeast. Failure of this QC checkpoint releases structurally and functionally defective ribosomes into the translationally active pool, and the defective translational fidelity of these mutants culminated in destabilization of selected mRNAs and shortened telomeres (Sulima et al. 2014). Through compensation for their ribosomal deficits, these cells end up with changes in gene expression that ultimately undermine cellular homeostasis.

Future studies advancing our understanding of p53-dependent and p53-independent apoptotic pathways will likely reveal targets for effective cancer treatments as well as more insight into the pathogenesis of DBA.

7.4 Novel Treatment Strategies

Current mainstays of treatment are red blood cell transfusions, corticosteroid therapy, and hematopoietic stem cell transplantation (HSCT). According to the most recent DBAR report, about 80% of patients will initially respond to steroid therapy, but ultimately a third of DBA patients are transfusion dependent due usually to the inability to achieve a corticosteroid dose not leading to significant untoward effects. Chronic transfusions must be combined with iron chelation therapy to avoid iron overload leading to cardiac and liver dysfunction and premature death. The only current curative therapeutic option for the hematopoietic manifestations of DBA thus far for DBA patients is HSCT. The 3-year overall survival was found to be 64% (50–74%) upon analysis of 61 DBA patients reported to the International Bone Marrow Transplantation Registry between 1984 and 2000 (Roy et al. 2005). From the North American DBAR, as of 2009, survival for sibling HSCT performed prior to 9 years of age was 90 ± 9.5%, and those older than 9 years of age had a survival rate of 70 ± 11.6%. Survival for alternative donor transplant was 85.7 ± 13.2% since 2000 (Lipton et al. 2006). Transfusion therapy, corticosteroid therapy, and transplantation all carry a great risk of morbidity and mortality.

Over the years, numerous alternative therapies have been tried in the treatment of DBA, but few have been routinely successful (reviewed in Narla et al. (2011a)). IL-3 is known to promote cell cycle progression and survival of early erythroid progenitors and on clinical trials resulted in good response in about 10% of patients (Dunbar et al. 1991; Gillio et al. 1993; Bastion et al. 1994; Olivieri et al. 1991; Ball et al. 1995; Ganser et al. 1990). Some patients have responded to cyclosporine with (Tötterman et al. 1984; Williams et al. 1987) and without concomitant steroids (Seip and Zanussi 1988; Leonard et al. 1989; El-Beshlawy et al. 2002; Splain and Berman 1992; Monteserin et al. 1993; Alessandri et al. 2000; Bobey et al. 2003) or metoclopramide (Akiyama et al. 2005; Abkowitz et al. 2002), but the effects were mostly transient. There is a case report of a patient who developed complete remission after valproic acid treatment (Jabr et al. 2004) for seizures. Valproic acid is a histone deacetylase inhibitor and is known to induce the expression of fetal hemoglobin (Bradner et al. 2010), but given that DBA patients are known to undergo spontaneous remission, it is unknown if the putative response to valproate, reported as a single case report, was actual. The likelihood of entering remission is approximately 20% by 25 years of age (Narla et al. 2011a). Up to 17% of all patients with DBA enter remission, defined as treatment independence for at least 6 months with physiologically stable hemoglobin levels. The mechanism behind remission remains unknown, and around 15% of those who go into remission ultimately relapse (Vlachos et al. 2008; Lipton et al. 2006).

Considerable progress made in our understanding of the pathogenesis of DBA and the pathophysiology of ribosomopathies has led to

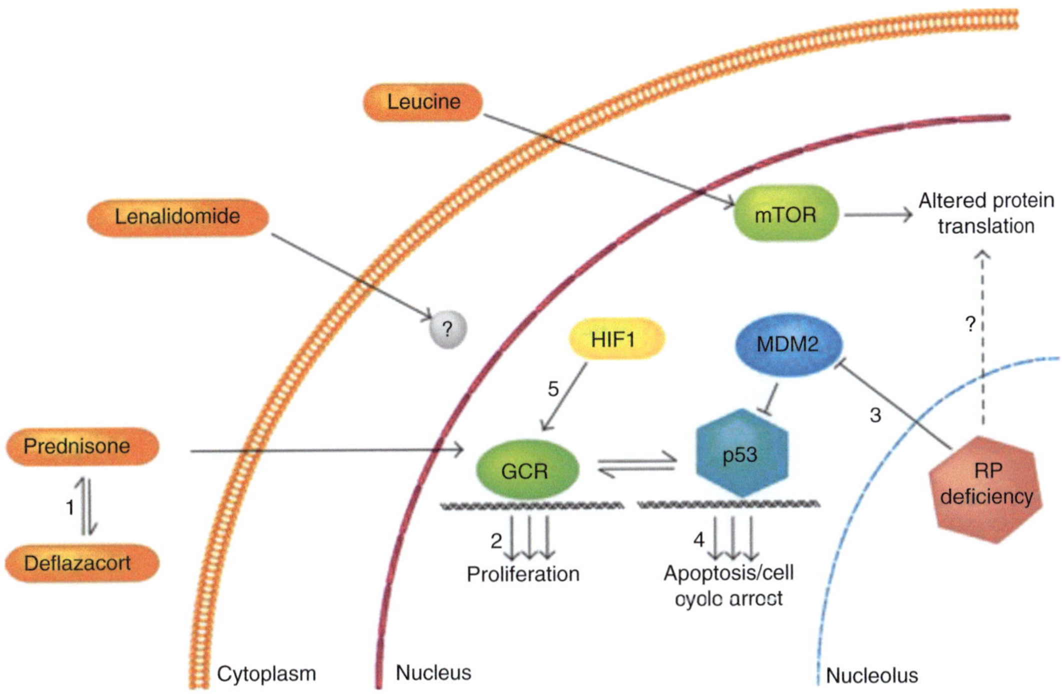

Fig. 7.2 Novel treatment strategies targeting pathways of DBA pathogenesis (adapted from Sjögren and Flygare (2012)). (1) Replacement of prednisone with a GC receptor agonist with fewer potential side effects, for example, deflazacort (DFZ). (2) Identification of genes involved in the therapeutic response to prednisone; identification of compounds that activate these genes. (3) Identification of genes and pathways involved in the mechanism by which nucleolar stress induces a p53 response. (4) Identification of genes that act downstream of p53 to enact the DBA phenotype. (5) Enhance the effect of GC in combination with other compounds, for example, stabilizers of HIF1α or PPAR α agonists

the development of novel treatment strategies for patients with DBA (Fig. 7.2) that may help direct future therapeutic approaches.

7.4.1 Gene Therapy

As the only curative option for patients with DBA is HSCT, one strategy for cure is by gene therapy using retroviral transduction of the patients' own hematopoietic stem cells to correct haploinsufficiency of ribosomal proteins. Treatment of RPS19-deficient CD34$^+$ bone marrow cells from DBA patients in vitro with retroviral vectors containing *RPS19* increased their proliferative capacity threefold compared to control DBA cells (Hamaguchi et al. 2002, 2003). Moreover, CD34$^+$ cells from RPS19-deficient DBA patients corrected via *RPS19* transduction had a proliferative advantage over nontransduced RPS19-deficient cells upon transplantation into immunodeficient mice (Flygare et al. 2008). Although still preliminary, gene therapy has great potential to ultimately cure DBA patients, and its success is largely dependent on the advancement of biomedical gene therapy techniques including viral vector optimization, primary hematopoietic stem cell transduction, and newer genome editing approaches.

7.4.2 Current Clinical Trials

Two novel mechanism-directed therapies using either leucine or Sotatercept are currently in clinical trial ("A Study, Safety, and Efficacy Study of Sotatercept in Adults with Transfusion-Dependent Diamond-Blackfan Anemia (ACE-011-DBA)" and "A Pilot, Phase I/II Study of the Amino Acid Leucine in the Treatment of Patients with Transfusion-Dependent Diamond-Blackfan Anemia") to evaluate their effect on transfusion dependence and macrocytic anemia in DBA.

7.4.2.1 Leucine

The use of the branched-chain amino acid leucine is based on a small cohort of patients from the Czech Republic (Pospisilova et al. 2007) and alleviation of anemia in mouse and zebrafish models of DBA. Leucine stimulates initiation of protein translation through activation of the mTOR complex. The hypothesis is that leucine will compensate for the decreased rate of protein translation caused by ribosomal protein deficiency. Current in vitro data is very promising, as leucine administration partially rescued the erythroid defects in RPS19-deficient mice, increased bone marrow cellularity, and alleviated stress hematopoiesis and was associated with decreased p53 activity (Jaako et al. 2012). Leucine was also successful in alleviating anemia and rescuing developmental and growth defects in DBA and del(5q) zebrafish models, as well as alleviating the anemia in human in vitro models of DBA and del(5q) MDS created by shRNA against *Rsp19* or *Rps14* in a human CD34+ cell culture system (Payne et al. 2012). This effect was abrogated by rapamycin, supporting that leucine acts through the mammalian target of rapamycin (mTOR) pathway and is a potential therapy for either del(5q) MDS or DBA.

7.4.2.2 Sotatercept

Sotatercept (ACE-011) is a recombinant chimeric protein ligand trap that binds to and inhibits members of the activin/TGFβ superfamily of cytokines. A murine orthologue of Sotatercept is effective in ameliorating the anemia in a mouse model of β-thalassemia intermedia (Dussiot et al. 2014), and Sotatercept has been shown to increase hemoglobin levels in a dose-dependent but non-Epo-dependent fashion by expanding late-stage erythropoiesis in healthy postmenopausal women (Ruckle et al. 2009). More recent studies demonstrate that the murine orthologue (RAP-011) ameliorates anemia in a zebrafish model of DBA by antagonizing lefty1 (Lft1), a member of the activin/TGFβ superfamily (Ear et al. 2015).

7.4.3 Alternatives to Glucocorticoids or Reduction in Steroid Dosage

Lenalidomide is a thalidomide derivative with immunomodulatory and antiangiogenic properties (a class of drugs called IMiDs) that is currently used to treat del(5q) syndrome, the subtype of MDS characterized by defective terminal erythroid differentiation due to loss of RPS14, which links the molecular pathophysiology of del(5q) syndrome to DBA (Ebert et al. 2008a). Although patients with the del(5q) syndrome have historically been maintained on chronic transfusions, in a phase II trial in low-risk MDS patients with 5q deletions, lenalidomide treatment decreased transfusion requirement in 76% of patients, and 61% of patients had a complete cytogenetic response (List et al. 2006). Given that ribosomal protein deficiency and p53 upregulation contribute to anemia in both del(5q) syndrome and DBA, DBA should respond to lenalidomide in a similar in fashion as del(5q) (Ebert et al. 2008b). Although recent anecdotal experience in adults suggests that that drug may not be suitable in DBA, other immunomodulatory analogues of thalidomide (IMiDs) should be investigated.

Narla et al. demonstrated that GC-induced proliferation of erythroid precursors was augmented when lenalidomide was combined with dexamethasone. Interestingly, dexamethasone stimulated proliferation of normal BFU-Es while lenalidomide mainly enhanced proliferation of CFU-Es (Narla et al. 2011b). The two compounds further upregulated a different set of genes, indicating that they act through two distinct mechanisms. The authors propose that a combinatory therapy could be an option for patients with poor response to normal GC treatment. In the event that lenalidomide has disqualifying toxicity, there is an abundance of IMiD compounds, such as pomalidomide, which could be efficacious.

Besides prednisone, there are several steroid and nonsteroid compounds that are potent GC receptor agonists. Some of these ligands only partially activate the GC receptor, so it is potentially possible to identify GC receptor agonists that retain the therapeutic effect in DBA patients without inducing significant side effects. While no such compounds are currently available, there have been attempts to test safer GC receptor agonists such as deflazacort (DFZ) in DBA. Deflazacort, a bulky derivative of prednisolone, is used as an alternative to prednisone in children with Duchenne muscular dystrophy (DMD) and has been used successfully in at least one DBA patient (Soker et al. 2004). DFZ is reported to have milder side effects on growth of the long bones in children treated for DMD at equivalent dosages of prednisolone, but it still remains to be seen if it results in less severe side effects compared to conventional corticosteroids in DBA.

Another group of drugs with the possibility to enhance the effect of GC are drugs that promote activation of hypoxia-inducible factor 1α(HIF1α), such as prolyl hydroxylase inhibitors (PHIs). Flygare et al. demonstrated in normal BFU-E that genes regulated by GC also contain binding sites for HIF1α, indicating that these transcription factors might synergize their functions. Indeed, co-treatment with prolyl hydroxylase inhibitors that inhibit HIF1α degradation increased the expression of GC-induced genes and boosted the proliferative capacity of GC treated BFU-E cells in vitro (Flygare et al. 2011). Interestingly, there are case reports of transfusion independence after starting iron chelation therapy in patients with myelodysplastic syndrome and DBA, resulting from a rapid increase in red cell production (Messa et al. 2008; Taher et al. 2009). Though this therapeutic response was hypothesized to occur because of decreased iron toxicity on bone marrow erythropoiesis, iron chelators are also potent HIF1α activators. One possible mechanism may be that increased red cell production could be attributed to HIF1α activation in BFU-E precursors (Flygare et al. 2011; Saletta et al. 2010; Wang and Semenza 1993). Therefore, if iron chelation also has an enhanced effect on HIF1α activation in DBA, patients with DBA on iron chelation could hypothetically be able to reduce their GC dosage and therefore reduce accompanying steroid side effects.

Activation of the peroxisome proliferator-activated receptor α (PPAR-α) by the PPAR-α agonist GW7647 also synergizes with the glucocorticoid receptor (GR) to promote BFU-E self-renewal, suggesting that targets downstream of GR or PPAR-α synergistic binding sites may also offer future novel treatment approaches. Lee and colleagues (Lee et al. 2015) showed that the PPAR-α agonist GW7647 facilitates recovery of wild-type but not *Ppar-α*$^{-/-}$ mice from phenylhydrazine-induced acute hemolytic anemia, improves recovery from anemia in a murine model of chronic hemolytic anemia and neonatal anemia (*Nan*) mice, and significantly increases the proliferation and survival of erythroid progenitors in human C34+ culture after RPS19 knockdown, recapitulating DBA in an in vitro model. PPAR-α co-occupies many chromatin sites with GR. When activated by PPAR-α agonists, additional PPAR-α is recruited to GR-adjacent sites and presumably facilitates GR-dependent BFU-E self-renewal. This synergy with steroids suggests that agonists like GW7647, already in clinical trials for erythropoietin-refractory anemias, may also improve the efficacy of corticosteroids in treatment of DBA or allow patients to lower their dose of steroids and thus lower associated side effects.

7.4.4 Future Approaches

Several murine modes offer promising future approaches to the treatment of ribosomopathies via modulation of the p53 pathway (Jones et al. 2008). Treacher-Collins syndrome is an autosomal dominant condition that includes severe craniofacial defects arising from diminished growth of the first and second pharyngeal arch, groove, and pouch (Sakai and Trainor 2009). *TCOF1*, encoding a protein called Treacle, was identified as the gene responsible for TCS (Dixon et al. 1996). Mice haploinsufficient for *Tcof1* have diminished production of ribosomes that correlates with decreased proliferation of both neural ectoderm and neural crest cells (Dixon et al. 2006). Interestingly, chemical and genetic inhibition of p53 activity in these mice prevents the craniofacial abnormalities (Jones et al. 2008). This offers a unique treatment strategy in diseases such as TCS or DBA where p53 or its downstream effectors could be targeted. There is precedence for targeting p53 in the successful reversible inhibition of p53 as a treatment strategy to prevent damage of normal tissues during treatment of p53-deficient tumors (Komarov et al. 1999). The compound pifithrin-α was identified for its ability to reversibly block p53-dependent transcriptional activation and apoptosis and subsequently protected mice from lethal genotoxic stress associated with gamma irradiation without promoting the formation of tumors. Further studies along this line, while considering the oncogenic potential of p53 inhibition, could offer new treatment strategies for stabilization of p53 activity in ribosomopathies like DBA.

Studies in mice with conditional inactivation of *rps6* offer another target by elucidating the mechanism of MDM2-mediated induction of p53 by ribosomal haploinsufficiency (Fumagalli et al. 2009). Conditional deletion of *Rps6* in murine liver inhibited 40S (but not 60S) ribosomal biogenesis and liver cells failed to proliferate after partial hepatectomy (Volarevic et al. 2000). Impaired ribosome biogenesis is normally attributed to nucleolar disruption and accumulation of 60S proteins such as Rpl11 into the nucleoplasm where they inhibit MDM2, leading to p53 activation and apoptosis. Free RPL11 generated by the loss of *Rps6* in these mice was found to be due to increased translation of RPL11 mRNAs through derepression of 5′-TOP mRNA translation (Fumagalli et al. 2009). This mechanism, Rpl11 accumulation via deregulated 5′-TOP mRNA translation, offers a novel pathway that could be targeted to alleviate the consequence of abortive ribosomal biogenesis without involving other necessary pathways downstream of p53.

In summary, our increasing understanding of the pathophysiology of DBA is leading to novel therapeutic approaches potentially involving the modulation of p53 and/or mTOR. Data from open trials with leucine, lenalidomide, and Sotatercept, as well as trials with HDAC inhibitors, prolyl hydroxylase inhibitors, or PPAR-α agonists in other anemias, may also provide useful insights that may direct future therapies.

References

Abkowitz JL, Schaison G, Boulad F, Brown DL, Buchanan GR, Johnson CA, Murray JC, Sabo KM (2002) Response of Diamond-Blackfan anemia to metoclopramide: evidence for a role for prolactin in erythropoiesis. Blood 100:2687

Akiyama M, Yanagisawa T, Yuza Y, Yokoi K, Ariga M, Fujisawa K, Hoshi Y, Eto Y (2005) Successful treatment of Diamond-Blackfan anemia with metoclopramide. Am J Hematol 78:295–298. https://doi.org/10.1002/ajh.20278

Alessandri AJ, Rogers PC, Wadsworth LD, Davis JH (2000) Diamond-Blackfan anemia and cyclosporine therapy revisited. J Pediatr Hematol Oncol 22:176–179

Alter BP, Greene MH, Velazquez I, Rosenberg PS (2003) Cancer in Fanconi anemia. Blood 101:2072. https://doi.org/10.1182/blood-2002-11-3597

Amsterdam A, Sadler KC, Lai K, Farrington S, Bronson RT, Lees JA, Hopkins N (2004) Many ribosomal protein genes are cancer genes in zebrafish. PLoS Biol 2:E139. https://doi.org/10.1371/journal.pbio.0020139

Bagby GC, Lipton JM, Sloand EM, Schiffer CA (2004) Marrow failure. Hematology Am Soc Hematol Educ Program 2004:318–336. https://doi.org/10.1182/asheducation-2004.1.318

Ball S, Tchernia G, Wranne L (1995) Is there a role for interleukin-3 in Diamond-Blackfan anaemia? Results of a European multicentre study. Br J Haematol 91(2):313–318

Barlow JL, Drynan LF, Hewett DR, Holmes LR, Lorenzo-Abalde S, Lane AL, Jolin HE, Pannell R, Middleton AJ, Wong SH, Warren AJ, Wainscoat JS, Boultwood J, McKenzie ANJ (2010) A p53-dependent mechanism underlies macrocytic anemia in a mouse model of human 5q- syndrome. Nat Med 16:59–66. https://doi.org/10.1038/nm.2063

Bastion Y, Bordigoni P, Debre M, Girault D, Leblanc T, Tchernia G, Ball S, McGuckin C, Gordon-Smith E, Bekassy A (1994) Sustained response after recombinant interleukin-3 in Diamond Blackfan anemia [letter; comment]. Blood 83:617

Bobey NAM, Carcao M, Dror Y, Freedman MH, Dahl N, Woodman RC (2003) Sustained cyclosporine-induced erythropoietic response in identical male twins with Diamond-Blackfan anemia. J Pediatr Hematol Oncol 25:914–918

Bradner JE, Mak R, Tanguturi SK, Mazitschek R, Haggarty SJ, Ross K, Chang CY, Bosco J, West N, Morse E, Lin K, Shen JP, Kwiatkowski NP, Gheldof

N, Dekker J, DeAngelo DJ, Carr SA, Schreiber SL, Golub TR, Ebert BL (2010) Chemical genetic strategy identifies histone deacetylase 1 (HDAC1) and HDAC2 as therapeutic targets in sickle cell disease. Proc Natl Acad Sci U S A 107:12617–12622. https://doi.org/10.1073/pnas.1006774107

Brooks CL, Gu W (2006) p53 ubiquitination: Mdm2 and beyond. Mol Cell 21:307–315. https://doi.org/10.1016/j.molcel.2006.01.020

Chakraborty A, Uechi T, Higa S, Torihara H, Kenmochi N (2009) Loss of ribosomal protein L11 affects zebrafish embryonic development through a p53-dependent apoptotic response. PLoS One 4:e4152. https://doi.org/10.1371/journal.pone.0004152

Clinton C, Gazda HT (1993) Diamond-Blackfan anemia. University of Washington, Seattle, WA

Cmejla R, Cmejlova J, Handrkova H, Petrak J, Petrtylova K, Mihal V, Stary J, Cerna Z, Jabali Y, Pospisilova D (2009) Identification of mutations in the ribosomal protein L5 (RPL5) and ribosomal protein L11 (RPL11) genes in Czech patients with Diamond-Blackfan anemia. Hum Mutat 30:321–327. https://doi.org/10.1002/humu.20874

Diamond LK, Blackfan K (1938) Hypoplastic anemia. Am J Dis Child 56:464

Dixon J, Edwards SJ, Gladwin AJ, Dixon MJ, Loftus SK, Bonner CA, Koprivnikar K, Wasmuth JJ, Wasmuth JJ (1996) Positional cloning of a gene involved in the pathogenesis of Treacher Collins syndrome. Nat Genet 12:130–136. https://doi.org/10.1038/ng0296-130

Dixon J, Jones NC, Sandell LL, Jayasinghe SM, Crane J, Rey J-P, Dixon MJ, Trainor PA (2006) Tcof1/Treacle is required for neural crest cell formation and proliferation deficiencies that cause craniofacial abnormalities. Proc Natl Acad Sci U S A 103:13403–13408. https://doi.org/10.1073/pnas.0603730103

Donati G, Peddigari S, Mercer CA, Thomas G (2013) 5S ribosomal RNA is an essential component of a nascent ribosomal precursor complex that regulates the Hdm2-p53 checkpoint. Cell Rep 4:87–98. https://doi.org/10.1016/j.celrep.2013.05.045

Draptchinskaia N, Gustavsson P, Andersson B, Pettersson M, Willig TN, Dianzani I, Ball S, Tchernia G, Klar J, Matsson H, Tentler D, Mohandas N, Carlsson B, Dahl N (1999) The gene encoding ribosomal protein S19 is mutated in Diamond-Blackfan anaemia. Nat Genet 21:169–175. https://doi.org/10.1038/5951

Dunbar CE, Smith DA, Kimball J, Garrison L, Nienhuis AW, Young NS (1991) Treatment of Diamond-Blackfan anaemia with haematopoietic growth factors, granulocyte-macrophage colony stimulating factor and interleukin 3: sustained remissions following IL-3. Br J Haematol 79:316–321

Dussiot M, Maciel TT, Fricot A, Chartier C, Negre O, Veiga J, Grapton D, Paubelle E, Payen E, Beuzard Y, Leboulch P, Ribeil J-A, Arlet J-B, Coté F, Courtois G, Ginzburg YZ, Daniel TO, Chopra R, Sung V, Hermine O, Moura IC (2014) An activin receptor IIA ligand trap corrects ineffective erythropoiesis in β-thalassemia. Nat Med 20:398–407. https://doi.org/10.1038/nm.3468

Ear J, Huang H, Wilson T, Tehrani Z, Lindgren A, Sung V, Laadem A, Daniel TO, Chopra R, Lin S (2015) RAP-011 improves erythropoiesis in zebrafish model of Diamond-Blackfan anemia through antagonizing lefty1. Blood 126:880–890. https://doi.org/10.1182/blood-2015-01-622522

Ebert BL, Pretz J, Bosco J, Chang CY, Tamayo P, Galili N, Raza A, Root DE, Attar E, Ellis SR, Golub TR (2008a) Identification of RPS14 as a 5q- syndrome gene by RNA interference screen. Nature 451:335–339. https://doi.org/10.1038/nature06494

Ebert BL, Galili N, Tamayo P, Bosco J, Mak R, Pretz J, Tanguturi S, Ladd-Acosta C, Stone R, Golub TR, Raza A (2008b) An erythroid differentiation signature predicts response to lenalidomide in myelodysplastic syndrome. PLoS Med 5:e35. https://doi.org/10.1371/journal.pmed.0050035

El-Beshlawy A, Ibrahim I, Rizk S, Eid K (2002) Study of 22 Egyptian patients with Diamond-Blackfan anemia, corticosteroids, and cyclosporin therapy results. Pediatrics 110:e44

Farrar JE, Nater M, Caywood E, McDevitt MA, Kowalski J, Takemoto CM, Talbot CC, Meltzer P, Esposito D, Beggs AH, Schneider HE, Grabowska A, Ball SE, Niewiadomska E, Sieff CA, Vlachos A, Atsidaftos E, Ellis SR, Lipton JM, Gazda HT, Arceci RJ, Arceci RJ (2008) Abnormalities of the large ribosomal subunit protein, Rpl35a, in Diamond-Blackfan anemia. Blood 112:1582–1592. https://doi.org/10.1182/blood-2008-02-140012

Flygare J, Olsson K, Richter J, Karlsson S (2008) Gene therapy of Diamond Blackfan anemia CD34+ cells leads to improved erythroid development and engraftment following transplantation. Exp Hematol 36:1428

Flygare J, Rayon Estrada V, Shin C, Gupta S, Lodish HF (2011) HIF1alpha synergizes with glucocorticoids to promote BFU-E progenitor self-renewal. Blood 117:3435–3444. https://doi.org/10.1182/blood-2010-07-295550

Fumagalli S, Di Cara A, Neb-Gulati A, Natt F, Schwemberger S, Hall J, Babcock GF, Bernardi R, Pandolfi PP, Thomas G (2009) Absence of nucleolar disruption after impairment of 40S ribosome biogenesis reveals an rpL11-translation-dependent mechanism of p53 induction. Nat Cell Biol 11:501–508. https://doi.org/10.1038/ncb1858

Ganser A, Lindemann A, Seipelt G, Ottmann O (1990) Effects of recombinant human interleukin-3 in aplastic anemia. Blood 76:1287

Gazda HT, Sheen MR, Vlachos A, Choesmel V, O'Donohue M-F, Schneider H, Darras N, Hasman C, Sieff CA, Newburger PE, Ball SE, Niewiadomska E, Matysiak M, Zaucha JM, Glader B, Niemeyer C, Meerpohl JJ, Atsidaftos E, Lipton JM, Gleizes P-E, Beggs AH (2008) Ribosomal protein L5 and L11 mutations are associated with cleft palate and abnormal thumbs in Diamond-Blackfan anemia patients.

Am J Hum Genet 83:769. https://doi.org/10.1016/j.ajhg.2008.11.004

Gillio A, Faulkner L, Alter B, Reilly L, Klafter R (1993) Treatment of Diamond-Blackfan anemia with recombinant human interleukin-3. Blood 82:744

Giri K, Tisdale F, Rivera S, Kim Y, Rick D (2000) Clinical and laboratory evidence for a trilineage haematopoietic defect in patients with refractory Diamond-Blackfan anaemia. Br J Haematol 108:167–175. https://doi.org/10.1046/j.1365-2141.2000.01796.x

Goudarzi KM, Lindström MS (2016) Role of ribosomal protein mutations in tumor development (Review). Int J Oncol 48:1313–1324. https://doi.org/10.3892/ijo.2016.3387

Gripp KW, Curry C, Olney AH, Sandoval C, Fisher J, Chong JX-L, UW Center for Mendelian Genomics, Pilchman L, Sahraoui R, Stabley DL, Sol-Church K (2014) Diamond-Blackfan anemia with mandibulofacial dystostosis is heterogeneous, including the novel DBA genes TSR2 and RPS28. Am J Med Genet A 164A:2240–2249. https://doi.org/10.1002/ajmg.a.36633

Hamaguchi I, Ooka A, Brun A, Richter J, Dahl N, Karlsson S (2002) Gene transfer improves erythroid development in ribosomal protein S19–deficient Diamond-Blackfan anemia. Blood 100:2724–2731. https://doi.org/10.1182/blood.V100.8.2724

Hamaguchi I, Flygare J, Nishiura H, Brun ACM, Ooka A, Kiefer T, Ma Z, Dahl N, Richter J, Karlsson S (2003) Proliferation deficiency of multipotent hematopoietic progenitors in ribosomal protein S19 (RPS19)-deficient Diamond-Blackfan anemia improves following RPS19 gene transfer. Mol Ther 7: 613–622

Horos R, Ijspeert H, Pospisilova D, Sendtner R, Andrieu-Soler C, Taskesen E, Nieradka A, Cmejla R, Sendtner M, Touw IP, von Lindern M (2012) Ribosomal deficiencies in Diamond-Blackfan anemia impair translation of transcripts essential for differentiation of murine and human erythroblasts. Blood 119:262–272. https://doi.org/10.1182/blood-2011-06-358200

Jaako P, Flygare J, Olsson K, Quere R, Ehinger M, Henson A, Ellis S, Schambach A, Baum C, Richter J, Larsson J, Bryder D, Karlsson S (2011) Mice with ribosomal protein S19 deficiency develop bone marrow failure and symptoms like patients with Diamond-Blackfan anemia. Blood 118:6087–6096. https://doi.org/10.1182/blood-2011-08-371963

Jaako P, Debnath S, Olsson K, Bryder D, Flygare J, Karlsson S (2012) Dietary L-leucine improves the anemia in a mouse model for Diamond-Blackfan anemia. Blood 120:2225–2228. https://doi.org/10.1182/blood-2012-05-431437

Jabr FI, Aoun E, Azar C, Taher A (2004) Diamond-Blackfan anemia responding to valproic acid. Blood 104:3415

James A, Wang Y, Raje H, Rosby R, DiMario P (2014) Nucleolar stress with and without p53. Nucleus 5:402–426. https://doi.org/10.4161/nucl.32235

Janov AJ, Leong T, Nathan DG, Guinan EC (1996) Diamond-Blackfan anemia. Natural history and sequelae of treatment. Medicine (Baltimore) 75:77–78

Jones NC, Lynn ML, Gaudenz K, Sakai D, Aoto K, Rey J-P, Glynn EF, Ellington L, Du C, Dixon J, Dixon MJ, Trainor PA (2008) Prevention of the neurocristopathy Treacher Collins syndrome through inhibition of p53 function. Nat Med 14:125–133. https://doi.org/10.1038/nm1725

Josephs HW (1936) Anaemia of infancy and early childhood. Medicine (Baltimore) 15:307–451

Keel SB, Doty RT, Yang Z, Quigley JG, Chen J, Knoblaugh S, Kingsley PD, De Domenico I, Vaughn MB, Kaplan J, Palis J, Abkowitz JL (2008) A heme export protein is required for red blood cell differentiation and iron homeostasis. Science 319:825–828. https://doi.org/10.1126/science.1151133

Komarov PG, Komarova EA, Kondratov RV, Christov-Tselkov K, Coon JS, Chernov MV, Gudkov AV (1999) A chemical inhibitor of p53 that protects mice from the side effects of cancer therapy. Science 285:1733

Lajtha L, Oliver R (1961) A kinetic model of the erythron. Proc R Soc Med 54:369–371

Lee H-Y, Gao X, Barrasa MI, Li H, Elmes RR, Peters LL, Lodish HF (2015) PPAR-α and glucocorticoid receptor synergize to promote erythroid progenitor self-renewal. Nature 522:474–477. https://doi.org/10.1038/nature14326

Lensch MW, Rathbun RK, Olson SB, Jones GR, Bagby GC (1999) Selective pressure as an essential force in molecular evolution of myeloid leukemic clones: a view from the window of Fanconi anemia. Leukemia 13:1784–1789

Leonard E, Raefsky E, Griffith P (1989) Cyclosporine therapy of aplastic anaemia, congenital and acquired red cell aplasia. Br J Haematol 72(2):278

Lipton JM, Ellis SR (2009) Diamond-Blackfan anemia: diagnosis, treatment, and molecular pathogenesis. Hematol Oncol Clin North Am 23:261–282. https://doi.org/10.1016/j.hoc.2009.01.004

Lipton JM, Ellis SR (2010) Diamond Blackfan anemia 2008-2009: broadening the scope of ribosome biogenesis disorders. Curr Opin Pediatr 22:12–19. https://doi.org/10.1097/MOP.0b013e328334573b

Lipton J, Kudisch M, Gross R, Nathan D (1986) Defective erythroid progenitor differentiation system in congenital hypoplastic (Diamond-Blackfan) anemia. Blood 67(4):962–968

Lipton JM, Atsidaftos E, Zyskind I, Vlachos A (2006) Improving clinical care and elucidating the pathophysiology of Diamond Blackfan anemia: an update from the Diamond Blackfan Anemia Registry. Pediatr Blood Cancer 46:558–564. https://doi.org/10.1002/pbc.20642

List A, Dewald G, Bennett J, Giagounidis A, Raza A, Feldman E, Powell B, Greenberg P, Thomas D, Stone R, Reeder C, Wride K, Patin J, Schmidt M, Zeldis J, Knight R (2006) Lenalidomide in the myelodysplastic syndrome with chromosome 5q deletion. N

Engl J Med 355:1456–1465. https://doi.org/10.1056/NEJMoa061292

Llanos S, Clark PA, Rowe J, Peters G (2001) Stabilization of p53 by p14ARF without relocation of MDM2 to the nucleolus. Nat Cell Biol 3:445–452. https://doi.org/10.1038/35074506

Ludwig LS, Gazda HT, Eng JC, Eichhorn SW, Thiru P, Ghazvinian R, George TI, Gotlib JR, Beggs AH, C a S, Lodish HF, Lander ES, Sankaran VG (2014) Altered translation of GATA1 in Diamond-Blackfan anemia. Nat Med 20:748–753. https://doi.org/10.1038/nm.3557

Matsson H, Davey EJ, Draptchinskaia N, Hamaguchi I, Ooka A, Levéen P, Forsberg E, Karlsson S, Dahl N (2004) Targeted disruption of the ribosomal protein S19 gene is lethal prior to implantation. Mol Cell Biol 24:4032–4037

Mercurio S, Aspesi A, Silengo L, Altruda F, Dianzani I, Chiabrando D (2016) Alteration of heme metabolism in a cellular model of Diamond-Blackfan anemia. Eur J Haematol 96:367–374. https://doi.org/10.1111/ejh.12599

Messa E, Cilloni D, Messa F, Arruga F, Roetto A, Saglio G (2008) Deferasirox treatment improved the hemoglobin level and decreased transfusion requirements in four patients with the myelodysplastic syndrome and primary myelofibrosis. Acta Haematol 120:70–74. https://doi.org/10.1159/000158631

Monteserin MC, Garcia Vela JA, Oña F, Lastra AM (1993) Cyclosporin A for Diamond-Blackfan anemia: a new case. Am J Hematol 42:406–407

Narla A, Vlachos A, Nathan DG (2011a) Diamond Blackfan anemia treatment: past, present, and future. Semin Hematol 48:117–123. https://doi.org/10.1053/j.seminhematol.2011.01.004

Narla A, Dutt S, McAuley JR, Al-Shahrour F, Hurst S, McConkey M, Neuberg D, Ebert BL (2011b) Dexamethasone and lenalidomide have distinct functional effects on erythropoiesis. Blood 118:2296

O'Donohue M-F, Choesmel V, Faubladier M, Fichant G, Gleizes P-E (2010) Functional dichotomy of ribosomal proteins during the synthesis of mammalian 40S ribosomal subunits. J Cell Biol 190:853

Olivieri NF, Grunberger T, Ben-David Y, Ng J, Williams DE, Lyman S, Anderson DM, Axelrad AA, Correa P, Bernstein A (1991) Diamond-Blackfan anemia: heterogenous response of hematopoietic progenitor cells in vitro to the protein product of the steel locus. Blood 78:2211–2215

Parrella S, Aspesi A, Quarello P, Garelli E, Pavesi E, Carando A, Nardi M, Ellis SR, Ramenghi U, Dianzani I (2014) Loss of GATA-1 full length as a cause of Diamond-Blackfan anemia phenotype. Pediatr Blood Cancer 61:1319–1321. https://doi.org/10.1002/pbc.24944

Payne EM, Virgilio M, Narla A, Sun H, Levine M, Paw BH, Berliner N, Look AT, Ebert BL, Khanna-Gupta A (2012) L-leucine improves the anemia and developmental defects associated with Diamond-Blackfan anemia and del(5q) MDS by activating the mTOR pathway. Blood 120:2214–2224. https://doi.org/10.1182/blood-2011-10-382986

Perdahl EB, Naprstek BL, Wallace WC, Lipton JM (1994) Erythroid failure in Diamond-Blackfan anemia is characterized by apoptosis. Blood 83:645–650

Pospisilova D, Cmejlova J, Hak J, Adam T, Cmejla R (2007) Successful treatment of a Diamond-Blackfan anemia patient with amino acid leucine. Haematologica 92:e66

Quarello P, Garelli E, Carando A, Brusco A, Calabrese R, Dufour C, Longoni D, Misuraca A, Vinti L, Aspesi A, Biondini L, Loreni F, Dianzani I, Ramenghi U (2010) Diamond-Blackfan anemia: genotype-phenotype correlations in Italian patients with RPL5 and RPL11 mutations. Haematologica 95:206–213. https://doi.org/10.3324/haematol.2009.011783

Quigley JG, Yang Z, Worthington MT, Phillips JD, Sabo KM, Sabath DE, Berg CL, Sassa S, Wood BL, Abkowitz JL (2004) Identification of a human heme exporter that is essential for erythropoiesis. Cell 118:757–766. https://doi.org/10.1016/j.cell.2004.08.014

Raiser DM, Narla A, Ebert BL (2014) The emerging importance of ribosomal dysfunction in the pathogenesis of hematologic disorders. Leuk Lymphoma 55:491–500. https://doi.org/10.3109/10428194.2013.812786

Rey MA, Duffy SP, Brown JK, Kennedy JA, Dick JE, Dror Y, Tailor CS (2008) Enhanced alternative splicing of the FLVCR1 gene in Diamond Blackfan anemia disrupts FLVCR1 expression and function that are critical for erythropoiesis. Haematologica 93:1617–1626. https://doi.org/10.3324/haematol.13359

Ries L, Melbert D, Krapcho M, Stinchcomb D, Howlader N, Horner M, Mariotto A, Miller B, Feuer E, Altekruse S, Lewis D, Clegg L, Eisner M, Reichman M, Edwards B (2004) SEER cancer statistics review 1975-2001. SEER Cancer statistics review 1975-2005. National Cancer Institute, Bethesda, MD. http://seer.cancer.gov/csr/1975_2005/results_merge.

Roy V, Pérez WS, Eapen M, Marsh JCW, Pasquini M, Pasquini R, Mustafa MM, Bredeson CN (2005) Bone marrow transplantation for Diamond-Blackfan anemia. Biol Blood Marrow Transplant 11:600–608. https://doi.org/10.1016/j.bbmt.2005.05.005

Ruckle J, Jacobs M, Kramer W, Pearsall AE, Kumar R, Underwood KW, Seehra J, Yang Y, Condon CH, Sherman ML (2009) Single-dose, randomized, double-blind, placebo-controlled study of ACE-011 (ActRIIA-IgG1) in postmenopausal women. J Bone Miner Res 24:744–752. https://doi.org/10.1359/jbmr.081208

Sakai D, Trainor PA (2009) Treacher Collins syndrome: unmasking the role of Tcof1/treacle. Int J Biochem Cell Biol 41:1229–1232. https://doi.org/10.1016/j.biocel.2008.10.026

Saletta F, Suryo Rahmanto Y, Noulsri E, Richardson DR (2010) Iron chelator-mediated alterations in gene expression: identification of novel iron-regulated molecules that are molecular targets of hypoxia-inducible factor-1 alpha and p53. Mol Pharmacol 77:443–458. https://doi.org/10.1124/mol.109.061028

Sankaran VG, Ghazvinian R, Do R, Thiru P, Vergilio JA, Beggs AH, Sieff CA, Orkin SH, Nathan DG, Lander ES, Gazda HT (2012) Exome sequencing identifies GATA1 mutations resulting in Diamond-Blackfan anemia. J Clin Invest 122:2439–2443. https://doi.org/10.1172/JCI63597

Seip M, Zanussi G (1988) Cyclosporine in steroid-resistant Diamond-Blackfan anaemia. Acta Paediatr Scand 77:464

Shimamura A, Alter BP (2010) Pathophysiology and management of inherited bone marrow failure syndromes. Blood Rev 24:101–122. https://doi.org/10.1016/j.blre.2010.03.002

Singh SA, Goldberg TA, Henson AL, Husain-Krautter S, Nihrane A, Blanc L, Ellis SR, Lipton JM, Liu JM (2014) p53-independent cell cycle and erythroid differentiation defects in murine embryonic stem cells haploinsufficient for Diamond Blackfan anemia-proteins: RPS19 versus RPL5. PLoS One 9:e89098. https://doi.org/10.1371/journal.pone.0089098

Sjögren SE, Flygare J (2012) Progress towards mechanism-based treatment for Diamond-Blackfan anemia. ScientificWorldJournal 2012:184362. https://doi.org/10.1100/2012/184362

Sloan KE, Bohnsack MT, Watkins NJ (2013) The 5S RNP couples p53 homeostasis to ribosome biogenesis and nucleolar stress. Cell Rep 5:237–247. https://doi.org/10.1016/j.celrep.2013.08.049

Soker M, Ayyildiz O, Isikdogan A (2004) Aase-Smith syndrome type II. Saudi Med J 25:2004

Splain J, Berman BW (1992) Cyclosporin A treatment for Diamond-Blackfan anemia. Am J Hematol 39:208–211

Sulima SO, Patchett S, Advani VM, De Keersmaecker K, Johnson AW, Dinman JD (2014) Bypass of the pre-60S ribosomal quality control as a pathway to oncogenesis. Proc Natl Acad Sci U S A 111:5640–5645. https://doi.org/10.1073/pnas.1400247111

Taher AT, Musallam KM, Koussa S, Inati A (2009) Transfusion independence in Diamond-Blackfan anemia after deferasirox therapy. Ann Hematol 88:1263–1264. https://doi.org/10.1007/s00277-009-0750-6

Torihara H, Uechi T, Chakraborty A, Shinya M, Sakai N, Kenmochi N (2011) Erythropoiesis failure due to RPS19 deficiency is independent of an activated Tp53 response in a zebrafish model of Diamond-Blackfan anaemia. Br J Haematol 152:648–654. https://doi.org/10.1111/j.1365-2141.2010.08535.x

Tötterman TH, Nisell J, Killander A, Gahrton G, Lönnqvist B (1984) Successful treatment of pure red-cell aplasia with cyclosporin. Lancet 2:693

Vlachos A, Muir E (2010) How I treat Diamond-Blackfan anemia. Blood 116:3715–3723. https://doi.org/10.1182/blood-2010-02-251090

Vlachos A, Ball S, Dahl N, Alter BP, Sheth S, Ramenghi U, Meerpohl J, Karlsson S, Liu JM, Leblanc T, Paley C, Kang EM, Leder EJ, Atsidaftos E, Shimamura A, Bessler M, Glader B, Lipton JM (2008) Diagnosing and treating Diamond Blackfan anaemia: results of an international clinical consensus conference. Br J Haematol 142:859–876. https://doi.org/10.1111/j.1365-2141.2008.07269.x

Vlachos A, Rosenberg PS, Atsidaftos E, Alter BP, Lipton JM (2012) Incidence of neoplasia in Diamond Blackfan anemia: a report from the Diamond Blackfan Anemia Registry. Blood 119:3815–3819. https://doi.org/10.1182/blood-2011-08-375972

Vlachos A, Farrar JE, Atsidaftos E, Muir E, Narla A, Markello TC, Singh SA, Landowski M, Gazda HT, Blanc L, Liu JM, Ellis SR, Arceci RJ, Ebert BL, Bodine DM, Lipton JM (2013) Diminutive somatic deletions in the 5q region lead to a phenotype atypical of classical 5q− syndrome. Blood 122:2487

Vlachos A, Blanc L, Lipton JM (2014) Diamond Blackfan anemia: a model for the translational approach to understanding human disease. Expert Rev Hematol 7:359–372. https://doi.org/10.1586/17474086.2014.897923

Volarevic S, Stewart MJ, Ledermann B, Zilberman F, Terracciano L, Montini E, Grompe M, Kozma SC, Thomas G (2000) Proliferation, but not growth, blocked by conditional deletion of 40S ribosomal protein S6. Science 288:2045–2047

Wang GL, Semenza GL (1993) Desferrioxamine induces erythropoietin gene expression and hypoxia-inducible factor 1 DNA-binding activity: implications for models of hypoxia signal transduction. Blood 82:3610–3615

Williams DL, Mageed AS, Findley H, Ragab AH (1987) Cyclosporine in the treatment of red cell aplasia. Am J Pediatr Hematol Oncol 9:314–316

Willig T-N, Niemeyer CM, Leblanc T, Tiemann C, Robert A, Budde J, Lambiliotte A, Kohne E, Souillet G, Eber S, Stephan J-L, Girot R, Bordigoni P, Cornu G, Blanche S, Guillard JM, Mohandas N (1999) Identification of New Prognosis Factors from the Clinical and Epidemiologic Analysis of a Registry of 229 Diamond-Blackfan Anemia Patients. Pediatr Res 46:553. https://doi.org/10.1203/00006450-199911000-00011

Xue S, Barna M (2012) Specialized ribosomes: a new frontier in gene regulation and organismal biology. Nat Rev Mol Cell Biol 13:355–369. https://doi.org/10.1038/nrm3359

Yadav GV, Chakraborty A, Uechi T, Kenmochi N (2014) Ribosomal protein deficiency causes Tp53-independent erythropoiesis failure in zebrafish. Int J Biochem Cell Biol 49:1–7. https://doi.org/10.1016/j.biocel.2014.01.006

Yang Z, Keel SB, Shimamura A, Liu L, Gerds AT, Li HY, Wood BL, Scott BL, Abkowitz JL (2016) Delayed globin synthesis leads to excess heme and the macrocytic anemia of Diamond Blackfan anemia and del(5q) myelodysplastic syndrome. Sci Transl Med 8:338ra67. https://doi.org/10.1126/scitranslmed.aaf3006

Yaris N, Erduran E, Cobanoglu U (2006) Hodgkin lymphoma in a child with Diamond Blackfan anemia. J Pediatr Hematol Oncol 28:234–236. https://doi.org/10.1097/01.mph.0000210413.63478.91

Shwachman-Diamond Syndrome

8

Kasiani C. Myers and Akiko Shimamura

Contents

8.1 Introduction

Shwachman-Diamond syndrome (SDS) is a rare autosomal recessive disorder classically characterized by exocrine pancreatic dysfunction, bone marrow failure, and a predisposition toward transformation to myelodysplasia (MDS) or acute leukemia, predominantly acute myeloid leukemia (AML). SDS is a multi-system disease in which the skeletal system, growth, liver, central nervous system, heart, and immune function can also be affected. Biallelic mutations in the Shwachman-Bodian-Diamond syndrome (*SBDS*) gene located on chromosome 7q11 are found in approximately 90% of individuals with SDS. The SBDS protein participates in ribosomal maturation but is also involved in several other functions including the stromal microenvironment (Raaijmakers et al. 2010; Nihrane et al. 2009) and mitosis (Austin et al. 2008). Reports of the incidence of SDS vary from 1/77,000 (Goobie et al. 2001) to 1/150–200,000 (Minelli et al. 2012; Kent et al. 1990; Cipolli 2001).

Although inheritance of SDS is largely monogenic with the majority of individuals carrying biallelic mutations in *SBDS*, individuals with SDS show notable phenotypic diversity both between individuals and over time within the same individual. This

K. C. Myers (✉)
Division of Bone Marrow Transplantation and Immune Deficiency, Cincinnati Children's Hospital Medical Center, Cincinnati, OH, USA
e-mail: kasiani.myers@cchmc.org

A. Shimamura
Division of Pediatric Hematology/Oncology, Boston Children's Hospital, Dana Farber Cancer Institute, Boston, MA, USA
e-mail: Akiko.Shimamura@childrens.harvard.edu

G. M. Kupfer et al. (eds.), *Bone Marrow Failure*, Pediatric Oncology,
https://doi.org/10.1007/978-3-319-61421-2_8

is especially intriguing given the relative limited genotypic diversity in mutations across individuals. The rarity of SDS has to this point limited our understanding of the natural history of the disease and potential disease modifiers. Similarly, clinical trials to evaluate therapeutic approaches in SDS are lacking. Clinical management currently is guided largely by small case series and expert consensus. Longitudinal cohort studies are necessary to further define diagnostic criteria, uncover the breadth of phenotypic diversity, and advance our understanding of the pathogenesis of SDS. These collaborative efforts are critical to identify risk factors for disease progression and complications to inform clinical screening practices as well as clinical trial development to advance therapeutic approaches.

This review will provide an overview of SDS and recent progress in our knowledge regarding the clinical manifestations and pathophysiology of SDS.

8.2 Clinical Phenotypes

Our understanding of the diversity of clinical phenotype in SDS continues to evolve. The classic clinical presentation of SDS includes exocrine pancreatic dysfunction and bone marrow failure as described in the most recent consensus guidelines and summarized in Table 8.1 (Dror et al. 2011). Recently, however, data from the North American SDS registry reveals a broader range of clinical presentation for SDS. In this cohort only 51% (19 of 37) individuals with biallelic SBDS mutations initially presented with the classic combination of neutropenia and steatorrhea. Not surprisingly neutropenia was the most common hematologic abnormality at presentation seen in 81% (30/37, 81%); however, five individuals (14%) had no history of cytopenias upon initial medical evaluation. Additionally normal fecal elastase levels, absence of pancreatic lipomatosis on ultrasound or computed tomography scan, and normal skeletal imaging did not rule out the diagnosis of SDS. In fact, SDS was diagnosed in two asymptomatic siblings of SDS probands. These data suggest that reliance on classic clinical criteria for SDS may miss or delay diagnosis of a considerable number of individuals with SDS. In this study clues to the diagnosis of SDS included cytopenias associated with a hypocellular marrow, myelodysplasia with clonal abnormalities frequently found in SDS, congenital anomalies (seen in 50%, Table 8.2), and family history.

Due to the rarity of SDS, our understanding of the complete clinical spectrum of this

Table 8.1 Molecular and clinical diagnostic features of Shwachman-Diamond syndrome

Biallelic mutations in *SBDS*		
or		
clinical Shwachman-Diamond syndrome: one criteria from category I and II		
Category I	Category II	Supporting features
Low trypsinogen (age < 3 years) *or*	Hypoproductive cytopenias	First- or second-degree blood relative with:
low pancreatic isoamylase (age > 3 years)	Neutropenia (ANC < 1500)	Shwachman-Diamond syndrome
	Anemia or idiopathic macrocytosis	
Low fecal elastase	Thrombocytopenia (< 150,000)	
Supportive features:		
	Bone marrow examination with any of the	Personal history of:
Pancreatic lipomatosis	following:	Height ≤ 3% of unclear etiology
	Hypocellularity for age	Congenital skeletal abnormalities
Elevated 72 h fecal fat excretion and	Cytogenetic abnormalities	consistent with chondrodysplasia or
absence of intestinal pathology	Myelodysplasia	a congenital thoracic dystrophy
	Leukemia	Deficiency in ≥2 fat-soluble vitamins
		(A, 25-OHD, and E)

ANC absolute neutrophil count

Table 8.2 Congenital anomalies identified in patients with Shwachman-Diamond syndrome in the North American Shwachman-Diamond syndrome registry[a]

Congenital anomalies	Number of patients 30/55
Cardiac	8 (15%)
VSD	3
PFO/ASD	4
PDA	5
Gastrointestinal	4 (7%)
Malrotation	2
Bilateral inguinal hernia	2
Imperforate anus	1
Musculoskeletal	22 (40%)
Thoracic dystrophy/rib abnormalities	11
Short arms/legs	2
Metaphyseal dysplasia	7
Other legs (knock knees, bowing legs)	4
Pelvic dysostosis - absent pubic ramus	1
Scoliosis	4
Slipped capital femoral epiphysis	1
Syn/clino/polydactaly/other digit	5
Club foot	2
Scaphocephaly	1
Neurologic	2 (4%)
Chiari malformation, type I	1
Ectopic posterior pituitary	1
Cerebellar tonsillar ectopia	1
Myopathy/hypotonia	1
Urologic	4 (7%)
Testicular atrophy	2
Undescended testicle	1
Vesicoureteral reflux	1
Micropenis	1
Hypospadias	1
Other	6 (11%)
Subglottic stenosis	1
Horseshoe kidney	1
Eye anomaly	1
Ear anomalies/hearing loss	5

[a]Updated from J Pediatr. 2014 Apr;164(4):866–70

complex multi-system disease remains limited. Hematologic manifestations of neutropenia and progression to aplastic anemia or malignant transformation continue to remain a significant source of morbidity and mortality for individuals with SDS. Additional important disease manifestations include those of the pancreas, liver, skeletal and nervous systems, and other organ systems.

8.2.1 Hematologic Phenotype

Cytopenias are frequent in individuals with SDS secondary to marrow failure. Neutropenia has long been considered a hallmark of SDS. Neutropenia, defined as an absolute neutrophil count <1500/mcL, is the most frequent cytopenia and has been reported in 88–100% of individuals; however neutropenia may be intermittent or persistent and variable in severity. Neutropenia may present later in life or may be absent in a small subset of individuals (Myers et al. 2014). Anemia and thrombocytopenia of variable severity are also frequently noted in individuals with SDS. Progression to severe aplastic anemia with trilineage cytopenia remains a risk for a subset of SDS individuals. In 102 genetically diagnosed individuals with SDS in the French Severe Chronic Neutropenia Registry, 41 individuals (40%) developed hematologic complications including transient severe cytopenias (Donadieu et al. 2012). Persistent severe cytopenias with hemoglobin <7 g/dL or platelets $<20 \times 10^9$/L were identified in 21 of these (20.6%), 9 of whom were classified as malignant, another 9 as nonmalignant, and an additional 3 who progressed from nonmalignant to malignant. Prognostic markers in this cohort with severe cytopenias included young age at diagnosis and hematologic parameters.

Risk of malignant transformation to MDS or AML in SDS varies by report, which may arise in part from lack of consensus regarding the definition of MDS in this context. Many reports do not distinguish between MDS and AML when reporting outcomes. The Severe Congenital Neutropenia International Registry (SCNIR) has previously reported an incidence of 8.1% of MDS/AML in SDS over 10 years ($n = 37$) with a rate of 1% per year (Rosenberg et al. 2006; Dale et al. 2006). In a cohort of 55 SDS individuals in the French Severe Chronic Neutropenia Registry transformation to MDS or AML occured at a median age of 19.1 years in 18.8% at 20 years and 36.1% at 30 years (Donadieu et al. 2005). Recently the Canadian Inherited Marrow Failure Registry reported a 20% risk by age 18 ($n = 40$) of hematologic disease progression including clonal or malignant myeloid transformation, acquisition of new or additional cytogenetic clones, or worsening in severity of cytopenias (Cada et al. 2015). Previously they had reported a cumulative rate of transformation to MDS/AML of 18% in SDS individuals at a median age of 20 years in their cohort ($n = 34$) (Hashmi et al. 2011). There are no reports of malignant transformation in smaller younger cohorts such as the NIH ($n = 17$) and the Israeli registry ($n = 3$), median ages of 14 and 4 years, respectively, suggesting that risk may increase with age. Comparison rates of transformation to MDS in Fanconi anemia (FA) and dyskeratosis congenita (DC) are 40% and 30% by age 50, respectively. Risk of AML in these groups is 15% and 20% respectively (Alter 2014; Alter et al. 2010). Malignant transformation in severe congenital neutropenia is 11.8% at 10 years of follow-up in the SCNIR. In contrast individuals with Diamond-Blackfan anemia are less likely to progress to AML with a cumulative incidence of 5% by age 46; however, similar incidence increases with age (Vlachos et al. 2012). Taken together these data support a significant risk of malignant transformation in individuals with SDS.

Reports of solid tumors in SDS remain rare. Case reports in the literature include a 20-year-old woman with a slowly progressive dermatofibrosarcoma, which had been present for 3 years prior to diagnosis, a 20-year-old woman bilateral breast cancer, an 18-year-old young man with a CNS large B-cell lymphoma, and a 38-year-old man with pancreatic adenocarcinoma. To date, none of the study subjects in the SDS registry have reported solid tumors. Whether SDS is associated with an increased risk of solid tumors remains to be ascertained.

Development and persistence of clonal hematopoietic changes have been well described in SDS individuals. Cytogenetic changes classically associated with SDS include del(20)(q11) and isochromosome 7q (i(7)(q10)) (Dror et al. 2011). Several reports suggest that isolated del(20)(q11) in the setting of SDS may not be associated with a high risk of malignant transformation (Crescenzi et al. 2009; Maserati et al. 2009). Included in the interstitial deletion in 20q is the region encoding the *EIF6* gene (Pressato et al. 2012). Decrease in EIF6 is hypothesized to improve ribosome biogenesis in the context of SBDS deficiency. Similarly isochromosome 7q may be transient or persist over years of time without transformation to MDS/AML (Cunningham et al. 2002). Minelli et al. noted eight individuals with SDS and i(7)(q10) all of whom had gained an additional copy of the c.[258 + 2T > C] allele which is believed to be a hypomorphic mutation suggesting potential beneficial effects (Austin et al. 2005; Minelli et al. 2009). This phenomenon has also been demonstrated via copy number loss of heterozygosity of chromosome 7 (Parikh et al. 2012) in one SDS individual but was not seen in another larger series of ten SDS individuals (Nacci et al. 2014). A recent study from the Canadian Inherited Marrow Failure Registry, however, raises the concern that additional cytogenetic changes may remain a significant risk over time for these individuals with three of four individuals with i(7)(q10) developing clonal progression and one of the two with del(20)(q11) transforming to AML (Cada et al. 2015). Additionally, in a retrospective evaluation of cytogenetic monitoring and progression in the Italian SDS registry and other studies, Pressato et al. noted that while i(7)(q10) and del(20)(q11) clones did not acquire additional cytogenetic changes, 22 of these patients acquired additional independent clones with disease progression to aplasia or MDS/AML in several (Pressato et al. 2015). Thus, continuing surveillance for disease progression in these individuals remains of high importance.

Recurrent bacterial, viral, and fungal infections have been reported in individuals with SDS (Dror 2005). This spectrum of viral infections is not typically associated with neutropenia alone. Our understanding of immunologic dysfunction in SDS remains unclear. Abnormalities of neutrophil chemotaxis have been reported; however, individuals with SDS maintain the ability to form empyema and abscesses in contrast to other disorders of neutrophil chemotaxis (Aggett et al. 1979; Rothbaum et al. 1982; Grinspan and Pikora 2005). Neutrophil oxidative burst remains normal in SDS (Rochowski et al. 2010). Quantitative and functional abnormalities of T and B lymphocytes in 11 SDS individuals were also reported by Dror et al. (Dror et al. 2001); however, these were not seen in a recent SDS cohort of 12 individuals evaluated by Giri et al. with normal lymphocyte subsets and immunoglobulins (Giri et al. 2015).

8.2.2 Gastrointestinal Phenotype

Exocrine pancreatic dysfunction resulting from severe depletion of pancreatic acinar cells is a classic manifestation of SDS, typically noted in the first 6 months of life (Shwachman et al. 1964; Aggett et al. 1980; Hill et al. 1982). Manifestations clinically vary considerably from severe dysfunction with significant steatorrhea and resultant malabsorption of nutrients and subsequent failure to thrive, to clinically asymptomatic. Several recent publications report the absence of diarrhea at presentation of SDS (Myers et al. 2014; Andolina et al. 2013). For reasons that are not well understood, these clinical symptoms resolve spontaneously with age in many individuals with SDS. As many as 50% of children with SDS are able to stop pancreatic enzyme supplementation by age 4 with normal fat absorption, although enzyme secretion remains deficient (Mack et al. 1996). Parotid acinar dysfunction in SDS has also been reported. One study comparing parotid acinar function in 16 individuals with SDS to 13 individuals with fibrosing pancreatitis or cystic fibrosis and 13 healthy individuals identified parotid acinar dysfunction in SDS (Stormon et al. 2010). Secreted parotid amylase levels were lower in SDS than in both healthy and disease individuals, who were comparable to each other. Both serum pancreatic and parotid isoamlyase levels were also lower in individuals with SDS compared with healthy individuals, while only pancreatic isoamylase was lower in other disease individuals compared to the healthy cohort.

In addition to acinar dysfunction, Shah and colleagues have previously described potential enteropathies in approximately 50% of 15 symptomatic individuals with genetically confirmed SDS (Shah et al. 2010). Histologic changes in mucosal biopsies in this study varied but included villous blunting and partial villous atrophy with duodenal inflammation. Similarly in a recent publication evaluating nutritional deficiencies in SDS, Pichler and colleagues describe a subset of children who also underwent endoscopic evaluation for chronic gastrointestinal symptoms, and 50% demonstrated similar histologic changes (Pichler et al. 2015). In this retrospective review of 21 individuals with SDS, they were able to identify deficiencies of vitamin A and selenium in 76% and 48% of individuals, respectively, as well as vitamin E, zinc, and copper deficiency in 19%, 33%, and 24%. This was despite 95% receiving enzyme supplementation and 57% receiving enteral feeds, suggesting that monitoring of trace elements in SDS may be important to optimize nutritional health. Together these data suggest a potential enteropathic contribution to gastrointestinal symptoms in addition to exocrine pancreatic insufficiency in some individuals with SDS.

In addition to the well-recognized pancreatic disease manifestations, individuals with SDS may present with liver abnormalities early in life (Toiviainen-Salo et al. 2009). Elevated transaminases, hyperbilirubinemia, and hepatomegaly are frequently seen in young individuals with SDS. These liver abnormalities resolve with age. A study of 12 Finnish individuals with SDS reported elevated bile acids in 58%, and 3 of these individuals had persistent or intermittent elevation in longitudinal bile acid measurements concerning for persistent cholestasis (Toiviainen-Salo et al. 2009). Hepatomegaly was identified only in SDS individuals under the age of 3 years. Of interest, all three older SDS subjects (>30 years) were noted to have hepatic microcysts easily seen by imaging. Recently one small series also reported two young infants presenting with elevated transaminases and initial evaluation consistent with autoimmune hepatitis along with enteropathy believed to be consistent with celiac disease but neither responsive to immunosuppression nor gluten-free diet, who were subsequently diagnosed with SDS, highlighting the need for a high index of suspicion in these children (Veropalumbo et al. 2015). Additionally hepatic failure of unclear etiology has be seen in older individuals with SDS, reported in a 15-year-old patient with fibrosis and cholestasis (Schaballie et al. 2013) and another individual in the sixth decade of life in the North American SDS registry.

8.2.3 Neurocognitive Phenotype

Patients with SDS have historically been shown to have changes in brain structure and variable neurocognitive impairment (Kent et al. 1990; Toiviainen-Salo et al. 2008). Kerr and colleagues performed neuropsychiatric testing in 32 individuals with SDS as well as 13 sibling controls and 20 age- and gender-matched individuals with cystic fibrosis. In this study overall SDS individuals had a wide range of cognitive abilities from severely impaired to superior in some areas evaluated compared to controls. Areas of significant weaknesses included higher-order language, intellectual reasoning, visual-motor skills, and academic achievement with approximately 20% of SDS individuals meeting the diagnostic criteria for intellectual disability (Kerr et al. 2010). Attention deficits were also more common in SDS individuals and their siblings than cystic fibrosis controls. Recently Perobelli et al. performed questionnaire-based psychological and quality of life assessments in 54 SDS individuals and age- and gender-matched cystic fibrosis controls. Again cognitive impairment varied widely in 76% of adults and 65% of younger individuals from mild to severe but was increased from cystic fibrosis (CF) controls (Perobelli et al. 2012). SDS individuals also reported more attention deficits at 29% versus 0% in CF, social problems at 31% versus 6% in CF, and somatic complaints 24% versus 12% in CF.

Using structural MRI Toiviainen-Salo et al. demonstrated decreased global brain volume (1.74 L vs. 1.94 L, $P = 0.019$) in both white and gray matter in nine SDS individuals over a broad range of ages, 7–37 years (Toiviainen-Salo et al. 2008). Similar findings were seen by Booij et al. in an additional six SDS individuals ages 12–26 years with decreased brain volumes most evident posteriorly and caudally (Booij et al. 2013). Additionally they were able to demonstrate a dysregulated dopaminergic system. Most recently Perobelli et al. were able to combine neuroimaging by MRI with cognitive assessments and demonstrate diffuse changes in both gray and white matter associated with cognitive impairment in nine SDS individuals compared to age- and gender-matched normal controls. It remains unclear whether these changes may represent a delay in neurocognitive development relative to healthy controls, a static change, or may progress over time.

8.2.4 Skeletal Phenotype

Skeletal dysplasias are also seen frequently in individuals with SDS, although the phenotypes and severity are highly variable between individuals, even within families. The classic skeletal manifestations of SDS include short stature, progressive metaphyseal dysplasia or thickening in the long bones and costochondral junctions, and thoracic abnormalities such as pectus, flared ribs, asphyxiating thoracic dystrophy, as well as delayed development of normally shaped epiphyses (Aggett et al. 1980). Makitie et al. described skeletal abnormalities of varying severity and location in all 15 individuals of a cohort of genetically confirmed individuals with SDS, which often evolved with age (Makitie et al. 2004).

Low-turnover osteoporosis is also associated with SDS as demonstrated by Toiviainen-Salo and colleagues (Toiviainen-Salo et al. 2007) in a cohort of 11 genetically confirmed SDS individuals in whom 10 were shown to have abnormalities of bone health. Significantly reduced bone mineral density was demonstrated by low *Z*-scores, with vertebral compression fractures present in three individuals. Additionally deficiencies of vitamins K and D were each seen in six subjects, three with secondary hyperparathyroidism, both of which are known to be important for bone health.

8.2.5 Other Phenotypes

Other disease manifestations of SDS have been described, including those of the cardiac and endocrine systems. In a retrospective review of the French Severe Chronic Neutropenia Registry, cardiac abnormalities were identified in 12 (11%) of 102 SDS individuals (Hauet et al. 2013). Half of these consisted of a variety of congenital heart defects, most of which required clinical intervention. Cardiomyopathy, sometimes associated with viral infection or radiation/cyclophosphamide therapy, was seen in the other half. Abnormalities in circumferential strain by echocardiography were also seen a third of SDS individuals in a small retrospective cohort despite normal shortening fraction, suggesting there may be subclinical systolic dysfunction (Ryan et al. 2015).

Evaluations of endocrine function in SDS have been limited consisting largely of single case reports of individuals with SDS diagnosed with growth hormone deficiency or type I diabetes (Mack et al. 1996; Kamoda et al. 2005; Rosendahl et al. 2006; Gana et al. 2011; Fatih Akdogan et al. 2011; Goeteyn et al. 1991; Kawashima et al. 2006; Terlizzi et al. 2014). Short stature, however, is a commonly recognized feature of SDS (Ginzberg et al. 1999). In a recent retrospective study, 56% of biallelic SBDS mutation carrying individuals had short stature with height Z-scores less than −1.8 (Myers et al. 2013). BMI, however, was less affected with only 16% of those with biallelic SBDS mutations noted to have Z-scores less than −1.5. Endocrine manifestations of SDS aside from growth appear to be heterogeneous in nature. Seven (28%) of these individuals did show at least one endocrine abnormality excluding short stature including thyroid and growth hormone deficiencies, diabetes, and partial gonadal impairment in one individual after bone marrow transplant.

8.3 Diagnosis and Clinical Management

The diagnosis of SDS by classic criteria such as feeding difficulties associated with failure to thrive, along with recurrent infections or cytopenias, often occurs quite early in life within the first year. Many individuals, however, may present later in childhood or even as adults. This is especially true for those with nonclassical phenotypes for whom a high index of suspicion may be required to make the diagnosis. Table 8.1 summarizes the diagnostic criteria for SDS proposed in a consensus guidance document (Dror et al. 2011). While approximately 90% of individuals with SDS harbor biallelic mutations in SDS, there remains a small proportion of individuals who lack causative gene mutations. In these individuals other diagnostic considerations may include other etiologies of pancreatic and marrow dysfunction including cystic fibrosis or Pearson's disease, both of which are associated with pancreatic dysfunction. Pearson syndrome is characterized by cytopenias, ring sideroblasts, and vacuoles in the marrow.

Individuals with SDS should undergo comprehensive screening at diagnosis and regular intervals thereafter for known disease complications as shown in Table 8.3. Systematic monitoring of blood counts and marrow evaluations to assess risk for progression to aplastic anemia or malignant

Table 8.3 Clinical assessment in individuals with Shwachman-Diamond syndrome[a]

	Interval
Hematologic	
CBC	Diagnosis, every 3–4 months or as clinically indicated
Bone marrow aspirate and biopsy	Diagnosis, yearly or as clinically indicated
Fe, folate, B12 levels	Diagnosis, as clinically indicated
IgG, IgA, IgM levels	Diagnosis, as clinically indicated
HLA testing	As clinically indicated
Gastrointestinal	
Pancreatic enzymes	Diagnosis, as clinically indicated
(trypsinogen, pancreatic isoamylase)	
Fat-soluble vitamins (A, D, E)	Diagnosis, 1 month after initiation of pancreatic
Prothrombin time (surrogate for vitamin K)	Enzyme therapy; then every 6–12 months
Liver panel	Diagnosis, yearly or as clinically indicated
Pancreatic imaging (ultrasound)	Diagnosis
Growth/skeletal	
Height, weight, head circumference	Yearly, as clinically indicated
Skeletal evaluation	Consider at diagnosis or as clinically indicated[b]
Densitometry	As clinically indicated, screen in adults
Neurodevelopmental	
Developmental/neuropsychological screening	Diagnosis and regular assessment at follow-up for school aged
	Children ages 6–8, 11–13, 15–17

CBC complete blood count

[a]Adapted from Dror et al. Ann N Y Acad Sci. 2011 Dec;1242:40–55

[b]Potential clinical benefits of skeletal X-rays in asymptomatic patient must be balanced by potential risks of ionizing radiation in this cancer-prone disorder

transformation is critical. Neutropenia while very common is often intermittent in nature and is often mild or moderate in severity. Most SDS individuals do not require regular treatment with granulocyte colony stimulating factor (G-CSF). Indications for G-CSF treatment include persistent severe neutropenia accompanied by recurrent or severe bacterial or fungal infections. Most patients respond to relatively low doses of G-CSF. Therapeutic requirements in SDS individuals may range from continuous daily therapy to intermittent G-CSF use. When feasible, a bone marrow evaluation including cytogenetics and FISH testing is recommended prior to initiating G-CSF treatment to avoid potentially promoting outgrowth of abnormal clones.

Hematopoietic stem cell transplant (HSCT) remains the only curative therapeutic option for individuals with severe aplastic anemia or malignant transformation. Historic outcomes using myeloablative preparative regimens were poor with very high treatment-related mortality including significant pulmonary and cardiac toxicity (Myers and Davies 2009). With the advent of newer reduced intensity regimens, transplant outcomes for severe aplastic anemia or MDS have significantly improved. Outcomes for individuals with AML, however, remain quite challenging, underscoring the importance of consistent surveillance with blood counts and bone marrow evaluations. Sustained remission with chemotherapy for those with SDS and AML has been elusive and can result in significant toxicity including profound and often intractable aplasia adding to transplant risk and highlighting the need for timely utilization of HSCT in this setting.

Regular assessments of nutrition and growth, bone health, and neurodevelopment are also important to allow for early identification of areas of concern and prompt intervention. Supportive care with pancreatic enzyme supplementation to treat pancreatic insufficiency is essential for growth and nutrition.

Genetic counseling for patients and family members should be offered. All siblings of a proband are at risk for SDS regardless of clinical symptoms (Myers et al. 2014).

8.4 Molecular Pathogenesis

The SBDS protein has been demonstrated to be involved in several important pathways including ribosomal maturation (Finch et al. 2011), mitosis (Austin et al. 2008; Orelio et al. 2009), and the stromal microenvironment (Raaijmakers et al. 2010; Nihrane et al. 2009).

Finch et al. elegantly demonstrated the critical role of the SBDS protein in ribosome biogenesis in murine models. SBDS couples the GTPase elongation factor-like 1 (EFL1) results to the release of EIF6 protein from the pre-60S ribosomal subunit (Finch et al. 2011). EIF6 sterically blocks the association of the 60S ribosomal subunit to the 40S subunit. Release allows the joining of the 60S and 40S subunits resulting formation of the translationally active 80S ribosome (Menne et al. 2007; Wong et al. 2011). In yeast, mutations in *Tif6*, the eIF6 ortholog, reverse the slow growth phenotype of yeast lacking *Sdo1*, the *SBDS* ortholog (Menne et al. 2007). SBDS in humans is shown to associate with the large 60S subunit but not mature polysomal ribosomes (Ganapathi et al. 2007). Polysome profiles in SBDS-deficient animal models reveal half-mers, a pattern resulting from defective ribosome joining of the 40S and 6S subunits (Finch et al. 2011). SDS patient cells do not demonstrate these half-mer patterns, likely due to some residual SBDS expression, but they do demonstrate impaired ribosome association in vitro (Burwick et al. 2012). Ribosome association was improved by EIF6 knockdown, in these SDS patient cells; however, hematopoietic colony formation of SBDS-deficient CD34+ cells was not enhanced.

SBDS has also been shown to have additional roles outside that of ribosomal maturation. SBDS localizes to the mitotic spindles of primary human marrow stromal cells (Austin et al. 2008). Austin and colleagues demonstrated that lymphocytes and fibroblasts from SDS individuals have increased numbers of multipolar spindles, resulting in increased genomic instability that can be rescued with addition of purified SBDS protein (Austin et al. 2008). Additional of recombinant SBDS protein promoted the polymerization of purified microtubules, which supports a direct effect of SBDS on microtubule stabilization. Hematopoietic progenitor colony formation of primary SDS bone marrow was improved by the addition of the microtubule-stabilizing agent taxol. Additionally SBDS has been shown to co-localize with the centromeres and microtubules of the mitotic spindle and the microtubule-organizing center in neutrophils in interphase (Orelio et al. 2009; Orelio and Kuijpers 2009).

Cell proliferation and differentiation of neutrophils were also different in SDS in vitro compared to controls. These findings suggest a SBDS may play an important role in cell division and proliferation particularly in the myeloid lineage, as reflected by the clinical manifestations of neutropenia and propensity toward myeloid malignant transformation in SDS individuals.

SBDS has also been demonstrated to have a role in a variety of other cellular functions. It has been implicated in Fas ligand-induced apoptosis (Rujkijyanont et al. 2008), increased production of reactive oxygen species (Ambekar et al. 2010), decreased mitochondrial membrane potential (Henson et al. 2013), and intensified cellular stress responses (Ball et al. 2009). SBDS may also play a role in marrow stromal function (Dror and Freedman 1999; Andre et al. 2012). SBDS knockdown cell lines demonstrate increased expression by microarray of vascular endothelial growth factor-A and osteoprotegerin, which are known to influence osteoclast differentiation, monocyte and macrophage migration, and angiogenesis (Nihrane et al. 2009). Targeted deletion of SBDS in murine osteoprogenitors resulted in bone marrow dysfunction including leukopenia, lymphopenia, and myelodysplasia in the setting of bony abnormalities (Raaijmakers et al. 2010). Recently Zambetti and colleagues demonstrated that targeted deletion of *Sbds* in osteoprogenitor cells mice results in genotoxic stress in hematopoietic cells in the form of mitochondrial dysfunction and oxidative stress. This is driven through p53-S100A8/9-TLR4 signaling which was predictive of evolution to MDS/AML in non-SDS subjects with low-risk MDS (Zambetti Noemi et al. 2016). These findings suggest that decreased SBDS expression in stromal cells may lead to changes in the hematopoietic microenvironment favoring the development of marrow failure, MDS, and acute leukemia. However, others have shown normal function in vitro in SBDS-deficient mesenchymal stem cells (Andre et al. 2012).

Animal models of SDS have been challenging historically because targeted deletion of murine SBDS results in early embryonic lethality (Zhang et al. 2006). Knockdown of murine Sbds with RNA interference in murine bone marrow followed by transplantation results in delayed in vitro myeloid differentiation, impaired homing of hematopoietic progenitors, and decreased short term engraftment (Rawls et al. 2007). Knockdown of SBDS with morpholinos in zebrafish recapitulated many feature of the human disease, including neutrophil loss, skeletal changes, and pancreatic hypoplasia (Provost et al. 2012). Organ-specific murine models have demonstrated findings similar to the clinical SDS phenotype. Tourlakis et al. generated a pancreas-specific murine knock-in model introducing a missense mutation in *SBDS* which resulted in mice with smaller overall size as well as smaller pancreata with hypoplastic acni with fatty infiltration with decreased zymogen granules but intact islet cells, very similar to findings in SDS individuals (Tourlakis et al. 2012). Most recently, Zambetti et al. created a novel murine model of SDS utilizing conditional *SBDS* knockout under the control of a CEBPα-Cre recombinase, allowing for transplantation of *SBDS*-deficient fetal liver cells into lethally irradiated wild-type recipients (Zambetti et al. 2015). These recipients then developed hypoplastic bone marrow with decreased neutrophils and profound peripheral neutropenia. They demonstrated a block in myeloid differentiation at the myelocyte stage with activation of TP53 suggesting that apoptotic pathways may mediate this phenotype. Malignant transformation was not observed; however, the follow-up of these animals was relatively short at 4 months. iPSC derived from individuals with SDS have also been developed by knockdown of *SBDS* in human embryonic stem cells and demonstrate defects in hematopoietic differentiation with enhanced apoptosis as well as exocrine pancreatic dysfunction (Tulpule et al. 2013).

Novel IPSC and animal models have significant potential to advance our understanding of SDS disease pathogenesis and the role of SBDS in important cellular pathways such as ribosome biogenesis, mitosis, and others. These exciting scientific tools may also provide a mechanism for testing potential therapeutic strategies to advance our approach to the care of individuals with SDS.

Acknowledgments This work was supported by NIH/NIDDK R24 DK099808-03 (A.S.).

References

Aggett PJ, Harries JT, Harvey BA, Soothill JF (1979) An inherited defect of neutrophil mobility in Shwachman syndrome. J Pediatr 94:391–394

Aggett P, Cavanagh N, Matthew D, Pincott J, Sutcliffe J, Harries J (1980) Shwachman's syndrome. A review of 21 cases. Arch Dis Child 55:331–347

Alter B (2014) Fanconi anemia and the development of leukemia. Best Pract Res Clin Haematol 27:214–221

Alter BP, Giri N, Savage SA et al (2010) Malignancies and survival patterns in the National Cancer Institute inherited bone marrow failure syndromes cohort study. Br J Haematol 150:179–188

Ambekar C, Das B, Yeger H, Dror Y (2010) SBDS-deficiency results in deregulation of reactive oxygen species leading to increased cell death and decreased cell growth. Pediatr Blood Cancer 55:1138–1144

Andolina JR, Morrison CB, Thompson AA et al (2013) Shwachman-Diamond syndrome: diarrhea, no longer required? J Pediatr Hematol Oncol 35:486–489

Andre V, Longoni D, Bresolin S et al (2012) Mesenchymal stem cells from Shwachman-Diamond syndrome patients display normal functions and do not contribute to hematological defects. Blood Cancer J 2:e94

Austin KM, Leary RJ, Shimamura A (2005) The Shwachman-Diamond SBDS protein localizes to the nucleolus. Blood 106:1253–1258

Austin KM, Gupta ML, Coats SA et al (2008) Mitotic spindle destabilization and genomic instability in Shwachman-Diamond syndrome. J Clin Invest 118:1511–1518

Ball HL, Zhang B, Riches JJ et al (2009) Shwachman-Bodian Diamond syndrome is a multi-functional protein implicated in cellular stress responses. Hum Mol Genet 18:3684–3695

Booij J, Reneman L, Alders M, Kuijpers TW (2013) Increase in central striatal dopamine transporters in patients with Shwachman–Diamond syndrome: additional evidence of a brain phenotype. Am J Med Genet A 161:102–107

Burwick N, Coats SA, Nakamura T, Shimamura A (2012) Impaired ribosomal subunit association in Shwachman-Diamond syndrome. Blood 120:5143–5152

Cada M, Segbefia CI, Klaassen R et al (2015) The impact of category, cytopathology and cytogenetics on development and progression of clonal and malignant myeloid transformation in inherited bone marrow failure syndromes. Haematologica 100:633–642

Cipolli M (2001) Shwachman-Diamond syndrome: clinical phenotypes. Pancreatology 1:543–548

Crescenzi B, La Starza R, Sambani C et al (2009) Totipotent stem cells bearing del(20q) maintain multipotential differentiation in Shwachman Diamond syndrome. Br J Haematol 144:116–119

Cunningham J, Sales M, Pearce A et al (2002) Does isochromosome 7q mandate bone marrow transplant in children with Shwachman-Diamond syndrome? Br J Haematol 119:1062–1069

Dale DC, Bolyard AA, Schwinzer BG et al (2006) The severe chronic neutropenia international registry: 10-year follow-up report. Support Cancer Ther 3:220–231

Donadieu J, Leblanc T, Bader Meunier B et al (2005) Analysis of risk factors for myelodysplasias, leukemias and death from infection among patients with congenital neutropenia. Experience of the French Severe Chronic Neutropenia Study Group. Haematologica 90:45–53

Donadieu J, Fenneteau O, Beaupain B et al (2012) Classification and risk factors of hematological complications in a French national cohort of 102 patients with Shwachman-Diamond syndrome. Haematologica 97(9):1312–1319

Dror Y (2005) Shwachman-Diamond syndrome. Pediatr Blood Cancer 45:892–901

Dror Y, Freedman MH (1999) Shwachman-Diamond syndrome: an inherited preleukemic bone marrow failure disorder with aberrant hematopoietic progenitors and faulty marrow microenvironment. Blood 94:3048–3054

Dror Y, Ginzberg H, Dalal I et al (2001) Immune function in patients with Shwachman-Diamond syndrome. Br J Haematol 114:712–717

Dror Y, Donadieu J, Koglmeier J et al (2011) Draft consensus guidelines for diagnosis and treatment of Shwachman-Diamond syndrome. Ann N Y Acad Sci 1242:40–55

Fatih Akdogan M, Altay M, Denizli N, Gucun M, Tanrikulu S, Duranay M (2011) A rare case: Shwachman-Diamond syndrome presenting with diabetic ketoacidosis. Endocrine 40:146–147

Finch AJ, Hilcenko C, Basse N et al (2011) Uncoupling of GTP hydrolysis from eIF6 release on the ribosome causes Shwachman-Diamond syndrome. Genes Dev 25:917–929

Gana S, Sainati L, Frau MR et al (2011) Shwachman-Diamond syndrome and type 1 diabetes mellitus: more than a chance association? Exp Clin Endocrinol Diabetes 119:610–612

Ganapathi KA, Austin KM, Lee CS et al (2007) The human Shwachman-Diamond syndrome protein, SBDS, associates with ribosomal RNA. Blood 110:1458–1465

Ginzberg H, Shin J, Ellis L et al (1999) Shwachman syndrome: phenotypic manifestations of sibling sets and isolated cases in a large patient cohort are similar. J Pediatr 135:81–88

Giri N, Alter BP, Penrose K et al (2015) Immune status of patients with inherited bone marrow failure syndromes. Am J Hematol 90:702–708

Goeteyn M, Oranje A, Vuzevski V, de Groot R, van Suijlekom-Smit L (1991) Ichthyosis, exocrine pancreatic insufficiency, impaired neutrophil chemotaxis, growth retardation, and metaphyseal dysplasia (Shwachman syndrome). Report of a case with extensive skin lesions (clinical, histological, and ultrastructural findings). Arch Dermatol 127:225–230

Goobie S, Popovic M, Morrison J et al (2001) Shwachman-Diamond syndrome with exocrine pancreatic dysfunction and bone marrow failure maps to the centromeric region of chromosome 7. Am J Hum Genet 68:1048–1054

Grinspan ZM, Pikora CA (2005) Infections in patients with Shwachman-Diamond syndrome. Pediatr Infect Dis J 24:179–181

Hashmi S, Allen C, Klaassen R et al (2011) Comparative analysis of Shwachman-Diamond syndrome to other inherited bone marrow failure syndromes and genotype-phenotype correlation. Clin Genet 79(5):448–458

Hauet Q, Beaupain B, Micheau M et al (2013) Cardiomyopathies and congenital heart diseases in Shwachman–Diamond syndrome: a national survey. Int J Cardiol 167:1048–1050

Henson AL, Moore Iv JB, Alard P, Wattenberg MM, Liu JM, Ellis SR (2013) Mitochondrial function is impaired in yeast and human cellular models of Shwachman Diamond syndrome. Biochem Biophys Res Commun 437:29–34

Hill RE, Durie PR, Gaskin KJ, Davidson GP, Forstner GG (1982) Steatorrhea and pancreatic insufficiency in Shwachman syndrome. Gastroenterology 83: 22–27

Kamoda T, Saito T, Kinugasa H et al (2005) A case of Shwachman-Diamond syndrome presenting with diabetes from early infancy. Diabetes Care 28:1508–1509

Kawashima H, Ushio M, Aritaki K et al (2006) Discordant endocrinopathy in a sibling with Shwachman-Diamond syndrome. J Trop Pediatr 52:445–447

Kent A, Murphy GH, Milla P (1990) Psychological characteristics of children with Shwachman syndrome. Arch Dis Child 65:1349–1352

Kerr EN, Ellis L, Dupuis A, Rommens JM, Durie PR (2010) The behavioral phenotype of school-age children with Shwachman Diamond syndrome indicates neurocognitive dysfunction with loss of Shwachman-Bodian-Diamond syndrome gene function. J Pediatr 156:433–438

Mack DR, Forstner GG, Wilschanski M, Freedman MH, Durie PR (1996) Shwachman syndrome: exocrine pancreatic dysfunction and variable phenotypic expression. Gastroenterology 111:1593–1602

Makitie O, Ellis L, Durie PR et al (2004) Skeletal phenotype in patients with Shwachman-Diamond syndrome and mutations in SBDS. Clin Genet 65:101–112

Maserati E, Pressato B, Valli R et al (2009) The route to development of myelodysplastic syndrome/acute myeloid leukaemia in Shwachman-Diamond syndrome: the role of ageing, karyotype instability, and acquired chromosome anomalies. Br J Haematol 145:190–197

Menne TF, Goyenechea B, Sanchez-Puig N et al (2007) The Shwachman-Bodian-Diamond syndrome protein mediates translational activation of ribosomes in yeast. Nat Genet 39:486–495

Minelli A, Maserati E, Nicolis E et al (2009) The isochromosome i(7)(q10) carrying c.258+2t>c mutation of the SBDS gene does not promote development of myeloid malignancies in patients with Shwachman syndrome. Leukemia 23:708–711

Minelli A, Nicolis E, Cannioto Z et al (2012) Incidence of Shwachman–Diamond syndrome. Pediatr Blood Cancer 59:1334–1335

Myers KC, Davies SM (2009) Hematopoietic stem cell transplantation for bone marrow failure syndromes in children. Biol Blood Marrow Transplant 15:279–292

Myers KC, Rose SR, Rutter MM et al (2013) Endocrine evaluation of children with and without Shwachman-Bodian-Diamond syndrome gene mutations and Shwachman-Diamond syndrome. J Pediatr 162:1235–1240.e1231

Myers KC, Bolyard AA, Otto B et al (2014) Variable clinical presentation of Shwachman–Diamond syndrome: update from the North American Shwachman–Diamond syndrome registry. J Pediatr 164:866–870

Nacci L, Danesino C, Sainati L et al (2014) Absence of acquired copy number neutral loss of heterozygosity (CN-LOH) of chromosome 7 in a series of 10 patients with Shwachman–Diamond syndrome. Br J Haematol 165:573–575

Nihrane A, Sezgin G, Dsilva S et al (2009) Depletion of the Shwachman-Diamond syndrome gene product, SBDS, leads to growth inhibition and increased expression of OPG and VEGF-A. Blood Cell Mol Dis 42:85–91

Orelio C, Kuijpers TW (2009) Shwachman-Diamond syndrome neutrophils have altered chemoattractant-induced F-actin polymerization and polarization characteristics. Haematologica 94:409–413

Orelio C, Verkuijlen P, Geissler J, van den Berg TK, Kuijpers TW (2009) SBDS expression and localization at the mitotic spindle in human myeloid progenitors. PLoS One 4:e7084

Parikh S, Perdigones N, Paessler M et al (2012) Acquired copy number neutral loss of heterozygosity of chromosome 7 associated with clonal haematopoiesis in a patient with Shwachman-Diamond syndrome. Br J Haematol 159(4):480–482

Perobelli S, Nicolis E, Assael BM, Cipolli M (2012) Further characterization of Shwachman–Diamond syndrome: psychological functioning and quality of life in adult and young patients. Am J Med Genet A 158A:567–573

Pichler J, Meyer R, Köglmeier J, Ancliff P, Shah N (2015) Nutritional status in children with Shwachman-Diamond syndrome. Pancreas 44:590–595

Pressato B, Valli R, Marletta C et al (2012) Deletion of chromosome 20 in bone marrow of patients with

Shwachman-Diamond syndrome, loss of the EIF6 gene and benign prognosis. Br J Haematol 157(4):503–505

Pressato B, Valli R, Marletta C et al (2015) Cytogenetic monitoring in Shwachman-Diamond syndrome: a note on clonal progression and a practical warning. J Pediatr Hematol Oncol 37:307–310

Provost E, Wehner KA, Zhong X et al (2012) Ribosomal biogenesis genes play an essential and p53-independent role in zebrafish pancreas development. Development 139:3232–3241

Raaijmakers MHGP, Mukherjee S, Guo S et al (2010) Bone progenitor dysfunction induces myelodysplasia and secondary leukaemia. Nature 464:852–857

Rawls AS, Gregory AD, Woloszynek JR, Liu F, Link DC (2007) Lentiviral-mediated RNAi inhibition of Sbds in murine hematopoietic progenitors impairs their hematopoietic potential. Blood 110:2414–2422

Rochowski A, Sun C, Glogauer M, Alter BP (2010) Neutrophil functions in patients with inherited bone marrow failure syndromes. Pediatr Blood Cancer 57(2):306–309

Rosenberg PS, Alter BP, Bolyard AA et al (2006) The incidence of leukemia and mortality from sepsis in patients with severe congenital neutropenia receiving long-term G-CSF therapy. Blood 107:4628–4635

Rosendahl J, Teich N, Mossner J, Edelmann J, Koch CA (2006) Compound heterozygous mutations of the SBDS gene in a patient with Shwachman-Diamond syndrome, type 1 diabetes mellitus and osteoporosis. Pancreatology 6:549–554

Rothbaum RJ, Williams DA, Daugherty CC (1982) Unusual surface distribution of concanavalin A reflects a cytoskeletal defect in neutrophils in Shwachman's syndrome. Lancet 2:800–801

Rujkijyanont P, Watanabe K-i, Ambekar C et al (2008) SBDS-deficient cells undergo accelerated apoptosis through the Fas-pathway. Haematologica 93:363–371

Ryan TD, Jefferies JL, Chin C et al (2015) Abnormal circumferential strain measured by echocardiography is present in patients with Shwachman–Diamond syndrome despite normal shortening fraction. Pediatr Blood Cancer 62:1228–1231

Schaballie H, Renard M, Vermylen C et al (2013) Misdiagnosis as asphyxiating thoracic dystrophy and CMV-associated haemophagocytic lymphohistiocytosis in Shwachman-Diamond syndrome. Eur J Pediatr 172:613–622

Shah N, Cambrook H, Koglmeier J et al (2010) Enteropathic histopathological features may be associated with Shwachman-Diamond syndrome. J Clin Pathol 63:592–594

Shwachman H, Diamond LK, Oski FA, Khaw KT (1964) The syndrome of pancreatic insufficiency and bone marrow dysfunction. J Pediatr 65:645–663

Stormon MO, Ip WF, Ellis L, Schibli S, Rommens JM, Durie PR (2010) Evidence of a generalized defect of acinar cell function in Shwachman-Diamond syndrome. J Pediatr Gastroenterol Nutr 51:8–13

Terlizzi V, Zito E, Mozzillo E, Raia V, Franzese A (2014) Can continuous subcutaneous insulin infusion improve health-related quality of life in patients with Shwachman–Bodian–Diamond syndrome and diabetes? Diabetes Technol Ther 17:64–67

Toiviainen-Salo S, Mayranpaa MK, Durie PR et al (2007) Shwachman-Diamond syndrome is associated with low-turnover osteoporosis. Bone 41:965–972

Toiviainen-Salo S, Makitie O, Mannerkoski M, Hamalainen J, Valanne L, Autti T (2008) Shwachman-Diamond syndrome is associated with structural brain alterations on MRI. Am J Med Genet A 146A:1558–1564

Toiviainen-Salo S, Durie PR, Numminen K et al (2009) The natural history of Shwachman-Diamond syndrome-associated liver disease from childhood to adulthood. J Pediatr 155:807–811.e802

Tourlakis ME, Zhong J, Gandhi R et al (2012) Deficiency of Sbds in the mouse pancreas leads to features of Shwachman-Diamond syndrome, with loss of zymogen granules. Gastroenterology 143(2):481–492

Tulpule A, Kelley James M, Lensch MW et al (2013) Pluripotent stem cell models of Shwachman-Diamond syndrome reveal a common mechanism for pancreatic and hematopoietic dysfunction. Cell Stem Cell 12:727–736

Veropalumbo C, Campanozzi A, De Gregorio F, Correra A, Raia V, Vajro P (2015) Shwachman-Diamond syndrome with autoimmune-like liver disease and enteropathy mimicking celiac disease. Clin Res Hepatol Gastroenterol 39:e1–e4

Vlachos A, Rosenberg PS, Atsidaftos E, Alter BP, Lipton JM (2012) The incidence of neoplasia in Diamond-Blackfan anemia: a report from the Diamond-Blackfan Anemia Registry. Blood 119(16):3815–3819

Wong CC, Traynor D, Basse N, Kay RR, Warren AJ (2011) Defective ribosome assembly in Shwachman-Diamond syndrome. Blood 118(16): 4305–4312

Zambetti Noemi A, Ping Z, Chen S et al (2016) Mesenchymal inflammation drives genotoxic stress in hematopoietic stem cells and predicts disease evolution in human pre-leukemia. Cell Stem Cell 19(5):613–627

Zambetti NA, Bindels EMJ, Van Strien PMH et al (2015) Deficiency of the ribosome biogenesis gene Sbds in hematopoietic stem and progenitor cells causes neutropenia in mice by attenuating lineage progression in myelocytes. Haematologica 100: 1285–1293

Zhang S, Shi M, Hui C, Rommens J (2006) Loss of the mouse ortholog of the Shwachman-Diamond syndrome gene (Sbds) results in early embryonic lethality. Mol Cell Biol 26:6656–6663

9 Hematopoietic Cell Transplantation for the Treatment of Patients with Bone Marrow Failure Syndromes

Andrew C. Dietz and Michael A. Pulsipher

Contents

9.1 Introduction

Over 80% of patients presenting with bone marrow failure (BMF) are eventually diagnosed with acquired severe aplastic anemia (SAA), which is thought to be caused in the majority of patients by autoimmune destruction of hematopoietic stem cells (Samarasinghe and Webb 2012; Scheinberg and Young 2012). The other approximately 20% of patients, some of whom may present with clinical signs and symptoms other than BMF, are grouped into a category of inherited bone marrow failure syndromes (IBMFS). While many rare conditions will sometimes include BMF as part of their phenotype, the most common IBMFS, for the purpose of this discussion, include Fanconi anemia (FA), dyskeratosis congenita (DC), Diamond-Blackfan anemia (DBA), Shwachman-Diamond syndrome (SDS), severe congenital neutropenia (SCN), congenital amegakaryocytic thrombocytopenia (CAMT),

A. C. Dietz (✉) · M. A. Pulsipher
Children's Center for Cancer and Blood Disorders, Children's Hospital Los Angeles, University of Southern California, Los Angeles, CA, USA
e-mail: mpulsipher@chla.usc.edu

G. M. Kupfer et al. (eds.), *Bone Marrow Failure*, Pediatric Oncology,
https://doi.org/10.1007/978-3-319-61421-2_9

and thrombocytopenia absent radii (TAR) (Alter 2007). Myelodysplasia (MDS) can sometimes present with a hypocellular phenotype and be confused with BMF, especially in children, where a pathological entity called refractory cytopenia of childhood (RCC) is being recognized more commonly (Hasle 2016). Because RCC and other forms of MDS are more often grouped with and treated similar to myeloid malignancies, we will not address these diseases in this chapter. Distinction between SAA and IBMFS or MDS is vital, as treatment options and efficacy of approaches vary significantly depending on the specific diagnosis.

9.2 Severe Aplastic Anemia (SAA)

The treatment algorithm for acquired SAA, particularly in children, is under evolution (Dietz et al. 2016). The two mainstays of treatment include immunosuppressive therapy (IST) and/or allogeneic HSCT. When a human leukocyte antigen (HLA)-matched sibling donor (MSD) is available, HCT from that donor is considered standard of care for newly diagnosed, younger patients. Reports show greater than 95% survival and minimal graft GVHD with current reduced intensity conditioning (RIC) regimens, much improved from previous myeloablative conditioning (MAC) regimens (Samarasinghe and Webb 2012; Scheinberg and Young 2012; Storb et al. 2001; Burroughs et al. 2012). The currently preferred regimen is cyclophosphamide with anti-thymocyte globulin (ATG) (Storb et al. 2001; Burroughs et al. 2012), with some groups utilizing fludarabine and lower cyclophosphamide dosing (Bacigalupo 2014). Importantly, the use of bone marrow as a source of stem cells is superior to peripheral blood stem cells in this patient population due to lower rates of GVHD (Bacigalupo et al. 2012).

Patients without an available MSD typically proceed to IST with horse ATG and cyclosporine (Samarasinghe and Webb 2012; Scheinberg and Young 2012). Response rates are approximately 70–80%, taking on average 3–6 months. However, relapse can occur up to 30% of the time (Schrezenmeier et al. 1993), and secondary clonal hematopoiesis occurs in up to an additional 20% of patients (Saracco et al. 2008; Socie et al. 2000; Kojima et al. 2000). Matched unrelated donor (MUD) HCT is indicated for those patients with refractory SAA, relapsed disease, or clonal evolution. Ideally, the decision to proceed with MUD HCT should happen within 4–6 months in the case of refractory disease. Figure 9.1 shows overall survival in a European cohort from 2005 to 2009 broken down by MSD and MUD (Bacigalupo et al. 2015). More recently, using fludarabine, cyclophosphamide, and alemtuzumab, survival was reported in 96% of patients, with only 4% graft rejection, 10% acute GVHD, and 19% chronic GVHD (Dufour et al. 2015). With fludarabine, low-dose cyclophosphamide, ATG, and low-dose total body irradiation (TBI), survival was reported at 97% of patients with only 12% graft rejection, 24% acute GVHD, and 22% chronic GVHD (Anderlini et al. 2015). Once again, the importance of bone marrow as the preferred stem cell source for unrelated donor transplantation has been clearly demonstrated, once again related to the lower rates of GVHD (Eapen et al. 2011).

Unfortunately, not all patients will have an available MSD or MUD. Small case reports and case series of the use of cord blood (Peffault de Latour et al. 2011; Yoshimi et al. 2008; Chan et al. 2008) and haploidentical donors (Clay et al. 2014; Gao et al. 2014; Ciceri et al. 2013; Jaiswal et al. 2015; Gupta et al. 2015; Im et al. 2015; Esteves et al. 2015) initially showed poor outcomes. More recent, optimized RIC approaches with fludarabine, low-dose cyclophosphamide, low-dose TBI, and ATG and using both cord blood and haploidentical donors (with post-HSCT cyclophosphamide used for haploidentical donors) have resulted in encouraging outcomes and are currently being studied in a multi-institutional trial in the United States (Dietz et al. 2016) (NCT02918292 on www.clinicaltrials.gov). Also under investigation is the use of MUD HCT as initial therapy, given the excellent results reported above. This is being done already in Europe (Dietz et al. 2016; Dufour et al. 2015; Mackarel et al. 2016) and is being tested in a pilot

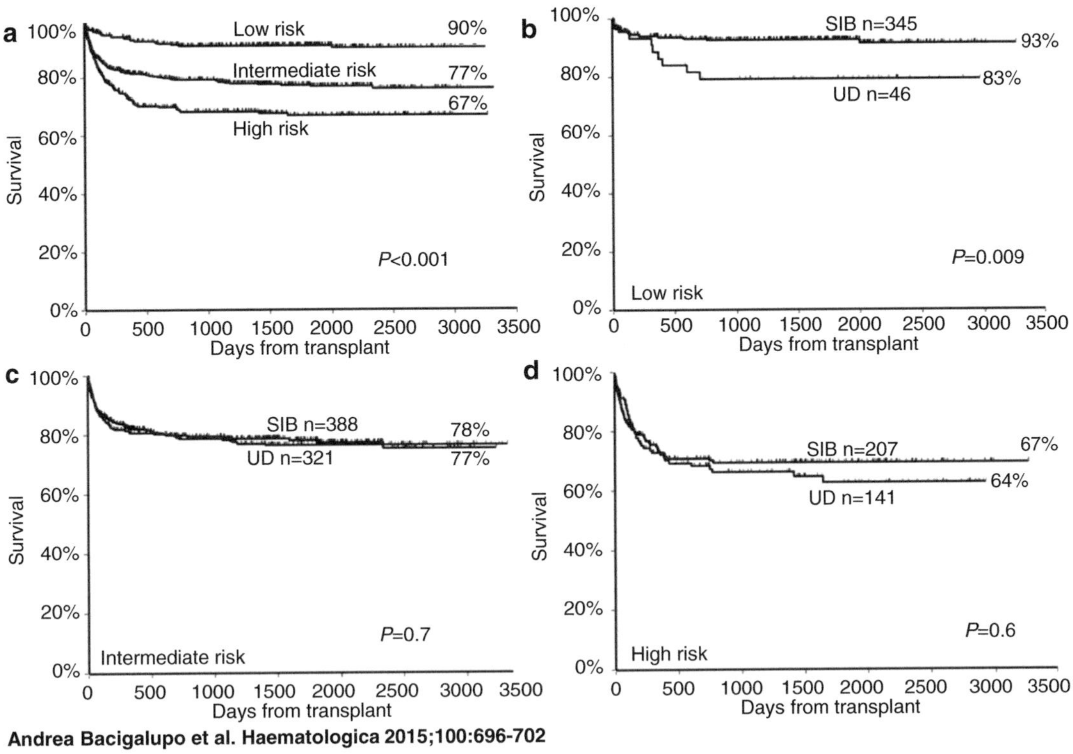

Fig. 9.1 Overall survival in low-risk SAA patients by donor type. SIB, matched sibling donor; UD, matched unrelated donor (Bacigalupo et al. 2015)

study randomizing patients to MUD HCT or IST (Dietz et al. 2016) (NCT02845596 on www.clinicaltrials.gov), in anticipation of a large phase III trial in children and young adults.

9.3 Fanconi Anemia (FA)

Given the complex and heterogeneous nature of FA, there are many important aspects to consider regarding current treatment options. The Fanconi Anemia Research Foundation has helped to sponsor and organize a set of clinical guidelines available in the book entitled *Fanconi Anemia: Guidelines for Diagnosis and Management* (http://fanconi.org/images/uploads/other/FA_Guidelines_4th_Edition_Revised_Names_in_Appendix.pdf). When specifically considering the BMF portion of this disorder, HCT offers cure related to the hematopoietic compartment. HCT, however, does not treat the other manifestations of FA and may in fact interact with the underlying disease process to magnify some risks, most notably head and neck squamous cell carcinoma (SCC) (Rosenberg et al. 2005). Due to the underlying chemotherapy and radiation therapy sensitivity of these patients, early MAC regimens resulted in significant mortality (Tan et al. 2006; Peffault de Latour et al. 2013). To date, this is the most studied IBMFS with respect to the use of allogeneic HCT.

The incorporation of fludarabine, reduction in alkylator doses, and elimination of TBI with use of a MSD have led to much improved outcomes, including some reports with 100% early survival (Tan et al. 2006; Peffault de Latour et al. 2013; Ayas et al. 2005, 2012, 2014; Smetsers et al. 2016; Stepensky et al. 2011; Kuşkonmaz et al. 2016; Benajiba et al. 2015; Shimada et al. 2012; Yabe et al. 2012). The preferred regimen today appears to be fludarabine with low doses of cyclophosphamide and ATG, with (Tan et al. 2006) or without (Smetsers et al. 2016; Ayas et al. 2012; Kuşkonmaz et al. 2016; Benajiba et al. 2015) ex vivo T-cell depletion to diminish the rates of GVHD. In the MUD setting, outcomes have generally been inferior, though much improved after studies showed success with reduction in alkylator and TBI doses and incorporation of fludarabine, which has reduced rates of rejection (Smetsers et al. 2016; Stepensky et al. 2011; Shimada et al. 2012; Wagner et al. 2007; MacMillan et al. 2015; Chao et al. 2015). While higher rates of GVHD are reported compared to MSD HCT, overall survival still is above 80–90% in most reports (Smetsers et al. 2016; MacMillan et al. 2015). The preferred regimen today appears to be fludarabine and ATG with lower doses of cyclophosphamide (though somewhat higher than in the MSD setting) and with (MacMillan et al. 2015) or without (Smetsers et al. 2016; Stepensky et al. 2011; Shimada et al. 2012) low-dose TBI. In the cord blood setting, similar preparative regimens to MUD HCT have been utilized (MacMillan et al. 2015; Jaing et al. 2014; Gluckman et al. 2007), though sometimes with higher rates of rejection (Gluckman et al. 2007). The importance of a higher cell dose has been clearly identified (Gluckman et al. 2007). Haploidentical HCT has been reported in very small numbers of patients undergoing transplantation with ex vivo T-cell depletion (Boulad et al. 2000; Dufort et al. 2012; Zecca et al. 2014) or reduced dose post-HCT cyclophosphamide (Thakar et al. 2012). These small studies have demonstrated early promising results. These approaches are under investigation at a limited number of centers.

As some patients will present with or have evolution to MDS or leukemia, the method for treating these patients prior to HCT has been a concern due to the underlying chemotherapy sensitivity of patients with FA. The largest study to date is a report from the CIBMTR on 113 patients that showed 55% survival at 3 years. Patients transplanted with a MSD and those with only abnormal cytogenetics rather than MDS or leukemia fared better (Ayas et al. 2013). Some reports suggest that pre-HCT chemotherapy made no clear difference and only led to toxicity (Mitchell et al. 2014), while others have successfully incorporated low-dose cytarabine as pre-HCT cytoreduction (Beier et al. 2015; Talbot et al. 2014; Peffault de Latour and Soulier 2016) or directly into the conditioning regimen (Aoki et al. 2016) with limited success. Ideally, HCT should occur before clonal evolution or before other significant complications such as iron overload, infection, bleeding events, and allosensitization but late enough to avoid early childhood morbidity from HCT.

With patients now living longer than previously, the need for a better understanding of long-term toxicities after HCT is becoming more apparent (Dietz et al. 2017a, b). Many patients have late endocrine abnormalities (Smetsers et al. 2016; Anur et al. 2016) that may be related to the underlying FA and may or may not be exacerbated by HCT. The presence of chronic GVHD is a major long-term toxicity for these patients, particularly given the association between GVHD and subsequent SCC above baseline levels seen in FA patients without HCT (Peffault de Latour et al. 2013; Smetsers et al. 2016; Anur et al. 2016; Bonfim et al. 2016). These malignant events contribute to significant late mortality (Smetsers et al. 2016; Bonfim et al. 2016). Aside from chronic GVHD, these studies also confirm that the use of radiation in the preparative regimen remains one of the leading factors for late effects including secondary malignancies.

Studies have demonstrated that the optimal timing to move to transplant is at presentation of significant BMF, preferably before starting chronic transfusion therapy. Patients who present with clear transformation to MDS or leukemia are also candidates for HCT. Regimens should be FA-specific RIC, with minimal to no radiation and alkylator exposure. These regimens should also balance the risk of mixed chimerism and the possibility of not eliminating all of the potential clones. A new question that arises for patients, families, and treating physicians in today's era of improved HCT outcomes is how early to move to transplantation. More recently some have suggested a role for preemptive HCT in FA (Khan et al. 2016), particularly in the highest-risk group with *BRCA2* mutations (Khan et al. 2015). If the assumption holds that regimens today have minimal TRM and little late carcinogenicity, younger patients may indeed benefit from this approach.

FA is mostly inherited in an autosomal recessive manner with more rare cases of autosomal dominant or X-linked inheritance. When choosing related donors for HCT, the genetic mutation should be known for the patient, and the donor should be screened to ensure they do not carry a pathogenic mutation pattern. There is little to no literature on the use of a carrier sibling in the event of an autosomal recessive pattern of inheritance. Notably, however, carriers of some pathogenic mutations such as *BRCA2/FANCD1*, *PALB2/FANCN*, and *RAD51C/FANCO* show increased rates of malignancy and should not be used as a donor for HCT purposes (Park et al. 2014). If the patient does not have a known genetic mutation, caution should be used when considering any related donors. Additional screening with chromosomal breakage studies should be conducted on all potential donors.

9.4 Dyskeratosis Congenita (DC)

Given the complex and heterogeneous nature of DC, there are many important aspects to consider regarding current treatment options. DC Outreach, a family support organization, has helped to sponsor and organize a set of clinical guidelines available in the book entitled *Dyskeratosis Congenita and Telomere Biology Disorders: Diagnosis and Management Guidelines* (https://www.dcoutreach.org/sites/default/files/DC%20%26%20TBD%20Diagnosis%20And%20Management%20Guidelines.pdf). When specifically considering the BMF portion of this disorder, HCT offers cure related to the hematopoietic compartment. HCT, however, does not treat the other manifestations of DC and may in fact interact with the underlying disease process to magnify risk of cancer, pulmonary fibrosis, and hepatic cirrhosis (Dietz et al. 2017b). Due to the underlying chemotherapy and radiation therapy sensitivity of these patients, early MAC transplantation resulted in significant early and late mortality with less than 30% of patients surviving (Dietz et al. 2011; Gadalla et al. 2013). The development of RIC protocols with fludarabine, lower doses of cyclophosphamide, lower doses of TBI, and serotherapy with ATG or alemtuzumab subsequently showed improved early outcomes with 9 patients out of 11 surviving, most of whom underwent MUD or cord blood HCT (Dietz et al. 2011; Brown et al. 2016; Nishio et al. 2011). A non-radiation preparative regimen with fludarabine, lower-dose melphalan, and alemtuzumab resulted in five of seven patients alive in early follow-up (Nelson et al. 2016). There has also been success utilizing haploidentical donors, with a similar RIC approach and the use of ex vivo T-cell depletion (Algeri et al. 2015). Survival outcomes separated by MSD and alternative donor after the year 2000 are shown in Fig. 9.2 (Barbaro and Vedi 2016).

Despite better early success with MSD HCT and RIC regimens, there is still a significant amount of late mortality, primarily from pulmonary complications, that may be a manifestation of underlying disease that is exacerbated by HCT (Gadalla et al. 2013). Pulmonary toxicity may be from infection, GVHD, or development of pulmonary fibrosis. Additionally, it is possible that multiple factors are involved, and it can be difficult to differentiate. In a systematic review of survival after HCT in patients with DC, 109 patients reported in the literature had an overall survival of 57% at 5 years and 23% at 10 years. This report confirmed improvement in early survival, but no change in long-term survival. While infection and graft failure dominate early causes of mortality, pulmonary disease dominates late mortality. The details of this pulmonary disease are not well described. These data demonstrate that HCT studies in patients with DC need to look beyond traditional 3–5 year time points and aim to understand and potentially prevent late mortality (Barbaro and Vedi 2016).

To further improve outcomes, some investigators are attempting to eliminate radiation and alkylating agents and use only fludarabine with ATG (Vuong et al. 2010) or alemtuzumab [ongoing multi-institution trial at Boston Children's Hospital (NCT01659606 on www.clinicaltrials.gov)]. Although there is some promise in early results with these approaches, larger numbers and longer follow-up will be needed to establish

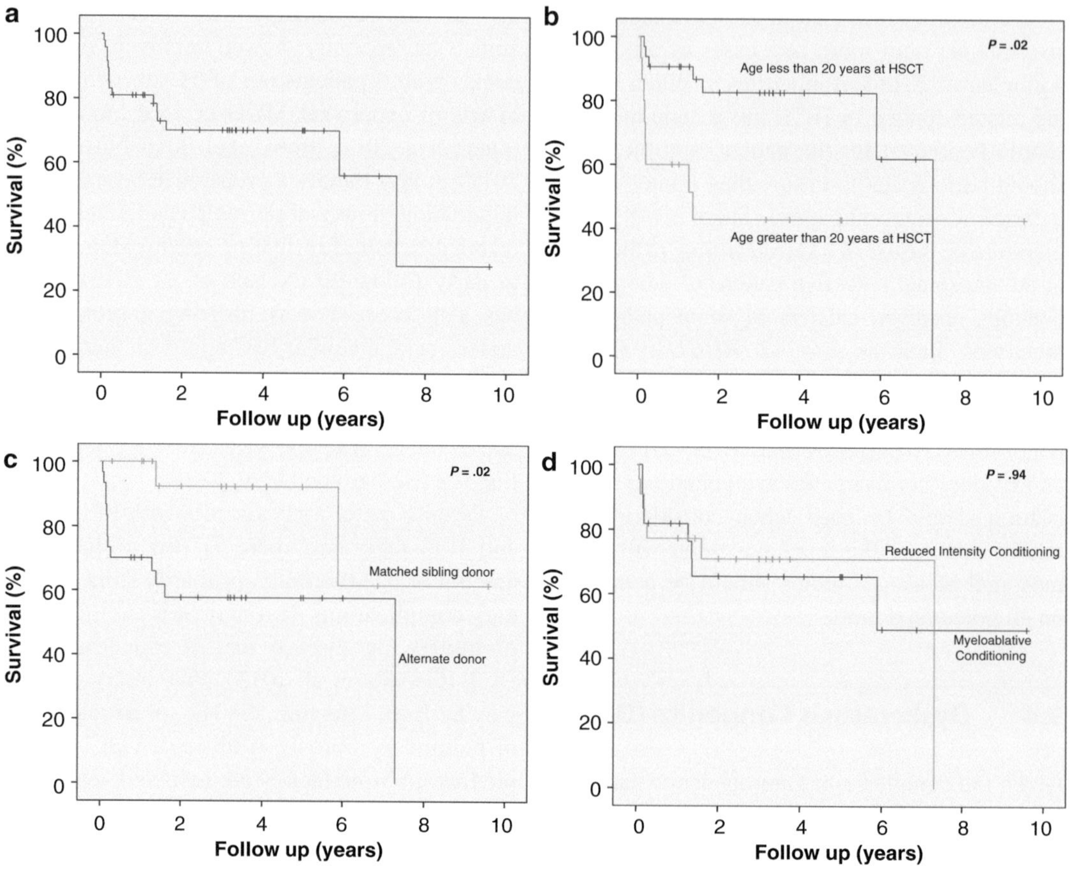

Fig. 9.2 Overall survival since 2000 in dyskeratosis congenita patients by donor type (Barbaro and Vedi 2016)

whether these approaches lead to improved outcomes. With these data in mind, most experts recommend waiting to proceed to HCT until patients develop significant BMF and preferably before they transform to MDS or leukemia. A challenge has been to determine what screening practices, such as bone marrow aspirate and biopsy evaluation at regular intervals, may permit such an approach. Regimens should be DC-specific RIC, with minimal to no radiation and reduced alkylator agent exposure.

DC can be inherited in an autosomal dominant, autosomal recessive, or X-linked manner. When choosing related donors for HCT, the genetic mutation should be known for the patient, and the donor should be screened to ensure they do not carry a pathogenic mutation pattern. There is little to no literature on the use of a carrier sibling in the event of an autosomal recessive pattern of inheritance. If the patient does not have a known genetic mutation, caution should be used when considering any related donors. Additional screening with telomere length should be conducted on all potential donors.

9.5 Diamond-Blackfan Anemia (DBA)

Good supportive care with transfusions and iron chelation is the mainstay of treatment for patients with DBA. About 80% will respond to steroids, though this therapy comes with significant short- and long-term side effects. Up to 20% of patients may experience a spontaneous remission. The remaining 80% or more of patients have an option of considering the only curative therapy with HCT (Vlachos and Muir 2010).

An early report from the DBA Registry in 2001 with 20 patients showed good survival of 87.5% after MSD HCT but a poor survival of only 14.1% after alternative donor HCT. These transplants were primarily MAC, with significant use of TBI in the alternative donor setting (Vlachos et al. 2001). A 2005 CIBMTR study of 61 patients all transplanted prior to 2001 and mostly with MAC regimens showed 64% survival at 3 years in all patients with 18% TRM by day 100, 9% graft failure, and 26% chronic GVHD. Again, those with a MSD fared much better with 76% survival compared to 39% from other transplants ($p = 0.05$) (Roy et al. 2005). The Japanese were among the first to show good outcomes in both MSD and MUD HCT when they reported on 19 patients in 2007, transplanted primarily with MAC. While the FFS was 100% in those patients with a MSD or MUD, cord blood transplants were not as successful with a FFS of 40% ($p = 0.002$), and survival for the entire cohort was 79% (Mugishima et al. 2007). The Italians similarly showed no difference between MSD and MUD HCT in a 2014 report of 30 patients that had a 5-year estimated survival of 74.4%, also primarily with MAC approaches (Fagioli et al. 2014).

More recent case reports of RIC regimens with fludarabine used in patients with DBA have shown success, but no larger studies of this approach have yet been reported (Asquith et al. 2015; Berndt et al. 2005; Gómez-Almaguer et al. 2003; Ostronoff et al. 2004). There are limited data about the use of cord blood donors, with a suggestion that outcomes are not as good as other stem cell sources to date (Bizzetto et al. 2011). In general, best outcomes will occur if children with transfusion-dependent DBA proceed with MSD or MUD transplantation before the age of 10 years prior to the development of significant comorbidities. For patients who develop significant BMF and/or progression to MDS or leukemia, transplantation is indicated with any donor, preferably after obtaining a remission.

DBA is inherited predominantly in an apparent autosomal dominant manner that is the result of haploinsufficiency. When choosing related donors for HCT, the genetic mutation should be known for the patient, and the donor should be screened to ensure they do not carry the mutation. Nonetheless, interpretation of the genetics even with a putative mutation should be taken with caution, since DBA may have variable penetrance. If the patient does not have a known genetic mutation, caution should be used when considering any related donors.

9.6 Shwachman-Diamond Syndrome (SDS)

Good supportive care with attention to pancreatic insufficiency issues and growth factor support for neutropenia is the mainstay of treatment for SDS patients. HCT offers a curative option for the bone marrow failure aspect of SDS (transplant indicated for mono-, bi-, or tri-lineage aplasia resulting in transfusion dependence or neutropenia) and if there are any signs of clonal evolution or transformation to leukemia. Reports of HCT in patients with SDS are primarily case reports and small series. There is no clear consensus on when to transplant these patients, though outcomes are clearly inferior when patients are transplanted after evolution to MSD or AML (Burroughs et al. 2009).

The largest series of 26 patients from Europe showed a high TRM rate of 35.5% that resulted in a survival rate of only 64.5%, mostly with the use of MAC (Cesaro et al. 2005). A similar 60% survival was reported from the French in ten patients who received MAC as well (Donadieu et al. 2005). Attempts to minimize transplant toxicity with agents such as treosulfan have shown success in three patients, two of whom are still alive (Sauer et al. 2007). More recently, the use of RIC using fludarabine, melphalan, and alemtuzumab was shown to be successful in seven patients, all of whom are alive with minimal GVHD, though with a significant incidence of bacterial and viral infections throughout the course of their transplants (Bhatla et al. 2008). This seems to be the most promising strategy to date, but this reflects only single-center transplant data. There are limited data with the use of cord blood donors. One series of the use of cord blood in three patients after a preparative regimen of melphalan, etoposide, total lymphoid irradiation, and ATG resulted in all patients being alive but all having developed acute GVHD and one having progressed to extensive chronic GVHD (Vibhakar et al. 2005). In general, patients should proceed to transplantation with a MSD or MUD when significant BMF or progression to MDS or leukemia occurs.

SDS is inherited predominantly in an autosomal recessive manner. When choosing related donors for HCT, the genetic mutation should be known for the patient, and the donor should be screened to ensure they do not carry two mutations. A carrier of one mutation should be unaffected, but little to no literature exists regarding the use of carrier donors. If the patient does not have a known genetic mutation, caution may still be warranted when considering any related donors.

9.7 Severe Congenital Neutropenia (SCN)

Good supportive care with growth factor stimulation is the mainstay of treatment in SCN patients. HCT offers a curative option for those patients not responsive to growth factor and those with evolution to MDS or leukemia. In general, there is a 1% per year rate of mortality due to sepsis, and evolution to MDS or leukemia in 8% of patients on growth factor will develop MDS or leukemia by 12 years of age. For those patients defined as unresponsive to growth factor, 14% died due to sepsis and 40% evolved to MDS or leukemia by 10 years (Rosenberg et al. 2006).

One of the first reviews of 37 HCT cases for SCN reported in the literature, including 7 additional patients transplanted in Sweden, showed reasonable survival of 76% (Carlsson et al. 2011). The next review (Connelly et al. 2012) increased the total to 18 reports with 65 patients transplanted prior to malignant transformation and 18 patients who underwent transplantation after transformation to MDS or leukemia. Survival was not good in patients transplanted after malignant transformation with only 8 of the 18 patients alive but was quite good at 89% in those transplanted prior to the development of MDS or leukemia. Most publications included in this review reported the use of MSD or cord blood. Graft rejection was more common after cord blood as a stem cell source. There was similar survival when either MAC or RIC was used, although the authors commented on a concern for more rejection and the unknown effects of mixed chimerism in this population of patients with a predisposition to malignant evolution (Connelly et al. 2012). The largest and most recent report is from the Europeans on 136 patients. Survival was good at 82%, TRM of 17%, graft failure of 10%, and chronic GVHD of 20% in the entire cohort. Most patients (87%) were transplanted using MAC and most without previous malignant transformation (84%). Those patients transplanted at a younger age and in the more recent era fared much better. There was no difference in overall outcome for those patients with MAC versus RIC, but those given bone marrow rather than peripheral blood stem cells did better (Fioredda et al. 2015).

While most of the early reports of cord blood used MAC, there has been more recent success of a RIC regimen consisting of fludarabine, melphalan, and low-dose TBI in three patients (Osone et al. 2016). Transplant is indicated using MSD, MUD, or cord blood transplantation in patients that are not responsive to growth factor support or in patients with progression to MDS or leukemia.

SCN can be inherited either in an autosomal dominant or autosomal recessive manner. When choosing related donors for HCT, the genetic mutation should be known for the patient. When the patient has an autosomal dominant mutation, the donor should be screened to ensure they do not carry the mutation. When the patient has an autosomal recessive mutation, the donor should be screened to ensure they do not carry two mutations. A carrier of one recessive mutation should be unaffected, but little to no literature exists regarding the use of carrier donors. If the patient does not have a known genetic mutation, caution should be used when considering any related donors.

9.8 Congenital Amegakaryocytic Thrombocytopenia (CAMT)

Due to lifelong bleeding risk and high rates of progression to complete BMF, HCT offers the only known cure for patients with CAMT. In the only major review, 52 patients were reported as having had HCT. MAC was most commonly used. Overall survival was good at 80% with TRM of 7.7% after MSD cases and 27.8% after MUD cases (Ballmaier and Germeshausen 2011). The use of cord blood has been successful in small case series including 5 of 5 patients alive in one single institution experience (Mahadeo et al. 2015) and 9 of 13 alive in the collective European experience (Bizzetto et al. 2011). More recent attempts have been made to use RIC with either cyclophosphamide, alemtuzumab, and low-dose TBI (Rao et al. 2015) or fludarabine, melphalan, and alemtuzumab (Woods et al. 2014), with good results. It appears to be reasonable to consider HCT using MSD, MUD, or cord blood transplantation in patients with marrow failure who are newly diagnosed with CAMT.

CAMT is inherited predominantly in an autosomal recessive manner. When choosing related donors for HCT, the genetic mutation should be known for the patient, and the donor should be screened to ensure they do not carry two mutations. A carrier of one mutation should be unaffected, and there is a case report with successful use of a carrier donor for HCT (Muraoka et al. 2005). If the patient does not have a known genetic mutation, caution may still be warranted when considering any related donors.

9.9 Thrombocytopenia Absent Radii (TAR)

Good supportive care with platelet transfusions and attention to orthopedic needs is the mainstay of treatment of patients with TAR. Often thrombocytopenia, the only typical hematologic abnormality, improves over time, and HCT is not typically utilized except in very unusual situations. Thus, the literature does not show significant experience with the use of HCT on this patient population (Geddis 2009).

9.10 Gene Therapy for IBMFS

There have been a number of attempts to correct specific genetic defects found in patients with IBMFS, utilizing gene editing or gene replacement therapies. If successful, these approaches would allow for cure of these patients without the risks associated with allogeneic HCT, including GVHD. The most work has been advanced in patients with FA (Osborn et al. 2015; Tolar et al. 2011, 2012; Adair et al. 2012; Williams et al. 2005; Kelly et al. 2007), though work is also underway to learn how to apply gene therapy to patients with DBA (Flygare et al. 2008; D'Allard and Liu 2016) and DC (Agarwal et al. 2010). There were early attempts of gene therapy in mice with CAMT, but it was shown to be technically difficult and unlikely to make the transfer to human trials (Ballmaier and Germeshausen 2011).

Some previous trials in FA have looked at lentiviral (Adair et al. 2012) and oncoretroviral-mediated (Kelly et al. 2007) ex vivo gene transfer in patients with complementation group A, which was found to be well tolerated with limited efficacy. Others have looked at the clustered regularly interspaced short palindromic repeats/Cas9 nuclease system to mediate gene correction in skin fibroblasts (Osborn et al. 2015). However, success to date has been limited largely by disease-specific characteristics such as limited number and quality of stem cells (Tolar et al. 2012; Williams et al. 2005). One approach for getting around the paucity of hematopoietic cells available for gene transfer approaches has been gene creation of induced pluripotent stem cells from patient fibroblasts or other sources followed by gene engineering and maturation to hematopoietic stem cells (Osborn et al. 2015). This has had limited technical feasibility to date, though basic investigation into this area is ongoing. There are only a few currently open clinical trials for gene therapy for patients with FA, most notably for patients with mutations in complementation group A (NCT01331018, NCT02931071, NCT02678533 on www.clinicaltrials.gov).

There are studies in DBA that have evaluated oncoretroviral vector transduction for *RPS19* gene transfer in mice (Flygare et al. 2008) as well as spliceosome-mediated mRNA trans-splicing to repair DBA stem cells (D'Allard and Liu 2016). Early work in DC has focused on reprograming to restore telomere elongation in patient-specific induced pluripotent stem cells to increase *TERC* expression (Agarwal et al. 2010). There are no currently open studies listed for DC, DBA, SDS, or SCN in clinicaltrials.gov.

9.11 Future of HCT for IBMFS

With significant improvements in the use of HCT for IBMFS, the next steps are to continue maximizing the benefit of HCT through efforts aimed at decreasing graft failure and GVHD while minimizing not only short-term toxicity but also late effects. Long-term surveillance consensus recommendations are being developed (Dietz et al. 2017b) and will further help to inform the evolution of HCT strategies in IBMFS. The impact that gene therapy will have on the field is yet to be determined until these strategies are able to be translated from the bench to the bedside successfully.

References

Adair JE, Zhao X, Chien S, Fang M, Wohlfahrt ME, Trobridge GD et al (2012) Cyclophosphamide promotes engraftment of gene-modified cells in a mouse model of Fanconi anemia without causing cytogenetic abnormalities. J Mol Med (Berl) 90(11):1283–1294. e-pub ahead of print 2012/06/03. https://doi.org/10.1007/s00109-012-0905-0

Agarwal S, Loh YH, McLoughlin EM, Huang J, Park IH, Miller JD et al (2010) Telomere elongation in induced pluripotent stem cells from dyskeratosis congenita patients. Nature 464(7286):292–296. https://doi.org/10.1038/nature08792

Algeri M, Comoli P, Strocchio L, Perotti C, Corbella F, Del Fante C et al (2015) Successful T-cell-depleted haploidentical hematopoietic stem cell transplantation in a child with dyskeratosis congenita after a fludarabine-based conditioning regimen. J Pediatr Hematol Oncol 37(4):322–326. https://doi.org/10.1097/MPH.0000000000000283

Alter BP (2007) Diagnosis, genetics, and management of inherited bone marrow failure syndromes. Hematology Am Soc Hematol Educ Program:29–39. e-pub ahead of print 2007/11/21. https://doi.org/10.1182/asheducation-2007.1.29

Anderlini P, Wu J, Gersten I, Ewell M, Tolar J, Antin JH et al (2015) Cyclophosphamide conditioning in patients with severe aplastic anaemia given unrelated marrow transplantation: a phase 1-2 dose de-escalation study. Lancet Haematol 2(9):e367–e375. https://doi.org/10.1016/S2352-3026(15)00147-7

Anur P, Friedman DN, Sklar C, Oeffinger K, Castiel M, Kearney J et al (2016) Late effects in patients with Fanconi anemia following allogeneic hematopoietic stem cell transplantation from alternative donors. Bone Marrow Transplant 51(7):938–944. https://doi.org/10.1038/bmt.2016.32

Aoki T, Koh K, Ikeda Y, Sekinaka Y, Akiyama K, Mori M et al (2016) Addition of high-dose cytarabine to fludarabine-based conditioning for hematopoietic stem cell transplantation for treating Fanconi anemia patients with advanced myeloid malignancy: a single-center experience and literature review. Biol Blood Marrow Transplant 22(9):1725–1728. e-pub ahead of print 2016/05/28. https://doi.org/10.1016/j.bbmt.2016.05.021

Asquith JM, Copacia J, Mogul MJ, Bajwa RP (2015) Successful use of reduced-intensity conditioning and matched-unrelated hematopoietic stem cell transplant in a child with Diamond-Blackfan anemia and cirrhosis. Pediatr Transplant 19(6):E157–E159. e-pub ahead of print 2015/06/23. https://doi.org/10.1111/petr.12547

Ayas M, Al-Jefri A, Al-Mahr M, Rifai S, Al-Seraihi A, Tbakhi A et al (2005) Stem cell transplantation for patients with Fanconi anemia with low-dose cyclophosphamide and antithymocyte globulins without the use of radiation therapy. Bone Marrow Transplant 35(5):463–466. https://doi.org/10.1038/sj.bmt.1704787

Ayas M, Al-Seraihi A, El-Solh H, Al-Ahmari A, Khairy A, Aldali A et al (2012) The Saudi experience in fludarabine-based conditioning regimens in patients with Fanconi anemia undergoing stem cell transplantation: excellent outcome in recipients of matched related stem cells but not in recipients of unrelated cord blood stem cells. Biol Blood Marrow Transplant 18(4):627–632. e-pub ahead of print 2011/08/24. https://doi.org/10.1016/j.bbmt.2011.08.015

Ayas M, Saber W, Davies SM, Harris RE, Hale GA, Socie G et al (2013) Allogeneic hematopoietic cell transplantation for fanconi anemia in patients with pretransplantation cytogenetic abnormalities, myelodysplastic syndrome, or acute leukemia. J Clin Oncol 31(13):1669–1676. e-pub ahead of print 2013/04/01. https://doi.org/10.1200/JCO.2012.45.9719

Ayas M, Siddiqui K, Al-Jefri A, El-Solh H, Al-Ahmari A, Khairy A et al (2014) Factors affecting the outcome of related allogeneic hematopoietic cell transplantation in patients with Fanconi Anemia. Biol Blood Marrow Transplant 20(10):1599–1603. e-pub ahead of print 2014/06/21. https://doi.org/10.1016/j.bbmt.2014.06.016

Bacigalupo A (2014) Bone marrow transplantation for acquired severe aplastic anemia. Hematol Oncol Clin North Am 28(6):1145–1155. e-pub ahead of print 2014/12/03. https://doi.org/10.1016/j.hoc.2014.08.004

Bacigalupo A, Socie G, Schrezenmeier H, Tichelli A, Locasciulli A, Fuehrer M et al (2012) Bone marrow versus peripheral blood as the stem cell source for sibling transplants in acquired aplastic anemia: survival advantage for bone marrow in all age groups. Haematologica 97(8):1142–1148. e-pub ahead of print 2012/02/09. https://doi.org/10.3324/haematol.2011.054841

Bacigalupo A, Socie G, Hamladji RM, Aljurf M, Maschan A, Kyrcz-Krzemien S et al (2015) Current outcome of HLA identical sibling vs. unrelated donor transplants in severe aplastic anemia: an EBMT analysis. Haematologica. e-pub ahead of print 2015/01/27. https://doi.org/10.3324/haematol.2014.115345

Ballmaier M, Germeshausen M (2011) Congenital amegakaryocytic thrombocytopenia: clinical presentation, diagnosis, and treatment. Semin Thromb Hemost 37(6):673–681. e-pub ahead of print 2011/11/18. https://doi.org/10.1055/s-0031-1291377

Barbaro P, Vedi A (2016) Survival after hematopoietic stem cell transplant in patients with dyskeratosis congenita: systematic review of the literature. Biol Blood Marrow Transplant 22(7):1152–1158. https://doi.org/10.1016/j.bbmt.2016.03.001

Beier R, Maecker-Kolhoff B, Sykora KW, Chao M, Kratz C, Sauer MG (2015) Minimal antileukaemic treatment followed by reduced-intensity conditioning in three consecutive children with Fanconi anaemia and AML. Bone Marrow Transplant 50(3):463–464. e-pub ahead of print 2014/12/22. https://doi.org/10.1038/bmt.2014.283

Benajiba L, Salvado C, Dalle JH, Jubert C, Galambrun C, Soulier J et al (2015) HLA-matched related-donor HSCT in Fanconi anemia patients conditioned with cyclophosphamide and fludarabine. Blood 125(2):417–418. https://doi.org/10.1182/blood-2014-10-605113

Berndt A, Helwig A, Ehninger G, Bornhäuser M (2005) Successful transplantation of CD34+ selected peripheral blood stem cells from an unrelated donor in an adult patient with Diamond-Blackfan anemia and secondary hemochromatosis. Bone Marrow Transplant 35(1):99–100. https://doi.org/10.1038/sj.bmt.1704700

Bhatla D, Davies SM, Shenoy S, Harris RE, Crockett M, Shoultz L et al (2008) Reduced-intensity conditioning is effective and safe for transplantation of patients with Shwachman-Diamond syndrome. Bone Marrow Transplant 42(3):159–165. e-pub ahead of print 2008/05/26. https://doi.org/10.1038/bmt.2008.151

Bizzetto R, Bonfim C, Rocha V, Socié G, Locatelli F, Chan K et al (2011) Outcomes after related and unrelated umbilical cord blood transplantation for hereditary bone marrow failure syndromes other than Fanconi anemia. Haematologica 96(1):134–141. e-pub ahead of print 2010/11/11. https://doi.org/10.3324/haematol.2010.027839

Bonfim C, Ribeiro L, Nichele S, Bitencourt M, Loth G, Koliski A et al (2016) Long-term survival, organ function, and malignancy after hematopoietic stem cell transplantation for Fanconi anemia. Biol Blood Marrow Transplant 22(7):1257–1263. https://doi.org/10.1016/j.bbmt.2016.03.007

Boulad F, Gillio A, Small TN, George D, Prasad V, Torok-Castanza J et al (2000) Stem cell transplantation for the treatment of Fanconi anaemia using a fludarabine-based cytoreductive regimen and T-cell-depleted related HLA-mismatched peripheral blood stem cell grafts. Br J Haematol 111(4):1153–1157

Brown M, Myers D, Shreve N, Rahmetullah R, Radhi M (2016) Reduced intensity conditioning regimen with fludarabine, cyclophosphamide, low dose TBI and alemtuzumab leading to successful unrelated umbilical cord stem cell engraftment and survival in two children with dyskeratosis congenita. Bone Marrow Transplant 51(5):744–746. https://doi.org/10.1038/bmt.2015.333

Burroughs L, Woolfrey A, Shimamura A (2009) Shwachman-Diamond syndrome: a review of the clinical presentation, molecular pathogenesis, diagnosis, and treatment. Hematol Oncol Clin North Am 23(2):233–248. https://doi.org/10.1016/j.hoc.2009.01.007

Burroughs LM, Woolfrey AE, Storer BE, Deeg HJ, Flowers ME, Martin PJ et al (2012) Success of allogeneic marrow transplantation for children with severe aplastic anaemia. Br J Haematol 158(1):120–128. e-pub ahead of print 2012/04/27. https://doi.org/10.1111/j.1365-2141.2012.09130.x

Carlsson G, Winiarski J, Ljungman P, Ringdén O, Mattsson J, Nordenskjöld M et al (2011) Hematopoietic stem cell transplantation in severe congenital neutropenia. Pediatr Blood Cancer 56(3):444–451. https://doi.org/10.1002/pbc.22836

Cesaro S, Oneto R, Messina C, Gibson BE, Buzyn A, Steward C et al (2005) Haematopoietic stem cell transplantation for Shwachman-Diamond disease: a study from the European Group for blood and marrow transplantation. Br J Haematol 131(2):231–236. https://doi.org/10.1111/j.1365-2141.2005.05758.x

Chan KW, McDonald L, Lim D, Grimley MS, Grayson G, Wall DA (2008) Unrelated cord blood transplantation in children with idiopathic severe aplastic anemia. Bone Marrow Transplant 42(9):589–595. https://doi.org/10.1038/bmt.2008.227

Chao MM, Kuehl JS, Strauss G, Hanenberg H, Schindler D, Neitzel H et al (2015) Outcomes of mismatched and unrelated donor hematopoietic stem cell transplantation in Fanconi anemia conditioned with chemotherapy only. Ann Hematol 94(8):1311–1318. https://doi.org/10.1007/s00277-015-2370-7

Ciceri F, Lupo-Stanghellini MT, Korthof ET (2013) Haploidentical transplantation in patients with acquired aplastic anemia. Bone Marrow Transplant 48(2):183–185. e-pub ahead of print 2013/01/08. https://doi.org/10.1038/bmt.2012.231

Clay J, Kulasekararaj AG, Potter V, Grimaldi F, McLornan D, Raj K et al (2014) Nonmyeloablative peripheral blood haploidentical stem cell transplantation for refractory severe aplastic anemia. Biol Blood Marrow Transplant 20(11):1711–1716. e-pub ahead of print 2014/07/13. https://doi.org/10.1016/j.bbmt.2014.06.028

Connelly JA, Choi SW, Levine JE (2012) Hematopoietic stem cell transplantation for severe congenital neutropenia. Curr Opin Hematol 19(1):44–51. https://doi.org/10.1097/MOH.0b013e32834da96e

D'Allard D, Liu J (2016) Towards RNA repair of Diamond-Blackfan anemia hematopoietic stem cells. Hum Gene Ther. e-pub ahead of print 2016/08/22. https://doi.org/10.1089/hum.2016.081

Dietz AC, Orchard PJ, Baker KS, Giller RH, Savage SA, Alter BP et al (2011) Disease-specific hematopoietic cell transplantation: nonmyeloablative conditioning regimen for dyskeratosis congenita. Bone Marrow Transplant 46(1):98–104. https://doi.org/10.1038/bmt.2010.65

Dietz AC, Lucchini G, Samarasinghe S, Pulsipher MA (2016) Evolving hematopoietic stem cell transplantation strategies in severe aplastic anemia. Curr Opin Pediatr 28(1):3–11. https://doi.org/10.1097/MOP.0000000000000299

Dietz AC, Duncan CN, Alter BP, Bresters D, Cowan MJ, Notarangelo L et al (2017a) The second pediatric blood and marrow transplant consortium international consensus conference on late effects after pediatric hematopoietic cell transplantation: defining the unique late effects of children undergoing hematopoietic cell transplantation for immune deficiencies, inherited marrow failure disorders, and hemoglobinopathies. Biol Blood Marrow Transplant 23(1):24–29. e-pub ahead of print 2016/10/11. https://doi.org/10.1016/j.bbmt.2016.10.004

Dietz AC, Mehta PA, Vlachos A, Savage SA, Bresters D, Tolar J et al (2017b) Current knowledge and priorities for future research in late effects after hematopoietic cell transplantation (HCT) for inherited bone marrow failure syndromes (IBMFS): consensus statement from the second pediatric blood and marrow transplant consortium international conference on late effects after pediatric HCT. Biol Blood Marrow Transplant. e-pub ahead of print 2017/01/20. https://doi.org/10.1016/j.bbmt.2017.01.075

Donadieu J, Michel G, Merlin E, Bordigoni P, Monteux B, Beaupain B et al (2005) Hematopoietic stem cell transplantation for Shwachman-Diamond syndrome: experience of the French neutropenia registry. Bone Marrow Transplant 36(9):787–792. https://doi.org/10.1038/sj.bmt.1705141

Dufort G, Pisano S, Incoronato A, Castiglioni M, Carracedo M, Pagés C et al (2012) Feasibility and outcome of haploidentical SCT in pediatric high-risk hematologic malignancies and Fanconi anemia in Uruguay. Bone Marrow Transplant 47(5):663–668. e-pub ahead of print 2011/07/18. https://doi.org/10.1038/bmt.2011.148

Dufour C, Veys P, Carraro E, Bhatnagar N, Pillon M, Wynn R et al (2015) Similar outcome of upfront-unrelated and matched sibling stem cell transplantation in idiopathic paediatric aplastic anaemia. A study on behalf of the UK Paediatric BMT Working Party, Paediatric Diseases Working Party and Severe Aplastic Anaemia Working Party of EBMT. Br J Haematol. e-pub ahead of print 2015/08/01. https://doi.org/10.1111/bjh.13614

Eapen M, Le Rademacher J, Antin JH, Champlin RE, Carreras J, Fay J et al (2011) Effect of stem cell source on outcomes after unrelated donor transplantation in severe aplastic anemia. Blood 118(9):2618–2621. e-pub ahead of print 2011/06/17. https://doi.org/10.1182/blood-2011-05-354001

Esteves I, Bonfim C, Pasquini R, Funke V, Pereira NF, Rocha V et al (2015) Haploidentical BMT and post-transplant Cy for severe aplastic anemia: a multicenter retrospective study. Bone Marrow Transplant 50(5):685–689. e-pub ahead of print 2015/03/03. https://doi.org/10.1038/bmt.2015.20

Fagioli F, Quarello P, Zecca M, Lanino E, Corti P, Favre C et al (2014) Haematopoietic stem cell transplantation for Diamond Blackfan anaemia: a report from the Italian Association of Paediatric Haematology and Oncology Registry. Br J Haematol 165(5):673–681. e-pub ahead of print 2014/02/24. https://doi.org/10.1111/bjh.12787

Fioredda F, Iacobelli S, van Biezen A, Gaspar B, Ancliff P, Donadieu J et al (2015) Stem cell transplantation in severe congenital neutropenia: an analysis from the European Society for Blood and Marrow Transplantation. Blood 126(16):1885–1892.; quiz 1970. e-pub ahead of print 2015/07/16. https://doi.org/10.1182/blood-2015-02-628859

Flygare J, Olsson K, Richter J, Karlsson S (2008) Gene therapy of Diamond Blackfan anemia CD34(+) cells leads to improved erythroid development and engraftment following transplantation. Exp Hematol 36(11):1428–1435. e-pub ahead of print 2008/08/19. https://doi.org/10.1016/j.exphem.2008.06.012

Gadalla SM, Sales-Bonfim C, Carreras J, Alter BP, Antin JH, Ayas M et al (2013) Outcomes of allogeneic hematopoietic cell transplantation in patients with dyskeratosis congenita. Biol Blood Marrow Transplant 19(8):1238–1243. e-pub ahead of print 2013/06/12. https://doi.org/10.1016/j.bbmt.2013.05.021

Gao L, Li Y, Zhang Y, Chen X, Zhang C, Liu Y et al (2014) Long-term outcome of HLA-haploidentical hematopoietic SCT without in vitro T-cell depletion for adult severe aplastic anemia after modified conditioning and supportive therapy. Bone Marrow Transplant 49(4):519–524. e-pub ahead of print 2014/01/28. https://doi.org/10.1038/bmt.2013.224

Geddis AE (2009) Congenital amegakaryocytic thrombocytopenia and thrombocytopenia with absent radii. Hematol Oncol Clin North Am 23(2):321–331. https://doi.org/10.1016/j.hoc.2009.01.012

Gluckman E, Rocha V, Ionescu I, Bierings M, Harris RE, Wagner J et al (2007) Results of unrelated cord blood transplant in fanconi anemia patients: risk factor analysis for engraftment and survival. Biol Blood Marrow Transplant 13(9):1073–1082. e-pub ahead of print 2007/07/20. https://doi.org/10.1016/j.bbmt.2007.05.015

Gómez-Almaguer D, Ruiz-Argüelles GJ, Tarín-Arzaga LC, González-Llano O, Jaime-Pérez JC, López-Martínez B et al (2003) Reduced-intensity stem cell transplantation in children and adolescents: the Mexican experience. Biol Blood Marrow Transplant 9(3):157–161. https://doi.org/10.1053/bbmt.2003.50004

Gupta N, Choudhary D, Sharma SK, Khandelwal V, Dhamija M (2015) Haploidentical hematopoietic SCT for acquired severe aplastic anemia using post-transplant high-dose CY. Bone Marrow Transplant 50:155–156

Hasle H (2016) Myelodysplastic and myeloproliferative disorders of childhood. Hematology Am Soc Hematol Educ Program 2016(1):598–604. https://doi.org/10.1182/asheducation-2016.1.598

Im HJ, Koh KN, Seo JJ (2015) Haploidentical hematopoietic stem cell transplantation in children and adolescents with acquired severe aplastic anemia. Korean J Pediatr 58(6):199–205. e-pub ahead of print 2015/07/28. https://doi.org/10.3345/kjp.2015.58.6.199

Jaing TH, Chen SH, Yang CP, Hung IJ, Chang TY, Hsueh C (2014) Successful hematopoietic reconstitution by unrelated donor cord blood transplantation in children with Fanconi anemia: report of 3 cases. J Pediatr Hematol Oncol 36(8):e553–e555. https://doi.org/10.1097/MPH.0000000000000215

Jaiswal SR, Chatterjee S, Mukherjee S, Ray K, Chakrabarti S (2015) Pre-transplant sirolimus might improve the outcome of haploidentical peripheral blood stem cell transplantation with post-transplant cyclophosphamide for patients with severe aplastic anemia. Bone Marrow Transplant 50:873–875

Kelly PF, Radtke S, von Kalle C, Balcik B, Bohn K, Mueller R et al (2007) Stem cell collection and gene transfer in Fanconi anemia. Mol Ther 15(1):211–219. https://doi.org/10.1038/sj.mt.6300033

Khan NE, Rosenberg PS, Lehmann HP, Alter BP (2015) Preemptive bone marrow transplantation for FANCD1/BRCA2. Biol Blood Marrow Transplant 21(10):1796–1801. https://doi.org/10.1016/j.bbmt.2015.07.006

Khan NE, Rosenberg PS, Alter BP (2016) Preemptive bone marrow transplantation and event-free survival in Fanconi anemia. Biol Blood Marrow Transplant 22(10):1888–1892. https://doi.org/10.1016/j.bbmt.2016.06.018

Kojima S, Horibe K, Inaba J, Yoshimi A, Takahashi Y, Kudo K et al (2000) Long-term outcome of acquired aplastic anaemia in children: comparison between immunosuppressive therapy and bone marrow transplantation. Br J Haematol 111(1):321–328 e-pub ahead of print 2000/11/25

Kuşkonmaz B, Ünal Ş, Bayhan T, Aytaç Eyüboğlu S, Tavil B, Çetin M et al (2016) Successful outcome with fludarabine-based conditioning regimen for hematopoietic stem cell transplantation from related donor in Fanconi anemia: a single center experience from Turkey. Pediatr Blood Cancer 63(4):695–700. e-pub ahead of print 2015/12/24. https://doi.org/10.1002/pbc.25844

Mackarel J, Iatan M, Kumar L, Storey L, O'Marcaigh A, Smith O (2016) In support of upfront stem cell transplantation as first-line therapy for paediatric patients with idiopathic severe aplastic anaemia who lack a sibling donor. Br J Haematol. e-pub ahead of print 2016/04/21. https://doi.org/10.1111/bjh.14097

MacMillan ML, DeFor TE, Young JA, Dusenbery KE, Blazar BR, Slungaard A et al (2015) Alternative donor hematopoietic cell transplantation for Fanconi anemia. Blood 125(24):3798–3804. e-pub ahead of print 2015/04/01. https://doi.org/10.1182/blood-2015-02-626002

Mahadeo KM, Tewari P, Parikh SH, Driscoll TA, Page K, Martin PL et al (2015) Durable engraftment and correction of hematological abnormalities in children with congenital amegakaryocytic thrombocytopenia following myeloablative umbilical cord blood transplantation. Pediatr Transplant 19(7):753–757. e-pub ahead of print 2015/09/14. https://doi.org/10.1111/petr.12577

Mitchell R, Wagner JE, Hirsch B, DeFor TE, Zierhut H, MacMillan ML (2014) Haematopoietic cell transplantation for acute leukaemia and advanced myelodysplastic syndrome in Fanconi anaemia. Br J Haematol 164(3):384–395. e-pub ahead of print 2013/10/30. https://doi.org/10.1111/bjh.12634

Mugishima H, Ohga S, Ohara A, Kojima S, Fujisawa K, Tsukimoto I et al (2007) Hematopoietic stem cell transplantation for Diamond-Blackfan anemia: a report from the Aplastic Anemia Committee of the Japanese Society of Pediatric Hematology. Pediatr Transplant 11(6):601–607. https://doi.org/10.1111/j.1399-3046.2006.00616.x

Muraoka K, Ishii E, Ihara K, Imayoshi M, Miyazaki S, Hara T et al (2005) Successful bone marrow transplantation in a patient with c-mpl-mutated congenital amegakaryocytic thrombocytopenia from a carrier donor. Pediatr Transplant 9(1):101–103. https://doi.org/10.1111/j.1399-3046.2005.00247.x

Nelson AS, Marsh RA, Myers KC, Davies SM, Jodele S, O'Brien TA et al (2016) A reduced-intensity conditioning regimen for patients with dyskeratosis congenita undergoing hematopoietic stem cell transplantation. Biol Blood Marrow Transplant 22(5):884–888. https://doi.org/10.1016/j.bbmt.2016.01.026

Nishio N, Takahashi Y, Ohashi H, Doisaki S, Muramatsu H, Hama A et al (2011) Reduced-intensity conditioning for alternative donor hematopoietic stem cell transplantation in patients with dyskeratosis congenita. Pediatr Transplant 15(2):161–166. https://doi.org/10.1111/j.1399-3046.2010.01431.x

Osborn MJ, Gabriel R, Webber BR, DeFeo AP, McElroy AN, Jarjour J et al (2015) Fanconi anemia gene editing by the CRISPR/Cas9 system. Hum Gene Ther 26(2):114–126. https://doi.org/10.1089/hum.2014.111

Osone S, Imamura T, Fukushima-Nakase Y, Kitamura-Masaki A, Kanai S, Imai T et al (2016) Case reports of severe congenital neutropenia treated with unrelated cord blood transplantation with reduced-intensity conditioning. J Pediatr Hematol Oncol 38(1):49–52. https://doi.org/10.1097/MPH.0000000000000487

Ostronoff M, Florencio R, Campos G, Arruda S, Matias C, Florencio M et al (2004) Successful nonmyeloablative bone marrow transplantation in a corticosteroid-resistant infant with Diamond-Blackfan anemia. Bone Marrow Transplant 34(4):371–372. https://doi.org/10.1038/sj.bmt.1704592

Park JY, Singh TR, Nassar N, Zhang F, Freund M, Hanenberg H et al (2014) Breast cancer-associated missense mutants of the PALB2 WD40 domain, which directly binds RAD51C, RAD51 and BRCA2, disrupt DNA repair. Oncogene 33(40):4803–4812. e-pub ahead of print 2013/10/21. https://doi.org/10.1038/onc.2013.421

Peffault de Latour R, Soulier J (2016) How I treat MDS and AML in Fanconi anemia. Blood 127(24):2971–2979. e-pub ahead of print 2016/03/28. https://doi.org/10.1182/blood-2016-01-583625

Peffault de Latour R, Purtill D, Ruggeri A, Sanz G, Michel G, Gandemer V et al (2011) Influence of nucleated cell dose on overall survival of unrelated cord blood transplantation for patients with severe acquired aplastic anemia: a study by eurocord and the aplastic anemia working party of the European group for blood and marrow transplantation. Biol Blood Marrow Transplant 17(1):78–85. e-pub ahead of print 2010/06/22. https://doi.org/10.1016/j.bbmt.2010.06.011

Peffault de Latour R, Porcher R, Dalle JH, Aljurf M, Korthof ET, Svahn J et al (2013) Allogeneic hematopoietic stem cell transplantation in Fanconi anemia: the European Group for Blood and Marrow Transplantation experience. Blood 122(26):4279–4286. https://doi.org/10.1182/blood-2013-01-479733

Rao AA, Gourde JA, Marri P, Galardy PJ, Khan SP, Rodriguez V (2015) Congenital amegakaryocytic thrombocytopenia: a case report of pediatric twins undergoing matched unrelated bone marrow transplantation. J Pediatr Hematol Oncol 37(4):304–306. https://doi.org/10.1097/MPH.0000000000000247

Rosenberg PS, Socié G, Alter BP, Gluckman E (2005) Risk of head and neck squamous cell cancer and death in patients with Fanconi anemia who did and did not receive transplants. Blood 105(1):67–73. https://doi.org/10.1182/blood-2004-04-1652

Rosenberg PS, Alter BP, Bolyard AA, Bonilla MA, Boxer LA, Cham B et al (2006) The incidence of leukemia and mortality from sepsis in patients with severe congenital neutropenia receiving long-term G-CSF therapy. Blood 107(12):4628–4635. e-pub ahead of print 2006/02/23. https://doi.org/10.1182/blood-2005-11-4370

Roy V, Pérez WS, Eapen M, Marsh JC, Pasquini M, Pasquini R et al (2005) Bone marrow transplantation for Diamond-Blackfan anemia. Biol Blood Marrow Transplant 11(8):600–608. https://doi.org/10.1016/j.bbmt.2005.05.005

Samarasinghe S, Webb DK (2012) How I manage aplastic anaemia in children. Br J Haematol 157(1):26–40. https://doi.org/10.1111/j.1365-2141.2012.09058.x

Saracco P, Quarello P, Iori AP, Zecca M, Longoni D, Svahn J et al (2008) Cyclosporin A response and dependence in children with acquired aplastic anaemia: a multicentre retrospective study with long-term observation follow-up. Br J Haematol 140:197–205

Sauer M, Zeidler C, Meissner B, Rehe K, Hanke A, Welte K et al (2007) Substitution of cyclophosphamide and busulfan by fludarabine, treosulfan and melphalan in a preparative regimen for children and adolescents with Shwachman-Diamond syndrome. Bone Marrow Transplant 39(3):143–147. e-pub ahead of print 2007/01/08. https://doi.org/10.1038/sj.bmt.1705553

Scheinberg P, Young NS (2012) How I treat acquired aplastic anemia. Blood 120(6):1185–1196. https://doi.org/10.1182/blood-2011-12-274019

Schrezenmeier H, Marin P, Raghavachar A, McCann S, Hows J, Gluckman E et al (1993) Relapse of aplastic anaemia after immunosuppressive treatment: a report from the European Bone Marrow Transplantation Group SAA Working Party. Br J Haematol 85(2):371–377 e-pub ahead of print 1993/10/01

Shimada A, Takahashi Y, Muramatsu H, Hama A, Ismael O, Narita A et al (2012) Excellent outcome of allogeneic bone marrow transplantation for Fanconi anemia using fludarabine-based reduced-intensity conditioning regimen. Int J Hematol 95(6):675–679. e-pub ahead of print 2012/04/22. https://doi.org/10.1007/s12185-012-1079-9

Smetsers SE, Smiers FJ, Bresters D, Sonnevelt MC, Bierings MB (2016) Four decades of stem cell transplantation for Fanconi anaemia in the Netherlands. Br J Haematol 174(6):952–961. e-pub ahead of print 2016/07/29. https://doi.org/10.1111/bjh.14165

Socie G, Rosenfeld S, Frickhofen N, Gluckman E, Tichelli A (2000) Late clonal diseases of treated aplastic anemia. Semin Hematol 37(1):91–101 e-pub ahead of print 2000/02/17

Stepensky P, Shapira MY, Balashov D, Trakhtman P, Skorobogatova E, Rheingold L et al (2011) Bone marrow transplantation for Fanconi anemia using fludarabine-based conditioning. Biol Blood Marrow Transplant 17(9):1282–1288. e-pub ahead of print 2011/01/08. https://doi.org/10.1016/j.bbmt.2011.01.001

Storb R, Blume KG, O'Donnell MR, Chauncey T, Forman SJ, Deeg HJ et al (2001) Cyclophosphamide and antithymocyte globulin to condition patients with aplastic anemia for allogeneic marrow transplantations: the experience in four centers. Biol Blood Marrow Transplant 7(1):39–44. e-pub ahead of print 2001/02/24. https://doi.org/10.1053/bbmt.2001.v7.pm11215697

Talbot A, Peffault de Latour R, Raffoux E, Buchbinder N, Vigouroux S, Milpied N et al (2014) Sequential treatment for allogeneic hematopoietic stem cell transplantation in Fanconi anemia with acute myeloid leukemia. Haematologica 99(10):e199–e200. e-pub ahead of print 2014/08/01. https://doi.org/10.3324/haematol.2013.098954

Tan PL, Wagner JE, Auerbach AD, Defor TE, Slungaard A, Macmillan ML (2006) Successful engraftment without radiation after fludarabine-based regimen in Fanconi anemia patients undergoing genotypically identical donor hematopoietic cell transplantation. Pediatr Blood Cancer 46(5):630–636. https://doi.org/10.1002/pbc.20538

Thakar MS, Bonfim C, Sandmaier BM, O'Donnell P, Ribeiro L, Gooley T et al (2012) Cyclophosphamide-based in vivo T-cell depletion for HLA-haploidentical transplantation in Fanconi anemia. Pediatr Hematol Oncol 29(6):568–578. e-pub ahead of print 2012/07/27. https://doi.org/10.3109/08880018.2012.708708

Tolar J, Adair JE, Antoniou M, Bartholomae CC, Becker PS, Blazar BR et al (2011) Stem cell gene therapy for fanconi anemia: report from the 1st international Fanconi anemia gene therapy working group meeting. Mol Ther 19(7):1193–1198. e-pub ahead of print 2011/05/03. https://doi.org/10.1038/mt.2011.78

Tolar J, Becker PS, Clapp DW, Hanenberg H, de Heredia CD, Kiem HP et al (2012) Gene therapy for Fanconi anemia: one step closer to the clinic. Hum Gene Ther 23(2):141–144. https://doi.org/10.1089/hum.2011.237

Vibhakar R, Radhi M, Rumelhart S, Tatman D, Goldman F (2005) Successful unrelated umbilical cord blood transplantation in children with Shwachman-Diamond syndrome. Bone Marrow Transplant 36(10):855–861. https://doi.org/10.1038/sj.bmt.1705142

Vlachos A, Muir E (2010) How I treat Diamond-Blackfan anemia. Blood 116(19):3715–3723. e-pub ahead of print 2010/07/22. https://doi.org/10.1182/blood-2010-02-251090

Vlachos A, Federman N, Reyes-Haley C, Abramson J, Lipton JM (2001) Hematopoietic stem cell transplantation for Diamond Blackfan anemia: a report from the Diamond Blackfan Anemia Registry. Bone Marrow Transplant 27(4):381–386. https://doi.org/10.1038/sj.bmt.1702784

Vuong LG, Hemmati PG, Neuburger S, Terwey TH, Vulliamy T, Dokal I et al (2010) Reduced-intensity conditioning using fludarabine and antithymocyte globulin alone allows stable engraftment in a patient with dyskeratosis congenita. Acta Haematol 124(4):200–203. https://doi.org/10.1159/000318721

Wagner JE, Eapen M, MacMillan ML, Harris RE, Pasquini R, Boulad F et al (2007) Unrelated donor bone marrow transplantation for the treatment of Fanconi anemia. Blood 109(5):2256–2262. e-pub ahead of print 2006/10/14. https://doi.org/10.1182/blood-2006-07-036657

Williams DA, Croop J, Kelly P (2005) Gene therapy in the treatment of Fanconi anemia, a progressive bone marrow failure syndrome. Curr Opin Mol Ther 7(5):461–466

Woods G, Bajwa RP, Rose MJ (2014) Reduced intensity transplantation for congenital amegakaryocytic thrombocytopenia: report of a case and review of the literature. Pediatr Transplant 18(1):E31–E34. e-pub ahead of print 2013/10/14. https://doi.org/10.1111/petr.12175

Yabe M, Shimizu T, Morimoto T, Koike T, Takakura H, Tsukamoto H et al (2012) Matched sibling donor stem cell transplantation for Fanconi anemia patients with T-cell somatic mosaicism. Pediatr Transplant 16(4):340–345. e-pub ahead of print 2012/03/08. https://doi.org/10.1111/j.1399-3046.2012.01669.x

Yoshimi A, Kojima S, Taniguchi S, Hara J, Matsui T, Takahashi Y et al (2008) Unrelated cord blood transplantation for severe aplastic anemia. Biol Blood Marrow Transplant 14(9):1057–1063. https://doi.org/10.1016/j.bbmt.2008.07.003

Zecca M, Strocchio L, Pagliara D, Comoli P, Bertaina A, Giorgiani G et al (2014) HLA-haploidentical T cell-depleted allogeneic hematopoietic stem cell transplantation in children with Fanconi anemia. Biol Blood Marrow Transplant 20(4):571–576. e-pub ahead of print 2014/01/22. https://doi.org/10.1016/j.bbmt.2014.01.015

10 Inherited Neutropenias and Their Insights into Cellular and Developmental Biology

Hrishikesh M. Mehta and Seth J. Corey

Contents

10.1 Introduction

Neutrophils are the indispensable first responders in defense against bacterial or fungal infections and form an essential component of innate immunity. The rate of neutrophil production at a one billion per day is second only to erythrocyte production rate. However in comparison with the 120-day life span of an erythrocyte, most recent estimates of neutrophil life span are only 5.4 days (Pillay et al. 2010). Previous estimates for neutrophil life span indicated 2 days. Thus with a life span of just 2–5 days, the neutrophil production requires a very high level of cell proliferation and intact differentiation. This is tightly regulated governed by expression of multiple genes encoding cytokines, transcription factors, and regulators of survival and metabolism.

H. M. Mehta · S. J. Corey (✉)
Division of Pediatric Hematology, Oncology, and Stem Cell Transplantation, Children's Hospital of Richmond, Massey Cancer Center, Virginia Commonwealth University, Richmond, VA, USA
e-mail: seth.corey@vcuhealth.org

G. M. Kupfer et al. (eds.), *Bone Marrow Failure*, Pediatric Oncology,
https://doi.org/10.1007/978-3-319-61421-2_10

Neutropenia is defined as an absolute neutrophil count below 1500/μL (1.5 × 10^9/L). Neutropenia is further categorized as mild (1000–1500/μL), moderate (500–1000/μL), and severe (less than 500/μL or 0.5 × 10^9/L) neutropenia. Neutropenia may also be classified as inherited (congenital) or acquired. Congenital neutropenia is due to genetic lesions that alter the process or survival of neutrophil production. Acquired neutropenia, more commonly observed in adults, is primarily associated with autoimmunity driven by anti-neutrophil autoantibodies or due to chemotherapy-induced neutropenia. Neutropenia alone is asymptomatic and may be detected due to failure to resolve bacterial infections or on screening complete blood counts with differentials. Lack of neutrophils predisposes neutropenic patients to extreme risk of bacterial or fungal infections. Severely neutropenic patients are prone to bacterial infections from the gut microflora. Antibiotic treatment may be ineffective, and thus primary cause of mortality in neutropenic patients is due to sepsis. Current therapy to treat congenital, chemotherapy-induced, or acquired symptomatic neutropenia is the cytokine granulocyte colony-stimulating factor (G-CSF, filgrastim).

10.2 Granulopoiesis

Granulopoiesis constitutes that subset of hematopoiesis specifically dealing with maturation from the granulocyte/monocyte progenitor (GMP), under the stimulation of cytokines IL3, G-CSF, and/or GMCSF. GMP are derived from the common myeloid progenitors (CMP), which arise from hematopoietic stem progenitor cells (HSPC). The HSPC give rise to common lymphoid progenitors (CLP) and CMP, which serves as precursor to GMP as well as the megakaryocytic/erythroid progenitor (MEP). An alternate hierarchy has been identified to suggest that cells of both the innate (neutrophils and macrophages) and adaptive (T and B cells) immune system are derived from a lymphoid/myeloid multipotent progenitor (LMPP) that does not give rise to megakaryocytes or erythrocytes (McKercher et al. 1996; Scott et al. 1994).

Maturation from GMP to neutrophils follows defined morphological changes. Differentiation from GMP to neutrophils is defined by four stages: myeloblasts (circular nucleus, highest nuclear to cytoplasmic (NC) ratio) → promyelocytes (largest cell in the series, high NC ratio, and presence of primary and azurophilic granules) → myelocyte/metamyelocyte (condensed nucleus, smaller NC ratio, presence of secondary granules) → bands/segmented cells (terminally differentiated, kidney shape, or multilobed nucleus). Promyelocytes give rise to neutrophilic, basophilic, and eosinophilic precursor cells (Mehta et al. 2015). Cell division continues through the promyelocyte stage. During episodes of stress such as infection, band cells can be found in the peripheral blood and are used as a measure of acute inflammation. Although the precise combination(s) of cytokines that lead to the production of a specific granulocyte remains incompletely understood, the decision to differentiate GMP into monocytes or neutrophils is largely governed by expression of the monocyte colony-stimulating factor (MCSF, gene nomenclature *CSF1*) and G-CSF (gene nomenclature *CSF3*). Granulocyte/macrophase colony-stimulating factor (GMCSF, gene nomenclature *CSF2*) functions early in maturation and promotes GMP formation. However, GMCSF is involved in monocyte maturation to a larger extent than in neutrophils, and it also participates to the production of dendritic cells.

10.2.1 Granulocyte Colony-Stimulating Factor Receptor

The most critical growth factor for granulopoiesis is G-CSF. The cognate receptor for G-CSF is G-CSFR (genomic nomenclature, *CSF3R*) Mice lacking either *Csf3* or *Csf3r* due to gene ablation have profound neutropenia and subsequent susceptibility to infection (Semerad et al. 1999; Seymour et al. 1997). The CSF3R is a member of the hematopoietin/cytokine receptor superfamily, which includes receptors for many of the interleukins, colony-stimulating factors (e.g., erythropoietin), cytokines (e.g., leptin), and hormones

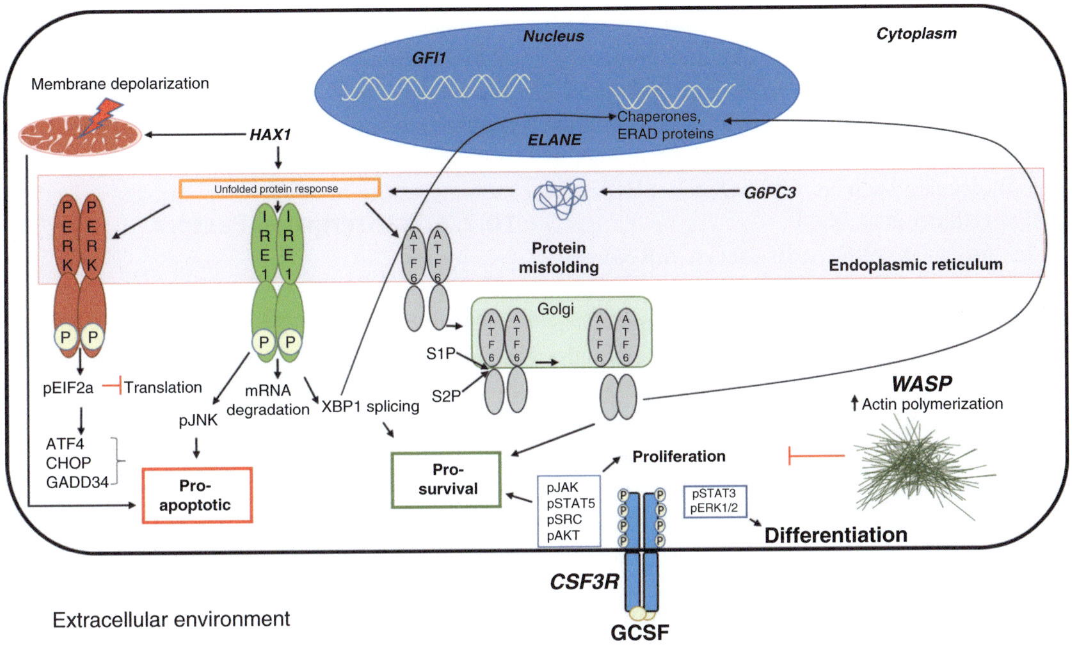

Fig. 10.1 Cartoon representation of genes and cellular processes in the pathogenesis of severe congenital neutropenia. The figure depicts the diversity of the genes that are mutated in congenital neutropenia and the diversity of the cellular processes that promote neutropenia via apoptosis. Congenital neutropenia is generally a result of block in differentiation and enhanced apoptosis of neutrophil precursors. Mutations in *GFI1*, impair its ability as a transcription factor to drive granulopoiesis. Mutations in *ELANE* result in misfolding of the expressed protein, which activates the unfolded protein response. The unfolded protein response has a dual role; the primary role is to halt translation and promote expression of chaperones and endoplasmic reticulum-associated degradation protein (ERAD) to resolve protein misfolding. Inability to resolve UPR activates the secondary role of UPR—promote cell death. *HAX1* mutations result in membrane depolarization but can also activate the unfolded protein response. Mutations in G6PC3 also promote the unfolded protein response and contribute to reactive oxygen species production in the ER. Neutropenia-associated *WASP* mutations promote excessive actin polymerization resulting in inhibition of proliferation. Treatment with G-CSF dimerizes its cognate receptor CSF3R, driving survival, proliferation, and differentiation of neutrophil progenitors. Neutropenia-associated germline *CSF3R* mutation results in an inactive receptor and thus comprehensively impaired G-CSF-mediated granulopoiesis

(e.g., prolactin). Upon ligand binding, the homodimeric CSF3R rapidly triggers changes in cellular phosphoprotein content. The external domain contains immunoglobulin-like and fibronectin type III domains. The cytoplasmic domain of the CSF3R contains two regions: a proximal region, which contains Box 1 and Box 2 and is conserved in the hematopoietin/cytokine receptor superfamily, and a distal region, which is involved in granulocytic maturation. Box 3, found also in the gp130 component of the IL-6 receptor complex, occurs between Y744 and Y764. Box 3 contains a dileucyl internalization motif that contributes to signal termination (Ward et al. 1999a). G-CSF binding results in rapid tyrosine phosphorylation and activation of the receptor as well as a number of substrates (Fig. 10.1). We and others have determined that JAK1, JAK2, and the Src kinase Lyn are involved in G-CSF signaling (Corey et al. 1994, 1998; Nicholson et al. 1994). Other tyrosine kinase-dependent signaling events include STAT3 and STAT5 activities (Tian et al. 1994; Nicholson et al. 1995, 1996). G-CSF activates the Ras-MAP kinase pathway in myeloid-derived cells (Bashey et al. 1994; Kuroki and O'Flaherty 1999). We have identified several PI3′kinase pathways in G-CSF signaling: CBL-PI3′kinase, GAB2-PI3′kinase, and PI3′kinase/AKT/ROS (Grishin et al. 2000; Wang et al. 2002; Zhu et al. 2004, 2006). These pathways are triggered in part by the recruitment of SH2-containing proteins to specific phosphotyrosine sites in the cytoplasmic domain of CSF3R. Besides being linked to granulocyte differentiation (Fukunaga et al. 1993), the C-terminus regulates the activation of critical negative regulatory molecules such as CIS/SOCS3, SHIP, and SHP-1 (Hunter et al. 2004).

In human myeloid cells, seven mRNA isoforms encoding the CSF3R have been isolated. The full-length, common form is known as Class I. The second most common form, the Class IV isoform lacks the C-terminal 87 amino acids and replaces them with a unique 34 amino acid stretch (Fukunaga et al. 1993; Ziegler et al. 1993). As a result, there is loss of the C-terminal tyrosine residues (Y729, Y744, and Y764) as well as the dileucyl motif required for receptor internalization. The Class IV isoform is differentiation-defective (Mehta et al. 2014; White et al. 2000). We and others have reported increased expression of the Class IV isoform in patients with myelodysplastic syndromes with or without monosomy 7 (Mehta et al. 2014; Sloand et al. 2006). Interestingly, monosomy 7 is the most common cytogenetic abnormality in inherited neutropenias, such as severe congenital neutropenia (SCN) or Shwachman-Diamond syndrome (SDS), which evolve to myelodysplastic syndrome/acute myeloid leukemia (MDS/AML). Of note, G-CSF promotes the outgrowth via upregulation of the Class IV isoform of monosomy 7 cells (Sloand et al. 2003). Also, pediatric patients with acute myeloid leukemia and who receive G-CSF have a higher incidence of relapse, when there is overexpression of the Class IV isoform (Ehlers et al. 2010). Recurrent missense mutations of *CSF3R* have recently been reported by us and others in hereditary chronic neutrophilia, chronic neutrophilic leukemia, atypical chronic myeloid leukemia, chronic myelomonocytic leukemia, and AML (Maxson et al. 2013; Pardanani et al. 2013; Beekman et al. 2013; Mehta et al. 2013). Somatic mutations in *CSF3R* were first discovered in patients with SCN, which had progressed to MDS/AML (Dong et al. 1994, 1995a, b; Awaya et al. 2002). Furthermore, in several large retrospective series of cancer and aplastic anemia patients, G-CSF use increased the risk of MDS (Smith et al. 2003; Lyman et al. 2010; Socie et al. 2007), but whether *CSF3R* variants contributed was not investigated.

10.2.2 Transcription Factors

Development of mature granulocytes from hematopoietic precursor cells is controlled by specific set of transcription factors that form gene regulatory networks. In particular, PU.1, CCAAT/enhancer-binding protein alpha (C/EBPα), C/EBP epsilon (ε), and GFI-1 are considered master regulators of myeloid development controlling granulocyte differentiation (Dahl et al. 2003; Friedman 2002; Laslo et al. 2008). Transcription factors PU.1 and GATA-1 oppose each other and are implicated in early determination of the LMPP or megakaryocyte erythrocyte progenitor (MEP) (Orkin et al. 1998; Arinobu et al. 2007). PU.1 is critical for myeloid cell fate determination during early stage of granulocyte/monocyte formation, by inactivating GATA-1 (Zhang et al. 2000). Further development of LMPP into GMP vs CLP is determined by both PU.1 and C/EBPα. C/EBPα expression is observed only in CMP and GMP vs CLP and MEP (Traver et al. 2001), and thus its expression directs the decision to generate GMP from LMPP. Determination of cell fate of GMP toward either monocytes or granulocytes is dependent on the interplay of C/EBPα and PU.1. High PU.1 expression drives expression of monocytic transcription factors *EGR1*, *EGR2*, and *NAB2* that promote expression of monocyte-specific genes and inhibition of neutrophil-specific genes (Dahl et al. 2003; Laslo et al. 2006). A critical regulator of neutrophil differentiation process is GFI-1. GFI-1 serves as secondary regulator of granulopoiesis, critical for later stages. C/EBPα serves as another primary regulator. The monocyte secondary regulators EGR2/NAB2 complex and GFI-1 can inhibit each other and serve as counteracting regulators to determine neutrophil vs monocyte lineage (Spooner et al. 2009). The secondary regulators along with the master regulators help make cell fate decisions between granulocytes and monocyte lineages (Spooner et al. 2009). GFI-1 and C/EBPε (epsilon) have been identified as regulators of terminal neutrophil differentiation.

10.3 Congenital Neutropenia

Congenital neutropenia is defined as the neutropenia presenting in newborn or infant children and is often due to monogenic lesions. Not discussed in this chapter are the inherited bone marrow failure syndromes associated with other cytopenias, e.g., Fanconi anemia, Dyskeratosis congenita, Shwachman-Diamond syndrome, and GATA2 deficiency. Monogenic-driven congenital neutropenia patients suffer from moderate to severe neutropenia throughout life. The most severe form of congenital neutropenia, SCN, formerly known as Kostmann syndrome, is driven by mutations in genes associated with neutrophil function or development, although they are not specific to the granulocyte lineage. Its inheritance could be autosomal recessive, autosomal dominant, or X-linked. SCN arises from at least six different genes. The most commonly affected (in over 50%) is *ELANE* (see below). Acquired neutropenia is more prominent in preterm neonates with low birth weight or due to development of infection at birth. With time neutropenia will resolve itself.

In addition to low counts, neutrophils present in many patients are functionally defective too. Bone marrow smears typically reveal an arrest at promyelocyte stage, which is the last cell in the granulocyte series to undergo cell division. Functional abnormalities include defective migration, bacterial killing, or increased apoptosis. Moderate congenital neutropenia is also observed in SDS and warts, hypogammaglobulinemia, immunodeficiency, myelokathexis (WHIM) syndrome.

Due to the profound deficiency of neutrophils, the individual is at risk for life-threatening infections. Pharmacologic administration of recombinant human GSCF has dramatically improved survival and the quality of life since its introduction in 1990. However, in a large series of 374 patients with SCN undergoing long-term G-CSF therapy, the predominant cause of death was secondary MDS/AML. The cumulative incidence after 15 years of follow-up was 21% (Rosenberg et al. 2006). Actuarial analysis suggests that lifetime risk is greater than 33%. This elevated risk (~31%) was confirmed in an independent survey of 231 patients enrolled in French Severe Chronic Neutropenia Study Group (Donadieu et al. 2005). A Swedish study also revealed a lifetime risk of 31% and strong association with *ELANE* mutation (Carlsson et al. 2012). A direct relationship exists between MDS/AML risk and the dose of G-CSF required to improve the neutropenia. The French Registry found that for patients with SCN or SDS, the MDS/AML risk strongly correlated with the total cumulative dose of G-CSF (Donadieu et al. 2005).

10.3.1 Neutrophil Elastase (ELANE)

A majority of SCN cases arises due to mutations in *ELANE* gene which encodes neutrophil elastase. Interestingly, SCN and cyclic neutropenia (CyN) occur due to spontaneous germline mutations in ELANE or can be inherited as autosomal dominant conditions. *ELANE* consists of five exons and encodes a 218 amino acid protein known as neutrophil elastase. ELANE targets bacterial virulence proteins and serves as the cell's first line of defense against bacterial infection. Mutations have been observed in all five exons. *ELANE* was the first gene that was identified to be mutated in patients with SCN and CyN (Horwitz et al. 1999; Dale et al. 2000). They identified that CyN mutations are closer to enzymatic active site of ELANE, whereas the opposite face mutations correlated with SCN. A more recent study identified a total of 116 different mutations in 162 SCN patients indicates the extent of heterogeneity and total number of *ELANE* mutations that drive neutropenia (Germeshausen et al. 2013). Nonsense and frameshift mutations affecting the carboxyl terminus correlate more often with SCN patients, while missense mutations and deletions are more common in cyclic neutropenia patients. However, there is considerable overlap of genotype with phenotype, even within families.

Multiple studies using different mutations identified that mutant ELANE expression triggers unfolded protein response (UPR). Upregulation of UPR markers BiP (a chaperone) and CHOP (a transcription factor) has been observed along with increased splicing of XBP1. A mouse model of mutant *Elane* showed increased expression of BiP and demonstrated transient neutropenia when given a single dose of bortezomib, a proteasome inhibitor (Nanua et al. 2011). Increased CHOP expression was observed after bortezomib injection, indicative of UPR. How G-CSF overcomes the UPR or promotes neutrophil production is not well understood. Protein misfolding in the endoplasmic reticulum (ER) triggers the UPR, activating the three pathways via three distinct sensor proteins IRE1, PERK, and ATF6 (Fig. 10.1). IRE1 and PERK are both membrane-bound Ser/Thr kinases that exist as inactive homodimers/oligomers which, when not bound by BiP, activate their kinase activity and drive phosphorylation of downstream proteins. IRE1 is a dual-function protein in that besides its kinase activity, it also has endoribonuclease activity. The endoribonuclease activity activated upon aggregation promotes nonspecific RNA degradation, thereby preventing further protein synthesis. However, IRE1 does result in specific processing of the *XBP1* transcript resulting in a spliced isoform sXBP1 which in turn serves as a transcription factor for expression of multiple ER chaperone proteins (Fig. 10.1). The second arm of UPR, PERK is also a Ser/Thr kinase, which phosphorylates and inhibits mRNA translation to make protein. The third arm of UPR involves ATF6, which upon activation, translocate to the Golgi and is cleaved by proteases S1P and S2P resulting in release of cytoplasmic fragment that acts as a transcription factor for ER chaperone proteins (Fig. 10.1). Thus, the three pathways help curb the production of protein to allow time for proper protein folding or its clearance via the ER associated degradation. An alternate function of UPR is to promote cell death in the event of prolonged ER stress. The IRE1 can promote activation of the JNK pathway driving cell death (Fig. 10.1). The PERK pathway also plays an important role in promoting cell death via enhanced expression of the pro-apoptotic transcription factor of the cEBP family, CHOP. GADD34 is the regulatory subunit of the protein phosphatase 1 PP1 holoenzyme. It associates with PP1 catalytic subunit (PP1c) targeting the complex to eIF2α and promoting eIF2α dephosphorylation, thus turning back on translation of proteins (Brush et al. 2003; Kojima et al. 2003). Although resolution of UPR would involve restarting translation, GADD34 is more strongly associated with apoptosis as opposed to cell survival. GADD34 induction associates with enhancement of CHOP expression (Kojima et al. 2003). Enhanced and prolonged expression of CHOP and ATF-4 mediate cell death (Fig. 10.1) by a mechanism involving oxidative stress and enhanced protein expression in cells undergoing UPR (Han et al. 2013; Marciniak et al. 2004).

An alternate hypothesis states neutropenia occurs due to mislocalization of ELANE. Mutations occurring in exon 1, especially the mutation of the start codon, have suggested a loss of the signal peptide. The first 29 aa of ELANE is the signal peptide that targets ELANE to the ER. In the case of mutations in exon 1, mutation in the signal peptide will lead to inefficient or defunct targeting of protein localization to the ER and through the secretory pathway. A recent study demonstrated that start site mutations in exon 1 can lead to alternative translation start sites for ELANE which would result in an N-terminally truncated ELANE (Tidwell et al. 2014).

As the disease progresses on G-CSF therapy, mutations in the *CSF3R* emerge. Particularly many of these mutations result in truncation of the CSF3R, most frequently resulting in a truncated 715 amino acid form of CSF3R (d715). More recent genomic studies have shown that sequential gain of mutations along the SCN → MDS → AML transitions with coexistence of mutations in *CSF3R* and *RUNX1* genes being highly recurrent (Skokowa et al. 2014; Beekman et al. 2012). An interesting observation made was that the clones with coexisting mutations were dependent on G-CSF treatment, further strengthening the role of *CSF3R* mutations in establishing clonal dominance, when high dose of G-CSF is used for treating the underlying neutropenia.

10.3.2 HCLS1-Associated Protein X-1 (HAX1)

Genome-wide linkage and candidate gene sequencing in three pedigrees from the original patients described by Kostmann led to the identification of *HAX1* mutations (Klein et al. 2007). *HAX1* mutations represent the second most common cases of SCN. The *HAX1* gene like the *CSF3R* gene is present on chromosome 1 and maps to 1q21.3. HAX1 is a ~35 kDa protein that was first identified as a binding partner for HS1, a SRC-associated substrate linked to the mitochondrion (Suzuki et al. 1997). Two isoforms of HAX1 have been identified that occur due to alternate splicing resulting in 231 aa or 279 aa long isoforms. Predominant cellular location for HAX1 is on the inner membrane of the mitochondria with some protein also found in the ER and nuclear envelope. First report identified nonsense mutations that introduce premature stop codons and protein truncation. Three mutations were identified: W44X, R86X, and G190X. Since mutations in *HAX1* have been identified to be autosomal recessive, it suggests that presence of a single copy is sufficient to promote normal function. Functionally, *HAX1* mutations associated with neutropenia have been identified to promote apoptotic cell death due to loss of inner mitochondrial membrane potential (Klein et al. 2007). HAX1 may also play a role in the UPR. In cardiac cells HAX1 reportedly interacts with phospholamban, which has an inhibitory effect on the sarcoplasmic reticulum Ca^{2+}-ATPase (SERCA2a). Alternatively, HAX1 has also been identified to directly bind to SERCA2, downregulating SERCA2 levels, resulting in reduced ER Ca^{2+} levels (Vafiadaki et al. 2009). SERCA is targeted by the chemical inducer of UPR, thapsigargin and is routinely used to study UPR in multiple cell types.

Similar to mouse model of mutant *Elane*, HAX1-deficient mice do not demonstrate any form of neutropenia. The mice however show increased apoptosis in lymphoid cells (Chao et al. 2008). Many SCN patients with *HAX1* mutations were also identified to have various neurological defects ranging from mild developmental delay to seizures (Rezaei et al. 2007). HAX1 deficiency in mice does phenocopy neurological abnormalities observed in humans. Unlike human HAX1, mice express only one form of HAX1. Alternate splicing of human *HAX1* results from alternate splicing of exon 2, resulting in isoform A (279 aa) and B (231 aa). Isoform B expression is observed in neuronal cells. Thus mutations in exon 2 only affect isoform A and are restricted to SCN, whereas mutations affecting both isoforms associate with both SCN and neurological impairment (Germeshausen et al. 2008; Carlsson et al. 2008).

10.3.3 Glucose-6-Phosphatase Catalytic Subunit 3 (G6PC3)

Glycogen storage disease, GSD-Ib, is characterized by signs of deficient metabolic alterations due to glycogen storage and by congenital neutropenia. The underlying mutations affect the endosomal transporter for glucose-6-phosphate (G6P), glucose-6-phosphate translocase (G6PT). G6PT is involved in transport of G6P from the cytosol to the ER lumen. The G6P is then hydrolyzed to give glucose and free phosphate. The hydrolysis is carried out by the catalytic subunit G6PC3. G6PT and G6PC3 are considered to be essential components of the G6Pase enzyme complex. Autosomal recessive mutations in *G6PC3* gene were described in SCN patients, revealed homozygous missense mutation in exon 6 that abolished the enzymatic activity (Boztug et al. 2009). Patient neutrophils with *G6PC3* mutations demonstrated increased neutrophil apoptosis. Myeloid precursors were identified to be susceptible to ER stress resulting in enlargement of the ER. Neutrophil counts are severely affected in these patients. Patients also demonstrated defects of cardiovascular system such as type 2 atrial septal defect. *G6pc3−/−* mice, unlike the *Elane*$^{-/-}$ and the *Elane G183X* mice, phenocopy the neutropenia observed in humans (McDermott et al. 2010; Gautam et al. 2013). The finding suggests G6PC3 function is conserved between humans and mice in the process of neutrophil development. Multiple mechanisms have been identified for the neutropenia in the knockout mice. Deficiency in glucose metabolism, UPR, and faulty neutrophil mobilization due to increased CXCR4 expression have been observed in the knockout mice. Gain-of-function mutations in CXCR4 associate with neutropenia observed in WHIM syndrome (Hernandez et al. 2003).

10.3.4 Growth Factor Independent-1 (GFI1)

Originally, SCN was suspected to be primarily due to defective neutrophil maturation. Research into mechanism has identified the defective maturation is generally due to increased apoptosis of neutrophil progenitors, mainly promyelocytes. GFI1 is a transcriptional repressor which acts as a secondary master regulator of neutrophil differentiation. Heterozygous dominant-negative mutations in the zinc finger domain of GFI1 have also been identified in a family with congenital neutropenia and in a sporadic case of congenital neutropenia (Person et al. 2003). The importance of GFI1 as a master regulator of granulopoiesis is evident from the fact that *Gfi*-knockout mice are severely neutropenic and accumulate immature monocytic cells in blood and bone marrow (Zarebski et al. 2008). Similar to G6PC3, GFI1 is also functionally conserved in granulopoiesis.

10.3.5 Wiskott-Aldrich Syndrome Protein (WASP)

Mutations in Wiskott-Aldrich syndrome protein (WASP) are generally characterized by X-linked microthrombocytopenia, lymphoid and myeloid immunodeficiency, and eczema (Thrasher 2002). The mutations associated with Wiskott-Aldrich syndrome are due to a loss of function in *WAS*, leading to decreased actin polymerization. Congenital neutropenia results from gain-of-function mutations, which promotes increased actin polymerization (Ancliff et al. 2006; Devriendt et al. 2001). In addition to the decrease in neutrophil, patients also show a reduction in their T and NK cell counts (Beel et al. 2009). Neutropenia-associated mutations in WAS results in increased apoptosis of progenitor cells. Studies using constitutive active WASP caused enhanced apoptosis coupled with decreased proliferation due to enhanced and delocalized actin polymerization throughout the cell (Moulding et al. 2007).

10.3.6 CSF3R

Germline mutations in *CSF3R* are observed in patients with SCN (Sinha et al. 2003; Ward et al. 1999b; Druhan et al. 2005). These mutations are different from the acquired somatic mutations in SCN patients. Mutations in *CSF3R* have been reported as missense or frameshift mutation. The missense mutation results in defective glycolysis and transport to the cell surface, whereas the frameshift mutations result in truncation. Since the *CSF3R* is being mutated, these patients tend to be unresponsive to G-CSF treatment (Triot et al. 2014).

10.3.7 Jagunal Homolog 1 (JAGN1)

A recently identified gene for SCN is *JAGN1*, which maps to 3p25.3. JAGN1 is a 183 amino acid ER resident protein, so mutation in *JAGN1* is implicated in ER stress. *JAGN1*-mutant granulocytes are characterized by ultrastructural defects, a paucity of granules, aberrant N-glycosylation of multiple proteins and increased incidence of apoptosis. JAGN1 is also important in the trafficking of CSF3R (Boztug et al. 2014).

10.4 Cyclic Neutropenia

CyN presents one of the most interesting disease phenotypes. Unlike SCN where neutrophil counts are consistently below 500/μL, in CyN the neutrophil counts fluctuate with a nadir every 21 days. *ELANE* mutations are found in over 90% of the CyN. The dual nature of *ELANE* mutations is not well understood. The cyclical nature of the disease is theoretically explained by suggesting disruption of a feedback loop (Horwitz et al. 2007). Neutrophils are hypothesized to produce a signal that regulates differentiation of myeloid progenitors. The inhibitory signal is the mutant ELANE. The mutant ELANE mislocalizes between the granules and plasma membrane. The "chalone" hypothesis is used to explain the cycling phenotype (Horwitz et al. 2007). Studies performed in gray collie dogs that develop neutropenia have provided critical clues to CyN. The cyclic nature of neutropenia in these animals was identified due to mutation in *AP3B1* resulting in reduced levels of the protein. The human gene is implicated in Hermansky-Pudlak syndrome type 2, a disease of defective intracellular trafficking. Some of these patients have neutropenia. Defect in trafficking is observed for transport or proteins from the Golgi to lysosomes, a route required for correct transport of granule proteins during granulopoiesis (Horwitz et al. 2007). Some *ELANE* mutations in CyN differ from those in SCN, in that they introduce a cryptic splice site. The mutations result in alternate splicing of the *ELANE* resulting in deletion mutants (Horwitz et al. 1999). It is not known why point mutations give rise to more severe disease as compared to the ten amino acid deletion. Alternate splicing might reduce the amount of mutant protein, and thus a pseudogene dosage may be implicated.

10.5 Benign Neutropenia

Benign neutropenia is observed in certain individuals with ethnic backgrounds such as North African, South Asian, and Middle Eastern descent. Highest frequency of neutropenia was observed in children of North Africa descent (~15%), followed by Middle Eastern and South Asian children (~7–10%) (Denic et al. 2016). Knowledge of the individual ethnicity is thus important in diagnosis of neutropenia. Termed "benign ethnic neutropenia," this form of neutropenia represents the most common variant of neutropenia. Genetic studies in people of African descent have identified a polymorphism in the gene encoding the Duffy antigen receptor for chemokines (*DARC*) (Reich et al. 2009).This polymorphism termed as Duffy null polymorphism (SNPrs2814778) associates with resistance to *Plasmodium vivax* malaria and correlates strongly with ethnic neutropenia. The mechanism for neutropenia remains elusive.

Conclusion

The congenital isolated neutropenias result from a diversity of affected genes that either target (*GFI1*, *G6PC3*, *JAGN1*, *HAX1*) or are targeted by (*ELANE*) diverse cellular processes such as transcription (GFI1), splicing [*ELANE* (CyN), *HAX1*], proteostasis [*ELANE* (SCN), *JAGN1*, *G6PC3*], energy homeostasis (*G6PC3*, *HAX1*), and endosomal and lysosomal trafficking [ELANE (SCN, CyN), *JAGN1*, *AP3B1*). It is thus important to determine how the diverse mutations and the cellular processes converge to promote isolated neutropenia. Although there is no clear consensus on a single mechanism/process, unfolded protein response and cellular trafficking are both implicated across the different genes. By elucidating how these diverse mutated genes cause neutropenia, we will understand more completely the normal physiology of neutrophils and granulopoiesis.

References

Ancliff PJ, Blundell MP, Cory GO et al (2006) Two novel activating mutations in the Wiskott-Aldrich syndrome protein result in congenital neutropenia. Blood 108(7):2182–2189

Arinobu Y, Mizuno S, Chong Y et al (2007) Reciprocal activation of GATA-1 and PU.1 marks initial specification of hematopoietic stem cells into myeloerythroid and myelolymphoid lineages. Cell Stem Cell 1(4):416–427

Awaya N, Uchida H, Miyakawa Y et al (2002) Novel variant isoform of G-CSF receptor involved in induction of proliferation of FDCP-2 cells: relevance to the pathogenesis of myelodysplastic syndrome. J Cell Physiol 191(3):327–335

Bashey A, Healy L, Marshall CJ (1994) Proliferative but not nonproliferative responses to granulocyte colony-stimulating factor are associated with rapid activation of the p21ras/MAP kinase signalling pathway. Blood 83(4):949–957

Beekman R, Valkhof MG, Sanders MA et al (2012) Sequential gain of mutations in severe congenital neutropenia progressing to acute myeloid leukemia. Blood 119(22):5071–5077

Beekman R, Valkhof M, van Strien P et al (2013) Prevalence of a new auto-activating colony stimulating factor 3 receptor mutation (CSF3R-T595I) in acute myeloid leukemia and severe congenital neutropenia. Haematologica 98(5):e62–e63

Beel K, Cotter MM, Blatny J et al (2009) A large kindred with X-linked neutropenia with an I294T mutation of the Wiskott-Aldrich syndrome gene. Br J Haematol 144(1):120–126

Boztug K, Appaswamy G, Ashikov A et al (2009) A syndrome with congenital neutropenia and mutations in G6PC3. N Engl J Med 360(1):32–43

Boztug K, Jarvinen PM, Salzer E et al (2014) JAGN1 deficiency causes aberrant myeloid cell homeostasis and congenital neutropenia. Nat Genet 46(9):1021–1027

Brush MH, Weiser DC, Shenolikar S (2003) Growth arrest and DNA damage-inducible protein GADD34 targets protein phosphatase 1 alpha to the endoplasmic reticulum and promotes dephosphorylation of the alpha subunit of eukaryotic translation initiation factor 2. Mol Cell Biol 23(4):1292–1303

Carlsson G, van't Hooft I, Melin M et al (2008) Central nervous system involvement in severe congenital neutropenia: neurological and neuropsychological abnormalities associated with specific HAX1 mutations. J Intern Med 264(4):388–400

Carlsson G, Fasth A, Berglof E et al (2012) Incidence of severe congenital neutropenia in Sweden and risk of evolution to myelodysplastic syndrome/leukaemia. Br J Haematol 158(3):363–369

Chao JR, Parganas E, Boyd K et al (2008) Hax1-mediated processing of HtrA2 by Parl allows survival of lymphocytes and neurons. Nature 452(7183):98–102

Corey SJ, Burkhardt AL, Bolen JB et al (1994) Granulocyte colony-stimulating factor receptor signaling involves the formation of a three-component complex with Lyn and Syk protein-tyrosine kinases. Proc Natl Acad Sci U S A 91(11):4683–4687

Corey SJ, Dombrosky-Ferlan PM, Zuo S et al (1998) Requirement of Src kinase Lyn for induction of DNA synthesis by granulocyte colony-stimulating factor. J Biol Chem 273(6):3230–3235

Dahl R, Walsh JC, Lancki D et al (2003) Regulation of macrophage and neutrophil cell fates by the PU.1:C/EBP[alpha] ratio and granulocyte colony-stimulating factor. Nat Immunol 4(10):1029–1036

Dale DC, Person RE, Bolyard AA et al (2000) Mutations in the gene encoding neutrophil elastase in congenital and cyclic neutropenia. Blood 96(7):2317–2322

Denic S, Narchi H, Al Mekaini LA et al (2016) Prevalence of neutropenia in children by nationality. BMC Hematol 16:15

Devriendt K, Kim AS, Mathijs G et al (2001) Constitutively activating mutation in WASP causes X-linked severe congenital neutropenia. Nat Genet 27(3):313–317

Donadieu J, Leblanc T, Bader Meunier B et al (2005) Analysis of risk factors for myelodysplasias, leukemias and death from infection among patients with congenital neutropenia. Experience of the French Severe Chronic Neutropenia Study Group. Haematologica 90(1):45–53

Dong F, Hoefsloot LH, Schelen AM et al (1994) Identification of a nonsense mutation in the granulocyte-colony-stimulating factor receptor in severe congenital neutropenia. Proc Natl Acad Sci U S A 91(10):4480–4484

Dong F, van Paassen M, van Buitenen C et al (1995a) A point mutation in the granulocyte colony-stimulating factor receptor (G-CSF-R) gene in a case of acute myeloid leukemia results in the overexpression of a novel G-CSF-R isoform. Blood 85(4):902–911

Dong F, Brynes RK, Tidow N et al (1995b) Mutations in the gene for the granulocyte colony-stimulating-factor receptor in patients with acute myeloid leukemia preceded by severe congenital neutropenia. N Engl J Med 333(8):487–493

Druhan LJ, Ai J, Massullo P et al (2005) Novel mechanism of G-CSF refractoriness in patients with severe congenital neutropenia. Blood 105(2):584–591

Ehlers S, Herbst C, Zimmermann M et al (2010) Granulocyte colony-stimulating factor (G-CSF) treatment of childhood acute myeloid leukemias that overexpress the differentiation-defective G-CSF receptor isoform IV is associated with a higher incidence of relapse. J Clin Oncol 28(15):2591–2597

Friedman AD (2002) Transcriptional regulation of granulocyte and monocyte development. Oncogene 21(21):3377–3390

Fukunaga R, Ishizaka-Ikeda E, Nagata S (1993) Growth and differentiation signals mediated by different regions in the cytoplasmic domain of granulocyte colony-stimulating factor receptor. Cell 74(6):1079–1087

Gautam S, Kirschnek S, Gentle IE et al (2013) Survival and differentiation defects contribute to neutropenia in glucose-6-phosphatase-beta (G6PC3) deficiency in a model of mouse neutrophil granulocyte differentiation. Cell Death Differ 20(8):1068–1079

Germeshausen M, Grudzien M, Zeidler C et al (2008) Novel HAX1 mutations in patients with severe congenital neutropenia reveal isoform-dependent genotype-phenotype associations. Blood 111(10):4954–4957

Germeshausen M, Deerberg S, Peter Y et al (2013) The spectrum of ELANE mutations and their implications in severe congenital and cyclic neutropenia. Hum Mutat 34(6):905–914

Grishin A, Sinha S, Roginskaya V et al (2000) Involvement of Shc and Cbl-PI 3-kinase in Lyn-dependent proliferative signaling pathways for G-CSF. Oncogene 19(1):97–105

Han J, Back SH, Hur J et al (2013) ER-stress-induced transcriptional regulation increases protein synthesis leading to cell death. Nat Cell Biol 15(5):481–490

Hernandez PA, Gorlin RJ, Lukens JN et al (2003) Mutations in the chemokine receptor gene CXCR4 are associated with WHIM syndrome, a combined immunodeficiency disease. Nat Genet 34(1):70–74

Horwitz M, Benson KF, Person RE et al (1999) Mutations in ELA2, encoding neutrophil elastase, define a 21-day biological clock in cyclic haematopoiesis. Nat Genet 23(4):433–436

Horwitz MS, Duan Z, Korkmaz B et al (2007) Neutrophil elastase in cyclic and severe congenital neutropenia. Blood 109(5):1817–1824

Hunter MG, Jacob A, O'Donnell LC et al (2004) Loss of SHIP and CIS recruitment to the granulocyte colony-stimulating factor receptor contribute to hyperproliferative responses in severe congenital neutropenia/acute myelogenous leukemia. J Immunol 173(8):5036–5045

Klein C, Grudzien M, Appaswamy G et al (2007) HAX1 deficiency causes autosomal recessive severe congenital neutropenia (Kostmann disease). Nat Genet 39(1):86–92

Kojima E, Takeuchi A, Haneda M et al (2003) The function of GADD34 is a recovery from a shutoff of protein synthesis induced by ER stress: elucidation by GADD34-deficient mice. FASEB J 17(11):1573–1575

Kuroki M, O'Flaherty JT (1999) Extracellular signal-regulated protein kinase (ERK)-dependent and ERK-independent pathways target STAT3 on serine-727 in human neutrophils stimulated by chemotactic factors and cytokines. Biochem J 341(Pt 3):691–696

Laslo P, Spooner CJ, Warmflash A et al (2006) Multilineage transcriptional priming and determination of alternate hematopoietic cell fates. Cell 126(4):755–766

Laslo P, Pongubala JM, Lancki DW et al (2008) Gene regulatory networks directing myeloid and lymphoid cell fates within the immune system. Semin Immunol 20(4):228–235

Lyman GH, Dale DC, Wolff DA et al (2010) Acute myeloid leukemia or myelodysplastic syndrome in randomized controlled clinical trials of cancer chemotherapy with granulocyte colony-stimulating factor: a systematic review. J Clin Oncol 28(17):2914–2924

Marciniak SJ, Yun CY, Oyadomari S et al (2004) CHOP induces death by promoting protein synthesis and oxidation in the stressed endoplasmic reticulum. Genes Dev 18(24):3066–3077

Maxson JE, Gottlib J, Pollyea DA et al (2013) Oncogenic CSF3R mutations in chronic neutrophilic leukemia and atypical CML. N Engl J Med 368:1781–1790

McDermott DH, De Ravin SS, Jun HS et al (2010) Severe congenital neutropenia resulting from G6PC3 deficiency with increased neutrophil CXCR4 expression and myelokathexis. Blood 116(15):2793–2802

McKercher SR, Torbett BE, Anderson KL et al (1996) Targeted disruption of the PU.1 gene results in multiple hematopoietic abnormalities. EMBO J 15(20):5647–5658

Mehta HM, Glaubach T, Long A et al (2013) Granulocyte colony stimulating factor mutant receptor T595I (T618I) confers ligand independence and enhanced signaling. Leukemia 27(12):2407–2410

Mehta HM, Futami M, Glaubach T et al (2014) Alternatively spliced, truncated GCSF receptor promotes leukemogenic properties and sensitivity to JAK inhibition. Leukemia 28:1041–1051

Mehta HM, Malandra M, Corey SJ (2015) G-CSF and GM-CSF in neutropenia. J Immunol 195(4):1341–1349

Moulding DA, Blundell MP, Spiller DG et al (2007) Unregulated actin polymerization by WASp causes defects of mitosis and cytokinesis in X-linked neutropenia. J Exp Med 204(9):2213–2224

Nanua S, Murakami M, Xia J et al (2011) Activation of the unfolded protein response is associated with impaired granulopoiesis in transgenic mice expressing mutant Elane. Blood 117(13):3539–3547

Nicholson SE, Oates AC, Harpur AG et al (1994) Tyrosine kinase JAK1 is associated with the granulocyte-colony-stimulating factor receptor and both become tyrosine-phosphorylated after receptor activation. Proc Natl Acad Sci U S A 91(8):2985–2988

Nicholson SE, Novak U, Ziegler SF et al (1995) Distinct regions of the granulocyte colony-stimulating factor receptor are required for tyrosine phosphorylation of the signaling molecules JAK2, Stat3, and p42, p44MAPK. Blood 86(10):3698–3704

Nicholson SE, Starr R, Novak U et al (1996) Tyrosine residues in the granulocyte colony-stimulating factor (G-CSF) receptor mediate G-CSF-induced differentiation of murine myeloid leukemic (M1) cells. J Biol Chem 271(43):26947–26953

Orkin SH, Shivdasani RA, Fujiwara Y et al (1998) Transcription factor GATA-1 in megakaryocyte development. Stem Cells 16(Suppl 2):79–83

Pardanani A, Lasho TL, Laborde RR et al (2013) *CSF3R* T618I is a highly prevalent and specific mutation in chronic neutrophilc leukemia. Leukemia 27(9):1870–1873

Person RE, Li FQ, Duan Z et al (2003) Mutations in proto-oncogene GFI1 cause human neutropenia and target ELA2. Nat Genet 34(3):308–312

Pillay J, den Braber I, Vrisekoop N et al (2010) In vivo labeling with 2H2O reveals a human neutrophil lifespan of 5.4 days. Blood 116(4):625–627

Reich D, Nalls MA, Kao WH et al (2009) Reduced neutrophil count in people of African descent is due to a regulatory variant in the Duffy antigen receptor for chemokines gene. PLoS Genet 5(1):e1000360

Rezaei N, Chavoshzadeh Z, O RA et al (2007) Association of HAX1 deficiency with neurological disorder. Neuropediatrics 38(5):261–263

Rosenberg PS, Alter BP, Bolyard AA et al (2006) The incidence of leukemia and mortality from sepsis in patients with severe congenital neutropenia receiving long-term G-CSF therapy. Blood 107(12):4628–4635

Scott EW, Simon MC, Anastasi J et al (1994) Requirement of transcription factor PU.1 in the devel-

opment of multiple hematopoietic lineages. Science 265(5178):1573–1577
Semerad CL, Poursine-Laurent J, Liu F et al (1999) A role for G-CSF receptor signaling in the regulation of hematopoietic cell function but not lineage commitment or differentiation. Immunity 11(2):153–161
Seymour JF, Lieschke GJ, Grail D et al (1997) Mice lacking both granulocyte colony-stimulating factor (CSF) and granulocyte-macrophage CSF have impaired reproductive capacity, perturbed neonatal granulopoiesis, lung disease, amyloidosis, and reduced long-term survival. Blood 90(8):3037–3049
Sinha S, Zhu QS, Romero G et al (2003) Deletional mutation of the external domain of the human granulocyte colony-stimulating factor receptor in a patient with severe chronic neutropenia refractory to granulocyte colony-stimulating factor. J Pediatr Hematol Oncol 25(10):791–796
Skokowa J, Steinemann D, Katsman-Kuipers JE et al (2014) Cooperativity of RUNX1 and CSF3R mutations in severe congenital neutropenia: a unique pathway in myeloid leukemogenesis. Blood 123(14): 2229–2237
Sloand EM, Mainwaring LA, Chen G et al (2003) Granulocyte-colony stimulating factor preferentially stimulates proliferation of monosomy 7 cells but does not foster development of this abnormality in cells with normal karyotype. Blood 102:Abstract 3395
Sloand EM, Yong AS, Ramkissoon S et al (2006) Granulocyte colony-stimulating factor preferentially stimulates proliferation of monosomy 7 cells bearing the isoform IV receptor. Proc Natl Acad Sci U S A 103(39):14483–14488
Smith RE, Bryant J, DeCillis A et al (2003) Acute myeloid leukemia and myelodysplastic syndrome after doxorubicin-cyclophosphamide adjuvant therapy for operable breast cancer: the National Surgical Adjuvant Breast and Bowel Project Experience. J Clin Oncol 21(7):1195–1204
Socie G, Mary JY, Schrezenmeier H et al (2007) Granulocyte-stimulating factor and severe aplastic anemia: a survey by the European Group for Blood and Marrow Transplantation (EBMT). Blood 109(7):2794–2796
Spooner CJ, Cheng JX, Pujadas E et al (2009) A recurrent network involving the transcription factors PU.1 and Gfi1 orchestrates innate and adaptive immune cell fates. Immunity 31(4):576–586
Suzuki Y, Demoliere C, Kitamura D et al (1997) HAX-1, a novel intracellular protein, localized on mitochondria, directly associates with HS1, a substrate of Src family tyrosine kinases. J Immunol 158(6):2736–2744
Thrasher AJ (2002) WASp in immune-system organization and function. Nat Rev Immunol 2(9):635–646
Tian SS, Lamb P, Seidel HM et al (1994) Rapid activation of the STAT3 transcription factor by granulocyte colony-stimulating factor. Blood 84(6):1760–1764
Tidwell T, Wechsler J, Nayak RC et al (2014) Neutropenia-associated ELANE mutations disrupting translation initiation produce novel neutrophil elastase isoforms. Blood 123(4):562–569
Traver D, Miyamoto T, Christensen J et al (2001) Fetal liver myelopoiesis occurs through distinct, prospectively isolatable progenitor subsets. Blood 98(3):627–635
Triot A, Jarvinen PM, Arostegui JI et al (2014) Inherited biallelic CSF3R mutations in severe congenital neutropenia. Blood 123(24):3811–3817
Vafiadaki E, Arvanitis DA, Pagakis SN et al (2009) The anti-apoptotic protein HAX-1 interacts with SERCA2 and regulates its protein levels to promote cell survival. Mol Biol Cell 20(1):306–318
Wang L, Rudert WA, Loutaev I et al (2002) Repression of c-Cbl leads to enhanced G-CSF Jak-STAT signaling without increased cell proliferation. Oncogene 21(34):5346–5355
Ward AC, van Aesch YM, Schelen AM et al (1999a) Defective internalization and sustained activation of truncated granulocyte colony-stimulating factor receptor found in severe congenital neutropenia/acute myeloid leukemia. Blood 93(2):447–458
Ward AC, van Aesch YM, Gits J et al (1999b) Novel point mutation in the extracellular domain of the granulocyte colony-stimulating factor (G-CSF) receptor in a case of severe congenital neutropenia hyporesponsive to G-CSF treatment. J Exp Med 190(4):497–507
White SM, Alarcon MH, Tweardy DJ (2000) Inhibition of granulocyte colony-stimulating factor-mediated myeloid maturation by low level expression of the differentiation-defective class IV granulocyte colony-stimulating factor receptor isoform. Blood 95(11):3335–3340
Zarebski A, Velu CS, Baktula AM et al (2008) Mutations in growth factor independent-1 associated with human neutropenia block murine granulopoiesis through colony stimulating factor-1. Immunity 28(3):370–380
Zhang P, Zhang X, Iwama A et al (2000) PU.1 inhibits GATA-1 function and erythroid differentiation by blocking GATA-1 DNA binding. Blood 96(8):2641–2648
Zhu QS, Robinson LJ, Roginskaya V et al (2004) G-CSF-induced tyrosine phosphorylation of Gab2 is Lyn kinase dependent and associated with enhanced Akt and differentiative, not proliferative, responses. Blood 103(9):3305–3312
Zhu QS, Xia L, Mills GB et al (2006) G-CSF induced reactive oxygen species involves Lyn-PI3-kinase-Akt and contributes to myeloid cell growth. Blood 107(5):1847–1856
Ziegler SF, Bird TA, Morella KK et al (1993) Distinct regions of the human granulocyte-colony-stimulating factor receptor cytoplasmic domain are required for proliferation and gene induction. Mol Cell Biol 13(4):2384–2390

Inherited Thrombocytopenias

11

Taizo Nakano and Jorge Di Paola

Contents

11.1 Introduction

Although many inherited bone marrow failure syndromes (IBMFS) exhibit reduced production of all hematopoietic cell lines, a few are characterized by the predominant deficiency of a single cell line. This chapter focuses on inherited disorders that manifest by ineffective megakaryopoiesis and thrombopoiesis leading to low platelet counts.

T. Nakano · J. Di Paola (✉)
Center for Cancer and Blood Disorders, Children's Hospital Colorado, University of Colorado School of Medicine, Aurora, CO, USA
e-mail: taizo.nakano@childrenscolorado.org; Jorge.DiPaola@ucdenver.edu

G. M. Kupfer et al. (eds.), *Bone Marrow Failure*, Pediatric Oncology,
https://doi.org/10.1007/978-3-319-61421-2_11

Platelets play a vital role in primary hemostasis as their activation is required to build a stable clot at the site of vessel injury. Megakaryocyte maturation and differentiation and the subsequent production of platelets are tightly regulated by thrombopoietin (TPO) and multiple key transcription factors. Mutations in the genes involved in these pathways result in a wide range of quantitative and qualitative platelet defects. We will review the inherited thrombocytopenia disorders and specifically expand upon two disorders, congenital amegakaryocytic thrombocytopenia (CAMT) and thrombocytopenia absent radius (TAR), which have been traditionally classified as inherited bone marrow failure syndromes.

Inherited thrombocytopenias commonly present in the newborn period with petechiae, easy bruising, mucosal bleeding, and prolonged, severe isolated thrombocytopenia. It can be difficult to differentiate these rare congenital disorders from the vastly more common causes of acquired thrombocytopenia in infancy including drug-induced infection and immune-mediated thrombocytopenia. Most times, a newborn with severe thrombocytopenia is evaluated and treated for auto- and alloimmune thrombocytopenia well before the consideration of a congenital disorder. Accurate and timely diagnosis of an inherited thrombocytopenia disorder is critical to provide targeted therapy, monitor for known complications of disease, and provide appropriate counseling to patients and their families (Geddis 2013). Clinicians should evaluate important factors that may increase suspicion for an inherited thrombocytopenia disorder including duration of the thrombocytopenia, response to therapy, associated physical abnormalities, pattern of inheritance, and platelet morphology (Table 11.1).

Family history: Patient families should be closely evaluated to identify any members with a history of thrombocytopenia. Inheritance patterns for these disorders include autosomal dominant, X-linked, and autosomal recessive. When multiple family members are involved, suspicion for a congenital thrombocytopenia disorder should be high. It is additionally important to document family history of autoimmunity and known autoimmune rheumatologic syndromes including lupus and juvenile idiopathic arthritis since many of these autoimmune disorders are associated with antibody-mediated thrombocytopenia.

Associated features: Patient and family members should be evaluated for congenital physical and functional anomalies including absence of radii, high-tone hearing loss, renal failure, bifid uvula, right-sided aortic arch, neonatal hematochezia, eczema, severe infections, platelet dysfunction, and family history of leukemia (Cines et al. 2004). The association of congenital hand or arm anomalies with bone marrow failure has been established in a number of IBMFS including Fanconi anemia, Diamond-Blackfan anemia, and TAR syndrome (Alter 1992). It is important to consider these in the differential diagnosis of inherited thrombocytopenias.

Peripheral blood morphology: Platelet number, size, shape, and granule content can provide diagnostic clues toward specific congenital thrombocytopenia disorders. In addition to the mean platelet volume (MPV) provided on standard laboratory blood count analysis, visual inspection of the peripheral blood smear remains the gold standard to assess platelet morphology. It is important to specifically note the presence of very small or very large/giant platelets and document their overall granule content and color. This can also be coupled with transmission electron microscopy (TEM) of platelets to assess for ultrastructural abnormalities.

Bone marrow morphology: With prolonged thrombocytopenia and increasing clinical suspicion for a congenital thrombocytopenia disorder, bone marrow aspirate and biopsy should be performed. It is important to document overall bone marrow cellularity, evaluate for dysplastic cell growth, and screen patients for cytogenetic abnormalities.

Response to therapy: Infants with congenital thrombocytopenias, as opposed to those with immune-mediated disease, are often refractory to immunosuppressive and immune-modulating therapies prescribed in an attempt to increase the platelet count. Agents commonly utilized include intravenous immunoglobulin (IVIG), intravenous anti-D, splenectomy, rituximab, and steroids. Many patients will have been exposed to a combination of these interventions prior to the suspicion of an inherited platelet disorder.

Table 11.1 Classification of the most common inherited thrombocytopenia disorders by platelet size

Platelet size	Disease	Inheritance	Gene (OMIM ID)	Associated features
Small	Wiskott-Aldrich syndrome (WAS)	X-linked	*WAS (300392)*	Abnormal aggregation, severe immunodeficiency, eczema, autoimmunity, lymphoma
	X-linked thrombocytopenia (XLT)	X-linked	*WAS (300392)*	Mild immunodeficiency
Normal	Congenital amegakaryocytic thrombocytopenia (CAMT)	AR	*MPL (601977)*	Reduced-absent megakaryocytes, progressing to bone marrow failure, myelodysplastic syndrome, increased TPO
	Amegakaryocytic thrombocytopenia with radioulnar synostosis (ATRUS)	AD	*HOXA11 (142958)* *MECOM* (EVI1)	Reduced-absent megakaryocytes, radioulnar synostosis, restricted pronation of forearm, hip dysplasia, progressing to bone marrow failure
	Thrombocytopenia with absent radii (TAR)	AR (complex)	*1q21.1 Del (RBM8A) (274000)*	Thrombocytopenia that improves with age, bilateral radial aplasia with thumbs present, milk protein allergy, renal malformations
	TH2 thrombocytopenia	AD	*ANKRD26 (610855)*	Platelets normal to microcytic in size, decreased alpha-granules
	Paris-Trousseau syndrome	AD	*11q23 Del FLI1 (193067)*	Cardiac defects, neurologic defects, syndactyly, hand defects. Large alpha-granules, abnormal aggregation
	ETV6-associated thrombocytopenia	AD	*ETV6 (600618)*	Dyserythropoiesis, increased risk of acute lymphoblastic leukemia
	Familial platelet disorder with propensity for myeloid malignancy (FPD-PMM)	AD	*RUNX1 (601399)*	Abnormal aggregation, increased risk of acute myeloid leukemia, and myelodysplastic syndrome
Large	Bernard-Soulier syndrome (BSS)	AR	*GPIBA (606672)* *GPIBB (138720)* *GP9 (173515)*	Defective GPIb-IX-V. Giant platelets. Decreased ristocetin-induced aggregation
	MYH9-related disorders (May-Hegglin anomaly, Fechtner syndrome, Epstein syndrome, Sebastian syndrome)	AD	*MYH9 (160775)*	Giant platelets. May-Hegglin anomaly, neutrophil inclusions. Renal disease, hearing loss, cataracts
	Gray platelet syndrome (GPS)	AR	*NBEAL2 (614169)*	Absent alpha-granules, abnormal aggregation, marrow fibrosis
	X-linked dyserythropoiesis with or without anemia	X-linked	*GATA1 (305371)*	Decreased alpha-granules, abnormal aggregation, dyserythropoiesis with or without anemia
	Autosomal dominant thrombocytopenia	AD	*ACTN1 (615193)*	Anisocytosis
	Macrothrombocytopenia with dyserythropoiesis	AD	*GFI1B (604383)*	Decreased alpha-granules, abnormal erythropoiesis
	Autosomal dominant macrothrombocytopenia	AD	*TUBB1 (613112)*	Macrothrombocytopenia, normal aggregation

AD autosomal dominant, *AR* autosomal recessive

Genetic defect: The genetic defects that underlie many of the inherited thrombocytopenias have been identified. Therefore, known associated genetic germline mutations can be screened to confirm the diagnosis. The inherited platelet disorders can generally be classified as defects of megakaryocyte production, defects of megakaryocyte maturation, and/or defects of platelet structure and function. However, many patients will not have an identified genetic defect, and they likely represent yet to be identified genetic mutations (Freson et al. 2014).

Prior to the regular use of platelet transfusions and hematopoietic stem cell transplant, many infants with an inherited thrombocytopenia disorder died from hemorrhagic complications. However, supportive care has improved significantly, allowing for sufficient time to make an accurate diagnosis and attempt definitive curative therapy.

11.1.1 Megakaryopoiesis and Thrombopoiesis

Megakaryopoiesis, the process of megakaryocyte maturation, and thrombopoiesis, the process of platelet biogenesis, define the complex sequential pathway toward platelet production from multipotent hematopoietic stem cells (HSCs). Significant advances have been made to identify the molecular events that lead to the differentiation of pluripotent HSCs to megakaryocytes, direct proplatelet formation, and, eventually, the release of 10^{11} platelets into the bloodstream per day in order to maintain a normal concentration of 150–400 × 10^9 platelets per liter of human blood (Thon and Italiano 2010). Over the last decade, a number of germline mutations have been found to disrupt the genes that encode for components of these pathways resulting in quantitative and qualitative platelet disorders (Song et al. 1999; Nichols et al. 2000; Monteferrario et al. 2014; Stevenson et al. 2015).

Multipotent HSCs have the ability to generate cells of all blood lineages. The traditional model of hematopoiesis involves the initial differentiation between common lymphoid progenitors (CLP) that lead to lymphocytic lineages and the common myeloid progenitors (CMP) that further divide into megakaryocyte-erythroid progenitors (MEPs) and subsequently megakaryocyte and erythroid progenitors. As megakaryocytes differentiate and mature in the bone marrow, they begin endomitotic cell cycles and become polyploid. These polyploid megakaryocytes increase the number of specialized granules and their cytoplasmic volume, extend cytoplasmic extensions, and develop a complex demarcation membrane system (Machlus and Italiano Jr. 2013) (Fig. 11.1). Pseudopodia elongate, branch, and eventually release proplatelets and preplatelets into the marrow space. These precursors undergo further remodeling in the circulation to form functional platelets (Thon et al. 2010).

The commitment of MEPs toward the final stages of megakaryocyte differentiation and subsequent thrombopoiesis is a highly regulated process that initially requires engagement of thrombopoietin (TPO) to its receptor, c-Mpl, triggering Janus kinase 2 (JAK2)-mediated signaling. TPO is the major cytokine responsible for initiating thrombopoiesis (Kaushansky 2008). It is a hematopoietic growth factor produced by the liver at a constant rate and is removed from the circulation by receptor-mediated uptake and destruction. TPO binding to the c-Mpl receptor stimulates both early- and late-phase megakaryopoiesis, increasing megakaryocyte number, size, and ploidy. TPO is not required for proplatelet formation and does not increase platelet shedding, but rather stimulates increased megakaryocyte progenitor production and is essential for the overall maintenance of HSCs (Alexander et al. 1996a, b; Savoia et al. 2007). More recently, it has been shown that the murine liver has a sensing mechanism that detects aged platelets, stimulating hepatic TPO production and subsequent megakaryopoiesis (Grozovsky et al. 2015).

The TPO receptor, c-Mpl, a member of the cytokine receptor superfamily, is found on the surface of platelets, early- and late-phase megakaryocytes, and CD34$^+$ hematopoietic stem cell precursors. c-Mpl is characterized by a conserved extracellular domain and an intracellular domain that interacts with components of the cellular signal transduction machinery (Alexander et al. 1996a, b). TPO engagement with the c-Mpl receptor results in homodimerization of the receptor and activation of the JAK2 pathway, which phosphorylate signal transducers and acti-

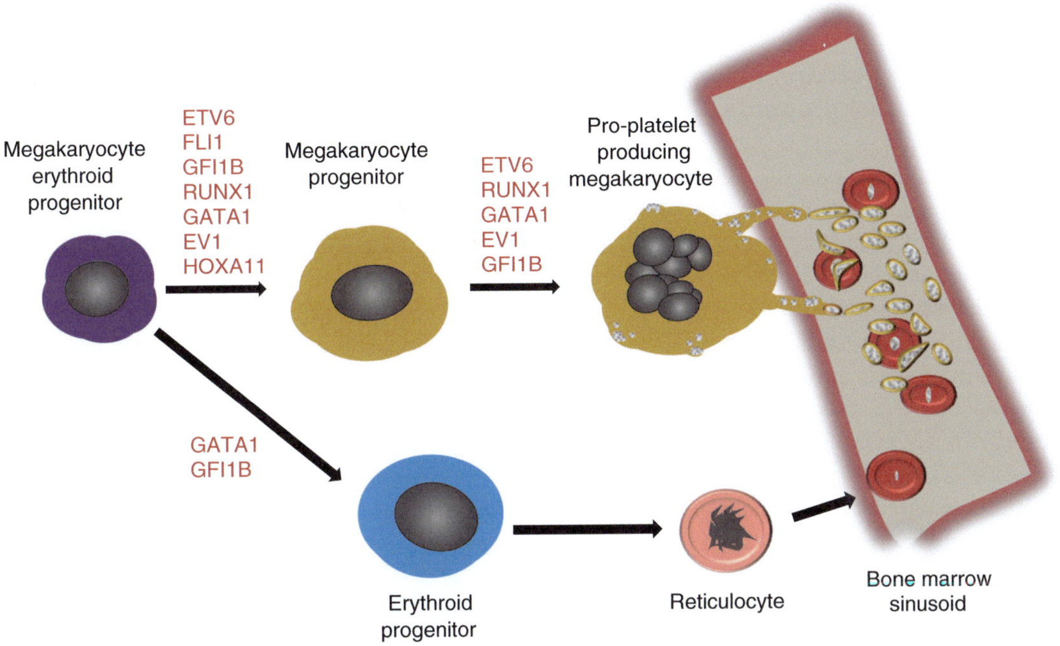

Fig. 11.1 Megakaryopoiesis and thrombopoiesis. Simplified cartoon of megakaryopoiesis and thrombopoiesis. Differentiation of MK progenitors likely occurs from a common megakaryocyte-erythroid progenitor. As MKs differentiate and mature in the bone marrow, they develop polyploidy, increase the numbers of specialized granules and their cytoplasmic volume, extend cytoplasmic extensions, and develop a complex demarcation membrane system. They will eventually extend long cytoplasmic arms (proplatelets) through fenestrations of the bone marrow sinusoidal blood vessels and deliver newly formed preplatelets (larger cytoplasmic units that will be remodeled into platelets in the circulation) and platelets into the circulation under physiologic flow. The erythroid progenitor will originate reticulocytes and mature red cells. All transcription factors involved in these processes are listed in dark red. Germline mutations in the genes that encode for these transcription factors cause hereditary thrombocytopenia

vators of transcription (STATs) including STAT5 and STAT3, which promote gene expression (Chen et al. 1995; Ezumi et al. 1995). TPO additionally stimulates the Ras/MAPK and PI3K signaling pathways. Megakaryocyte-erythroid differentiation is driven not only by lineage restricted transcription factors such as KLF1 for erythroid and FLI1 and ETS1 for megakaryocytic but also by a series of transcription factors (GATA1, GATA2, FOG, and GFI1b) that are shared by both lineages (Kerenyi and Orkin 2010) (Cheng et al. 2009; Foudi et al. 2014). Another critical transcription factor, RUNX1, affects megakaryocyte ploidy as well as proplatelet formation by regulating expression of other genes such as *MYH9*, *MYH10*, and *MYL9* (Jalagadugula et al. 2010; Bluteau et al. 2012; Lordier et al. 2012).

In addition to megakaryopoiesis, c-Mpl activation plays a role in erythropoiesis and is essential for hematopoietic stem cell maintenance and self-renewal. As evidence of its importance to HSCs, early studies on $MPL^{-/-}$ mice confirmed that the lack of TPO receptor expression resulted not only in significant decrease in marrow megakaryocytes and severe thrombocytopenia but also a marked reduction in the number of hematopoietic progenitors of multiple cell lineages. The number of neutrophils and granulocyte-macrophage, erythroid, bipotential, and mixed myeloid progenitor cells were found to all be reduced (Alexander et al. 1996a, b). Furthermore, mutations that impair *MPL* gene expression in humans not only cause thrombocytopenia but also progress to trilineage bone marrow failure (Geddis 2013).

11.2 Amegakaryocytic Disorders

11.2.1 Congenital Amegakaryocytic Thrombocytopenia (CAMT)

Congenital amegakaryocytic thrombocytopenia (CAMT) is a rare autosomal recessive marrow failure syndrome characterized by severe thrombocytopenia and absent or greatly reduced megakaryocytes and megakaryocyte precursors in the bone marrow. This disorder of megakaryocyte production presents at birth or shortly thereafter with easy bruising and/or bleeding. Since it lacks any known association with congenital physical anomalies, it is often initially mistaken for more common acquired causes of thrombocytopenia, most notably neonatal alloimmune thrombocytopenia (NAIT). As the child fails to improve over time, demonstrates a refractoriness to immunosuppressive and immune-modulating therapies, and remains dependent on platelet transfusions, a bone marrow aspirate and biopsy are typically pursued. The lack of megakaryocytes, combined with the preservation of myeloid and erythroid lineages, helps to confirm the clinical diagnosis of CAMT. Although early reports described hemorrhagic complications as the primary cause of death, improved supportive care with transfused blood products has greatly improved outcomes. CAMT is caused by mutations in the *MPL* gene that result in abnormal expression of the TPO receptor c-Mpl on the surface of platelets, megakaryocytes, and hematopoietic stem cell precursors (Ballmaier et al. 2001). Without appropriate TPO signaling, the hematopoietic stem cell population is reduced, and megakaryocytes do not proliferate, which leads to severe thrombocytopenia. Ultimately, patients with CAMT progress to complete bone marrow aplasia. The type of genetic mutation has been demonstrated to directly correlate to the degree of thrombocytopenia and the rate of progression to full marrow aplasia (Germeshausen et al. 2006).

Pathophysiology: CAMT is characterized by the almost complete absence of the surface TPO receptor c-Mpl, a member of the cytokine receptor superfamily. Upon stimulation with TPO, downstream signaling promotes megakaryopoiesis and platelet production. In CAMT, the lack of TPO signaling results in absent or defective c-Mpl expression and impaired megakaryocyte and platelet production. Additionally, TPO is important to the maintenance of hematopoietic stem cells; therefore, lack of appropriate signaling results not only in thrombocytopenia but eventually pancytopenia secondary to progressive marrow aplasia (Alexander et al. 1996a, b; Savoia et al. 2007). Impaired TPO signaling from reduced or absent c-Mpl receptors may lead to an exhaustion of the early progenitor cell pool within the first year of life (Ballmaier et al. 2001). Like most IBMFS, there is a slight increased risk of developing myelodysplasia or leukemia (Steinberg et al. 2007). Although the exact frequency has not been reported, many of the larger retrospective cohorts describe small groups of patients who have transformed to myelodysplastic or malignant disease.

Genetics: CAMT is an autosomal recessive disorder caused by mutations in *MPL*. Homozygous or compound heterozygous mutations involving the TPO receptor c-Mpl result in the inability of TPO to induce megakaryopoiesis. Familial cases of CAMT have been demonstrated mostly in consanguineous families (King et al. 2005). Clinically certified mutation analysis of *MPL* can now be obtained when clinical suspicion is high. There are children who fit the clinical picture of CAMT without an identified mutation in *MPL* implicating locus heterogeneity.

CAMT mutations can be classified based on the two major disease phenotypes observed, CAMT type I and type II (King et al. 2005). In CAMT type I, nonsense *MPL* mutations (stop codons, deletions, or frameshift mutations) result, if translated, in a premature terminated c-Mpl protein, which lacks a transmembrane and intracellular domain and completely eliminates c-Mpl receptor signaling. Patients are predisposed to early severe pancytopenia and bone marrow failure likely due to exhaustion of early progenitor stem cells. Patients demonstrate a median platelet count <21,000/μl, and complete marrow failure presents at a median age of 2 years. In CAMT type II, homozygous or compound heterozygous missense *MPL* mutations (splicing defects or substitutions) that affect the c-Mpl extracellular domain result in a less aggressive defect with some residual receptor signaling (Germeshausen et al. 2006). Patients with type II mutations demonstrate a transient improvement in platelet counts to near-normal levels during early infancy. Median platelet count is usually 35,000/μl, and complete marrow failure presents at a median age of 5 years (King et al. 2005; Geddis 2011). Of note, there have been reports of missense mutations that can also develop early bone marrow failure so that the general recommendation is to consider hematopoietic stem cell transplant at an early age in all patients (Savoia et al. 2007). Molecular investigations on the functionality of a particular missense mutation would need to be evaluated to better predict the clinical course. In addition to the loss-of-function *MPL* mutations that result in CAMT, gain-of-function *MPL* mutations have also been identified that clinically present with thrombocytosis (Moliterno et al. 2004).

Clinical presentation: Infants with CAMT present shortly after birth with unexplained purpura and petechiae and, upon initial laboratory evaluation, demonstrate severe thrombocytopenia (platelets <50,000/μl). Active bleeding may present as intracranial, gastrointestinal, pulmonary, or cutaneous hemorrhage. Platelets demonstrate normal morphology including normal size (normal mean platelet volume) and granule content. Overall, mean platelet count has been reported to be 21,000/μl (King et al. 2005). Infants with CAMT do not exhibit congenital skeletal abnormalities and demonstrate normal physical and mental development. Suspicion should remain high in the neonate with persistent, recurrent severe thrombocytopenia (thrombocytopenia that persists after 3 months) (Geddis 2011). CAMT is the inherited bone marrow failure syndrome most likely to present with symptomatic marrow failure in the neonatal period. CAMT patients carry some increased risk for MDS and AML as well (Alter 2002).

Diagnosis and genetic testing: The peripheral blood counts of patients with CAMT commonly demonstrate severe thrombocytopenia and red cell macrocytosis. The first challenge to diagnose CAMT in a neonate with thrombocytopenia is to rule out the significantly more common causes of acquired thrombocytopenia of infancy. The differential diagnoses include, but are not limited to, preeclampsia, placental insufficiency, intrauterine growth retardation, anoxic insult, infection, and maternal transfer of platelet allo- or autoantibodies, all common causes of thrombocytopenia in neonates. It is also important to note the time of onset, severity, and persistence of thrombocytopenia. When CAMT patients are treated with immune-modulating and immunosuppressing agents (like intravenous immunoglobulin or corticosteroids) under the assumption of an immune thrombocytopenia, they generally show poor response to treatment. Taking a good family history is critical to establish the diagnosis of an inherited thrombocytopenia disorder and to evaluate genetic inheritance pattern (Cines et al. 2004). A thorough physical exam is required to ensure appropriate evaluation of forearms, thumbs, and skeletal structure.

Bone marrow evaluation should be considered in all children with persistent severe thrombocytopenia since birth. Early in the disease course, evaluation of the bone marrow often demonstrates normal marrow cellularity with severely reduced or absent megakaryocytes and small or immature megakaryocytes (King et al. 2005). Serial bone marrow aspirates and biopsies are usually necessary to confirm the diagnosis and monitor progression toward a more hypocellular marrow with increased lymphocytes and plasma cells, similar to the marrow morphology of any severe aplastic anemia patient. Cytogenetic analysis should be performed on marrow aspirates including chromosome karyotyping and FISH evaluation for chromosomal rearrangements commonly seen in myelodysplastic syndromes.

If the bone marrow evaluation demonstrates reduced number or absent megakaryocytes, screening for *MPL* gene mutations should be performed since homozygous or compound heterozygous mutations in *MPL* result in clinical CAMT. *MPL* genetic analysis is readily available at multiple laboratories including GeneDx and PreventionGenetics. Bidirectional sequencing of the coding regions and splice sites of exons 1–12 of the *MPL* gene can be obtained. Specimens are taken as a single sample with 1.5 ml whole blood in ethylenediaminetetraacetic acid (EDTA), buccal brushes as alternative samples, or 10 ml of amniotic fluid (Test Information Sheet. GeneDX DNA Diagnostic Experts. *MPL* gene analysis in congenital amegakaryocytic thrombocytopenia. www.genedx.com).

If left untreated, infants with CAMT will progress toward a more hypocellular bone marrow and nearly all go on to develop trilineage bone marrow failure within the first decade of life (Ihara et al. 1999). In one of the largest reviews of CAMT patients, King et al. report that the median age of onset of pancytopenia is 38 months. In the setting of pancytopenia and early evidence of marrow failure, one should consider excluding the diagnosis of Fanconi anemia through chromosome breakage analysis and dyskeratosis congenita by screening telomere lengths.

There are a number of adjuvant laboratory studies to help confirm the diagnosis of CAMT. Absent surface expression of the TPO receptor c-Mpl can be assessed by flow cytometry (Ihara et al. 1999). Unable to appropriately bind to the absent or abnormal receptor, TPO serum levels are significantly elevated as they often demonstrate a tenfold increase above normal controls (Muraoka et al. 1997; Ballmaier et al. 2001). Non-transfused or minimally transfused CAMT patients will have a negative antiplatelet antibody screening. Although difficult to obtain in the clinical setting, cells from CAMT patients will demonstrate defective signal and response to TPO in megakaryocyte colony formation assays (Muraoka et al. 1997) and will also exhibit absent surface expression of c-Mpl (Ihara et al. 1999). These tests are mostly based in research laboratories; therefore when suspected, genetic testing for CAMT should be performed.

Therapy: Early attempts to stimulate megakaryopoiesis were performed with a number of cytokines including interleukin (IL)-3, IL-11, and granulocyte-macrophage colony-stimulating factor (GM-CSF). However, responses were inconsistent and transient, and some of these treatments exhibited significant toxicity (Guinan et al. 1993).

From the initial presentation through the diagnostic evaluation, supportive care measures should be taken to manage and prevent disease complications. Caesarean section should be considered for children considered high risk for inheriting CAMT to reduced risk of cerebral hemorrhage. Once the diagnosis of CAMT is established, patients should be monitored with frequent examinations and have their platelet count monitored periodically to be aware of the severity of thrombocytopenia. Leukocyte reduced, irradiated random donor platelet transfusions are indicated for any patient with signs of active bleeding and could also be considered as a preventative measure in the asymptomatic neonate that demonstrates severe thrombocytopenia. In the older child, platelet transfusions are reserved for the setting of symptomatic bleeding to avoid unnecessary risk of developing platelet alloimmunization.

For minor bleeding, oral or intravenous antifibrinolytics (aminocaproic acid and tranexamic acid) can be effective to stabilize clot formation. The use of desmopressin (1-deamino-8-D-arginine vasopressin or DDAVP) is not recommended in small infants given the increased risk of dilutional hyponatremia, but can be considered in older children. Medications with antiplatelet effects including nonsteroidal anti-inflammatory and aspirin should be avoided.

Hematopoietic stem cell transplant (HSCT) remains the only curative therapy for CAMT. Transplant should be considered early in life in all patients and is indicated as soon as an infant develops pancytopenia and becomes transfusion dependent. The risks associated with transplant are often outweighed by the potential risk of bleeding, transfusions, progression to marrow failure, and, more importantly, potential clonal evolution of the disease. Early transplant also avoids the development of platelet antibodies from the repeated platelet transfusions. The evaluation, donor choice, and preparation regimen resembles that of patients with severe aplastic anemia (sAA) and other inherited bone marrow failure syndromes. HLA typing of the patient and full siblings should be obtained at time of diagnosis.

Matched sibling donor HSCT is the treatment of choice with case series collectively reporting an overall survival greater than 90% (Henter et al. 1995; Al-Ahmari et al. 2004; Frangoul et al. 2010). Transplant conditioning regimens often include busulfan (BU), cyclophosphamide (CY), and antithymocyte globulin (ATG). Heterozygous sibling donor transplant has been reported (Frangoul et al. 2010). Transplant with matched unrelated donors has less favorable outcome secondary to a higher rate of rejection, graft-versus-host disease (GVHD), infection, delayed engraftment, and regimen-related toxicity. A recent case series proposed the use of T-cell-depleted hematopoietic stem cells to reduce rates of GVHD associated with matched unrelated donor HSCT (Tarek et al. 2012).

Historically, the majority of CAMT patients received fully myeloablative preparative regimens including the use of total body irradiation. Myeloablative regimens were associated with increased acute graft-versus-host disease, transplant-related morbidity (23%), and mortality and graft failure (Tarek et al. 2012). Reduced-intensity preparative regimens have recently been attempted in a few cases without significant complications (Woods et al. 2014). Reduced-intensity regimens similar to those used in other IBMFS like Fanconi anemia, dyskeratosis congenita, severe aplastic anemia, and hemoglobinopathies are now being utilized given the reduced risk of organ toxicity (Myers and Davies 2009).

TPO receptor agonists, romiplostim and eltrombopag, are now approved for the treatment of adult and children greater than 1 year of age with chronic immune thrombocytopenia. The advent of these TPO receptor agonists has created a potential opportunity to activate mutated c-Mpl receptors with residual activity (CAMT type II mutations). Specific type II CAMT mutations involving the extracellular domain of the c-Mpl receptor have demonstrated increased stimulation from novel TPO agonists that was not seen with native TPO (Fox et al. 2010). However, the utility of TPO agonists appears to be limited to a minority of patients that carry these specific low impact mutations.

CAMT is a monogenetic defect, making it an ideal target for gene therapy with the theoretical potential for cure if able to induce expression of an intact *MPL* gene. Attempts have been made to study vector-mediated expression of artificial TPO receptors in stem cells to convey a growth advantage of cells able to mature and produce platelets (Richard and Blau 2003; Wicke et al. 2010). A notable risk remains in that mutations that result in constitutive *MPL* activation have been correlated to myeloproliferative disease in patients, and overexpression of *MPL* in mice has been shown to induce leukemias or hyperproliferative erythropoiesis (Cocault et al. 1996; Pikman et al. 2006; Wicke et al. 2010).

Outcome: Before HSCT, CAMT patients progressed to complete marrow aplasia and carried a poor survival rate. The prognosis of CAMT is worse when trilineage marrow aplasia has already developed. Historically, cause of death has been secondary to hemorrhagic complications (30%) and now complications of the HSCT (20%) (Al-Ahmari et al. 2004; King et al. 2005). In patients who do not undergo HSCT, CAMT is a fatal disease with mortality at a young age often secondary to hemorrhages or the clonal transformation to myelodysplasia or leukemia (Maserati et al. 2008). Solid tumors have not been reported in CAMT patients.

11.2.2 Thrombocytopenia Absent Radius (TAR)

Thrombocytopenia absent radius (TAR) is a rare IBMFS with complex inheritance and has an estimated prevalence of ~1:240,000 (Martinez-Frias et al. 1998; Houeijeh et al. 2011). The diagnosis of TAR is suggested by the finding of isolated, severe thrombocytopenia at birth or shortly thereafter secondary to severe amegakaryocytosis, along with the evident congenital physical anomaly of bilateral absent or abnormally formed radii sparing the presence of both thumbs (Hall 1987). The combination of thrombocytopenia and absent radii was first described by Greenwald and Sherman in 1929. The term TAR as a multiple anomaly syndrome was coined by Hall et al. in 1969, reporting these clinical findings in a cohort of 40 patients (Greenwald and Sherman 1929;

Hall et al. 1969). The physical anomalies in TAR syndrome are not limited to absent radii and often involve additional orthopedic abnormalities of the ulna, humerus, and tibia and other cardiac, renal, genitourinary, cerebral, and facial congenital malformations of variable expressivity. Infants with TAR often present with hemorrhagic manifestations including petechiae and bloody diarrhea (secondary to thrombocytopenia and associated milk protein intolerance) in the first few weeks to months of life.

Genetics: The inheritance pattern for TAR syndrome is complex and most commonly reported as either autosomal recessive or de novo. Even though the molecular defect associated with TAR is now better understood, the mechanism of action for the disease is not yet completely defined. In 2007, Klopocki et al. studied 30 patients with TAR and reported a consistent association with a 1q21.1 microdeletion (Klopocki et al. 2007). The roughly 200 kb microdeletion was inherited paternally in 5 cases, maternally in 12 cases, and de novo in 5 cases. Given that unaffected parents carried the deletion and some unaffected controls were also found to carry the deletion, the authors rightly concluded that the 1q21.1 variant is required, but not sufficient alone to be the sole causative defect in TAR syndrome (Klopocki et al. 2007). A subsequent study confirmed the presence of the 1q21.1 microdeletions in 14 TAR patients with variable clinical phenotypes (Houeijeh et al. 2011). Inherited from a healthy parent, the deletion was present in family members with minor congenital anomalies (Khincha and Savage 2013) suggesting incomplete penetrance and variable expressivity.

The 1q21.1 microdeletion encompasses at least 12 known genes including the *RBM8A* gene. In 2013, Albers et al. using high-throughput sequencing identified low-frequency noncoding single nucleotide polymorphisms (SNP) in the 5′ UTR or first intron of *RBM8A* in 53 out of 55 TAR patients with the microdeletion (Albers et al. 2013). The authors concluded unequivocally ($p < 5 \times 10^{-228}$) that the compound (biallelic) inheritance of these noncoding SNPs together with a null mutation in *RBM8A* causes TAR syndrome (Fig. 11.2). The mechanism by which these co-inherited molecular defects reduce *RBM8A* transcription and protein expression is not known.

Pathophysiology: Despite the progress made in the genetic elucidation of the disease, the molecular basis of TAR syndrome is not yet fully understood. Recent advances have pointed to defective TPO receptor signaling resulting in poor maturation and maintenance of megakaryocytes (Strippoli et al. 1998; Dreyfus and Tchernia 2000). The 1q21.1 microdeletion previously mentioned contains multiple genes that have been proposed to influence pathophysiology of the disease. *PIAS3* is contained within the defect, and it has been hypothesized that dysfunctional *PIAS3* could interrupt the TPO signaling pathway and result in impaired megakaryopoiesis (Klopocki et al. 2007). *RBM8A* is contained within the defect and, as previously mentioned, is now thought to play a significant role in the pathophysiology of TAR. *RBM8A* encodes an RNA-binding protein 8A (also known as Y14), which is thought to be involved in mRNA and snRNA biogenesis. Y14, predominantly found in the nucleus, is one of the four components of the core exon-junction complex (EJC) which impacts nuclear export, subcellular localization of specific transcripts, translational enhancement, and nonsense-mediated RNA decay (Bottillo et al. 2013). Platelet levels of Y14 are decreased in patients with TAR syndrome (Albers et al. 2013). There is, however, no clear mechanism to explain how Y14 deficiency directly affects megakaryocyte maturation and how it may influence skeletal and other nonhematologic features of the syndrome. Complete loss of Y14 protein is presumed lethal given its widespread involvement in basic cellular functions (Albers et al. 2013).

Clinical presentation: TAR syndrome is clinically characterized by the association of severe thrombocytopenia at birth or shortly thereafter and bilateral absence of the radii with the presence of both thumbs (Hall et al. 1969; Hedberg and Lipton 1988; Toriello 2011). Although the thumbs may themselves have dysmorphic features (wider and flatter) and tend to have limited function, their presence distinguishes TAR syndrome from other IBMFS most notably Fanconi

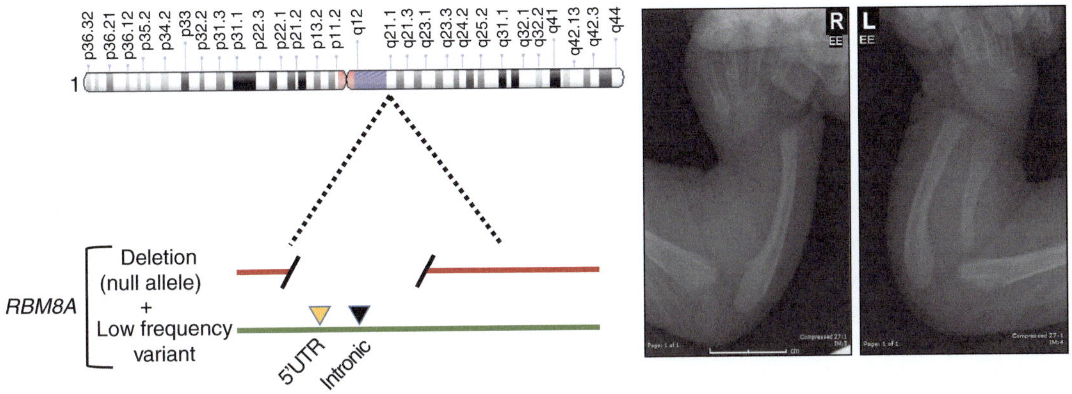

Fig. 11.2 Genetics of thrombocytopenia absent radius (TAR) syndrome. The genetics of TAR syndrome are characterized by compound heterozygosity. The gene *RBM8A*, located in the q21.1 region of chromosome 1, is always included in the microdeletion that almost universally characterizes this disease (red bar). However, in order to exhibit the phenotype, an affected individual has to co-inherit a low-frequency regulatory variant on the other allele of *RBM8A* (green bar). These variants are single nucleotide polymorphisms (SNPs) located either in the 5′ UTR (yellow triangle) or in the first intron of the gene (black triangle). The consequences of the genetic defect are seen on the right of the figure. The forearm X-rays of a child affected with TAR show complete absence of the radius in the right arm (R) and radial hypoplasia in the left forearm (L)

anemia (Goldfarb et al. 2007). There is a slight female predominance in TAR syndrome (Hall et al. 1969; Greenhalgh et al. 2002; Klopocki et al. 2007).

Hematologic findings: Variable thrombocytopenia at birth and in the first few months of life place the infant at increased risk of intracranial hemorrhage and gastrointestinal bleeding. Platelets are of normal size and have normal granule content. The platelet count is typically below 50,000/μl, and patients can present with gastrointestinal or intracerebral hemorrhage. Bone marrow aspirate in patients with TAR syndrome demonstrates normal erythroid and myeloid maturation with absent or severely reduced and immature megakaryocytes. Transient leukocytosis or leukemoid reactions have been documented with white blood cell counts exceeding 35,000/μl. Interestingly, most patients with TAR syndrome spontaneously improve their platelet count to near-normal levels after the first year of life. These patients do not typically develop other cytopenias and do not progress to bone marrow failure. Patients who survive any bleeding complications that occur in the first year of life carry an excellent clinical prognosis and demonstrate platelet levels adequate to tolerate any necessary orthopedic procedures. Some reports have shown a mild increased risk of leukemia (AML and ALL) associated with TAR syndrome (Fadoo and Naqvi 2002). However, the evidence remains anecdotal with only case series that have reported this association and without strong enough evidence that proves a causative relationship (Camitta and Rock 1993; Symonds et al. 1995).

Skeletal findings: Bilateral radial hypo−/aplasia with presence of the thumbs is a consistent feature of the syndrome. Classification of the radial deficiency is based on the amount of residual radius present. Type I anomalies demonstrate a short distal radius. In type II, there is a small radius with proximal and distal growth plates. In type IIII, there is a small proximal radius. In type IV, which remains the most common presentation, there is complete absence of the radius. The extent of upper limb abnormalities greatly varies from isolated radial aplasia to the additional finding of severe humeral and ulnar shortening with phocomelia. Patients with more severe presentations of upper limb phocomelia are more likely to demonstrate diffuse skeletal abnormalities especially in the shoulder girdle and the lower limbs (Greenhalgh et al. 2002; Houeijeh et al.

2011; Bottillo et al. 2013). Shoulder abnormalities include absent or hypoplastic glenoid fossa, acromion, scapula, clavicle, or a combination of these (Al Kaissi et al. 2015). Hands are often severely radially deviated. Fingers may demonstrate syndactyly and fifth finger clinodactyly. Abnormalities of the lower limbs are less frequent, but may consist of patella subluxation, hip dislocation or dysplasia, absence of the tibiofibular joint, bowing of the legs, and lower limb phocomelia (Toriello 2011). Children with TAR syndrome tend toward shorter stature.

Extraskeletal abnormalities: Cognitive development does not appear to be impacted in TAR syndrome. Facial dysmorphism including micrognathia, low-set and posteriorly rotated ears, hypertelorism, and cleft palate has been observed (Houeijeh et al. 2011). Common cardiac abnormalities include tetralogy of fallot, atrial septal defect, and patent ductus arteriosus (Hall 1987). Renal anomalies, found in approximately 25% of patients, include duplicated ureter, horseshoe kidney, small kidneys, and dilatation of the renal pelvis (Toriello 2011). Cow's milk intolerance has been described to be present in as high as 47% of TAR patients in some studies (Geddis 2009). Persistent diarrhea may result in malnutrition and failure to thrive. Additionally, the introduction of cow's milk has been linked to induce episodes of thrombocytopenia that can be improved through the elimination of cow's milk from the diet (Greenhalgh et al. 2002).

Diagnosis and testing: The diagnosis of TAR syndrome is based on a combination of clinical features. Neonatal-onset thrombocytopenia, with platelet counts below 50,000/μl, persists often despite immune-modulating agents. Bilateral absence or hypoplasia of radii and presence of thumbs can be confirmed by physical exam and plain film X-ray. Fetal ultrasound should identify radial anomalies to increase suspicion of TAR syndrome. Although mild normocellular anemia may result from blood loss, it is typically accompanied by reticulocytosis, indicating adequate marrow erythrocyte production. A leukocytosis or leukemoid reaction is commonly noted and, if present, almost always resolves within the first year of life. Although not commonly measured, serum TPO levels are often elevated. Bone marrow evaluation demonstrates normal overall marrow cellularity with absent or severely reduced megakaryocytes and normal to increased myeloid and erythroid cell lines. Bone marrow biopsy and aspirate should also be sent for cytogenetic analysis including chromosome karyotype and myelodysplastic panel. Additional screening radiography should include an echocardiogram to rule out cardiac anomalies, abdominal ultrasound to rule out genitourinary anomalies, and a cerebral ultrasound to rule out intracranial anomalies and hemorrhage.

Presently, molecular testing can be used for the diagnosis of TAR. As mentioned previously, the 1q21.1 microdeletion has been found in patients with TAR, and its identification supports the diagnosis in individuals who meet the clinical diagnosis of TAR. Perhaps, more specifically, identifying pathologic variants of the *RBM8A* gene represents the most accurate way to define TAR syndrome genetics (Klopocki et al. 2007; Albers et al. 2013). Deletion/duplication analysis of the *RBM8A* gene can be performed first to detect the 200 kb microdeletion at 1q21.1 that includes *RBM8A*. Sequence analysis of the coding and noncoding regions of *RMB8A* can follow in order to identify the second *RBM8A* hypomorphic mutation for confirmation of diagnosis or genetic counseling. In addition to diagnosing the patient, this molecular testing can be used to screen family members for carrier status and contribute to determine prenatal diagnosis (Toriello 1993). In the future, next-generation sequencing may present a more cost-effective method to simultaneously detect copy number variations and nucleotide substitutions of the *RBM8A* gene (Nicchia et al. 2016).

Differential diagnosis: Although the clinical diagnosis of TAR is not difficult, numerous other potential diagnoses should be considered. Fanconi anemia, Holt-Oram syndrome, VACTERL (vertebrae, anal atresia, cardiac defects, tracheoesophageal fistula, esophageal atresia, renal defects, limb defects) association, and Roberts syndrome to name a few. Therefore, a medical genetics consult is often recommended (Table 11.2).

Therapy: The treatment of TAR syndrome is primarily based on adequate supportive care. A

Table 11.2 Differential diagnosis for TAR syndrome

Disorder	Upper limb exam	Diagnostic evaluation	Molecular defect	Associated features
Thrombocytopenia absent radius (TAR)	Radial anomalies, thumbs intact	Clinical evaluation, X-ray, gene sequencing	*RBM8A*	Thrombocytopenia, absent radius with thumbs, milk protein allergy, cardiac and renal anomalies
Fanconi anemia (FA)	Radial anomalies, thumb anomalies,	Chromosome breakage studies, gene sequencing	17 FA or FA-like genes have been identified	Short stature, progression to pancytopenia and bone marrow failure, cancer predisposition
Holt-Oram syndrome (HOS)	Thumb anomalies (absent or hypoplastic), radial, thenar, or carpal bone anomalies	Clinical evaluation, X-ray, ECHO, gene sequencing	*TBX5*	Cardiac defects (atrial septal defect and first-degree heart block)
Roberts syndrome (RBS)	Absent/fused fingers	Clinical evaluation for prenatal growth retardation and limb malformations, cytogenetics for premature centromere separation gene sequencing	*ESCO2*	Prenatal growth retardation, craniofacial abnormalities, lower limbs involved
VACTERL association	Radial anomalies, thumb anomalies	Clinical evaluation for associated features	Multifactorial	Vertebral anomalies, anal atresia, cardiac defects, tracheoesophageal fistula, renal and radial anomalies, limb anomalies

baseline echocardiogram is recommended to assess for cardiac anomalies. Also, it is important to consider evaluation of renal structure and function. In infants with suspected cow's milk intolerance, the use of hydrolysate formulas is recommended. Dietary modifications to avoid milk protein exposure continue to be helpful in older children as well. A medical genetics consultation is helpful to confirm diagnosis in the proband and provide appropriate genetic counseling to the family. Parents of affected individuals are recommended to be evaluated including radiographs of the limbs and molecular screening for *RBM8A* pathologic variants.

Platelet transfusions: Once diagnosed, patients with TAR syndrome should be monitored with frequent examinations and have their platelet count monitored to be aware of the severity of thrombocytopenia. Peripheral blood counts should be obtained with any evidence of increased bleeding or bruising. Leukocyte reduced, irradiated random donor platelet transfusions are indicated for any patient with signs of active bleeding and should also be considered as a preventative measure in the asymptomatic neonate that demonstrates severe thrombocytopenia or undergoes invasive procedures. Patients typically demonstrate a robust response in platelet count after platelet transfusion and may require frequent transfusions in the first 4 months of life, mostly due to gastrointestinal bleeding. However, when possible, caution should be taken to limit unnecessary transfusions in order to reduce development of alloimmunization. Patients with TAR syndrome often face difficulties with venous access for phlebotomy and supportive care. The pain caused by repeated venipuncture impacts patient quality of life. Stable venous access may be required, and providers should consider placement of a central venous catheter to allow for the safe administration of blood products, intravenous medications, parenteral nutrition, and blood sampling (Coccia et al. 2012).

Orthopedic interventions: An orthopedic consultation should be obtained with evaluation of the upper and lower limbs. Many patients will have serious functional disability demonstrating difficulties with activities of daily living including dressing, feeding, and washing. The clinical goal is to maximize function of the limbs. Splinting of the wrist and stretching programs are utilized to passively correct the radial deviations and allow for improved ability to control fingers. After 3 years of age, splinting and stretching are less effective and more definitive surgical options are available (Al Kaissi et al. 2015). Surgical goals include alignment and stabilization of the wrist, rebalance of the musculotendinous forces around the wrist, and reversal of the ulnar forearm bow.

Physical therapy: Consultation with a physical therapist is recommended with the goal to increase muscle strength in the upper shoulders and upper limbs. At an early age, patients should consider instituting stretching protocols to correct the radial deviation.

Outcomes: Patients with TAR syndrome carry an overall good prognosis. Mortality is higher in children less than 2 years of age likely related to the higher incidence of severe thrombocytopenia in this age group. However, as most children experience complete resolution of thrombocytopenia after the first year of life, their risk of hemorrhage reduces concurrently. Long-term monitoring of patients for late recurrence of thrombocytopenia or rare transformation to leukemia is recommended (Camitta and Rock 1993; Fadoo and Naqvi 2002).

11.2.3 Amegakaryocytic Thrombocytopenia with Radioulnar Synostosis (ATRUS)

Amegakaryocytic thrombocytopenia with radioulnar synostosis (ATRUS, also referred to as RUSAT, radioulnar synostosis with amegakaryocytic thrombocytopenia) is a rare autosomal dominant disorder characterized by neonatal thrombocytopenia in association with proximal fusion of the radius and ulna (Thompson et al. 2001). Children with ATRUS demonstrate amegakaryocytosis of the bone marrow and, like CAMT, rapidly progress to complete marrow aplasia. Physical findings often include proximal radial ulnar synostosis that severely limits pronation and supination of the forearm. ATRUS is clinically suspected in the neonate with restricted pronation-supination movements. Other skeletal and extraskeletal abnormalities may include clinodactyly, syndactyly, hip dysplasia, and sensorineural hearing loss. Heterozygous point mutations in the homeobox gene *HOXA11* have been associated with this syndrome and were reported in the families initially described (Thompson and Nguyen 2000). Individuals with ATRUS who did not demonstrate a *HOXA11* mutation were recently found to have de novo missense mutations in *MECOM* (MDS1 and EVI1 complex locus gene), which encodes the transcription factors EVI1 and MDS-EVI1, transcribed from alternative transcription start sites (Niihori et al. 2015). These mutations clustered in the 8th zinc finger motif of EV1, which is required for dimerization with itself and RUNX1. Interestingly, and differently from patients with *HOXA11* mutations, these patients also presented with severe anemia at birth indicating a more complex role for EVI1 in hematopoiesis.

Initial therapy for ATRUS is primarily based on supportive care including platelet transfusions and orthopedic consultation. However, as children progress to complete marrow failure, they require consultation for hematopoietic stem cell transplant (see CAMT section for HSCT guidelines).

11.3 Disorders of Megakaryopoiesis and Thrombopoiesis

The disorders described in this section do not usually present with or progress to bone marrow failure but are part of the initial differential diagnosis of inherited thrombocytopenia. Therefore, we will describe them briefly in order to provide specific clues for their diagnosis.

11.3.1 Paris-Trousseau Thrombocytopenia

Paris-Trousseau thrombocytopenia is an autosomal dominant inherited thrombocytopenia disorder associated with varying degrees of thrombocytopenia, qualitative platelet dysfunction, congenital heart defects, and neurologic abnormalities (Geddis 2013). The disorder has been associated with a deletion of the terminal portion of chromosome 11 and is often considered a component of the broader disorder known as Jacobsen syndrome, which is characterized by cardiac and neurodevelopmental anomalies as well as distinctive facial features. The gene that encodes for FLI1, a member the E-twenty-six (ETS) family of transcription factors, is contained within this deleted region and has been hypothesized to contribute to the phenotypic presentation of the disease (Raslova et al. 2004; Di Paola 2015; Stevenson et al. 2015). FLI1 has previously been identified as a key regulator of megakaryopoiesis, and murine models of FLI1 deficiency demonstrate defective megakaryopoiesis (Hart et al. 2000).

In Paris-Trousseau syndrome, platelets appear normal in size, but demonstrate abnormal giant alpha-granules and a paucity of dense granules on electron microscopy. These structural defects result in a population of platelets that exhibit abnormal responses to thrombin and may predispose patients to bleeding. Bone marrow evaluation demonstrates two populations of megakaryocytes including both a normal megakaryocytes population and a micromegakaryocyte population thought to express the *FLI1* mutation (Di Paola 2015). Similar to other platelet function disorders, treatment is primarily based on supportive care and commonly involves use of periprocedural antifibrinolytics and DDAVP for minor procedures and platelet transfusions for more invasive surgical procedures or active bleeds. Thrombocytopenia often resolves in adolescence; however, the qualitative defects may persist and result in ongoing bleeding issues.

11.3.2 X-Linked Thrombocytopenia (XLT)

X-linked thrombocytopenia (XLT) is caused by defects in GATA1, mentioned earlier as a transcription factor important to megakaryocyte-erythroid differentiation (Geddis 2013). Mutations in the N-terminal zinc finger of GATA1 prevent appropriate interaction between GATA1 and its cofactor FOG1. The result is macrothrombocytopenia with platelets that exhibit decreased alpha-granule content (Ciovacco et al. 2008). Given that the defect impacts both megakaryocyte and erythroid lineages, individuals with XLT often demonstrate varying degrees of dyserythropoiesis.

11.3.3 Familial Platelet Disorder with Propensity for Myeloid Malignancy (FPD-PMM)

Familial platelet disorder with propensity for myeloid malignancy (FPD-PMM) is an autosomal dominant quantitative and qualitative inherited thrombocytopenia disorder caused by mutations in the runt-related transcription factor 1 (*RUNX1*) gene (Liew and Owen 2011). *RUNX1* is well known for its role in hematopoietic cell differentiation and its association with myeloid malignancies. However, *RUNX1* also plays an important role in megakaryocyte differentiation. Patients with FPD-PMM often demonstrate mild thrombocytopenia with normal-sized platelets that have normal granule content. However, they present with more severe clinical bleeding than expected, likely secondary to platelet dysfunction (Stockley et al. 2013). Importantly, *RUNX1* mutations associated with FPD-PMM also carry the risk of developing myelodysplastic or acute myeloid leukemia. Rate of malignant transformation in patients with germline *RUNX1* mutations has been reported to range from 20% to 65% (Geddis 2013). Although management of the platelet defects is mostly supportive with antifibrinolytic and platelet transfusions, FPD-PMM patients must be screened at regular intervals for the development of leukemia.

11.3.4 Wiskott-Aldrich Syndrome

Wiskott-Aldrich syndrome is an X-linked inherited thrombocytopenia that is characterized by severe thrombocytopenia, eczema dermatitis, and immunodeficiency. A cardinal feature of this syndrome is the presence of small-sized platelets. The MPV in affected individuals ranges from 3.5 to 5.0 fl. Mutations in the Wiskott-Aldrich syndrome gene (*WAS*) cause abnormalities in the Wiskott-Aldrich syndrome protein (WASp). Abnormal WASp function results in platelet cytoskeleton abnormalities. Additionally, WASp-deficient megakaryocytes demonstrate defective migration toward marrow sinusoids, which likely contributes to the mechanism of thrombocytopenia (Gothwal et al. 2014). Although thrombocytopenia and bleeding can be treated with supportive care measures, the risk of infection in WAS confers greater morbidity and mortality. Given the significant risk of life-threatening infection, patients with WAS and an appropriate marrow donor are recommended to undergo allogenic HSCT.

11.3.5 Gray Platelet Syndrome

Gray platelet syndrome (GPS) is an autosomal recessive inherited thrombocytopenia disorder characterized by thrombocytopenia with large platelets that are deficient in alpha-granules as evaluated by electron microscopy. Patients present with thrombocytopenia and mucosal membrane bleeding. The lack of alpha-granules makes the platelets appear pale or "gray" on the peripheral blood smear. These abnormal alpha-granules demonstrate decreased levels of fibrinogen, von Willebrand factor, thrombospondin, and factor V (Di Paola and Johnson 2011). Bleeding symptoms are moderate to severe, and treatment is primary through supportive care with antifibrinolytics and platelet transfusions. There are no major phenotypic abnormalities associated with GPS; however, marrow myelofibrosis and splenomegaly have been reported in a significant number of patients as they age (Gunay-Aygun et al. 2010).

GPS is caused by biallelic mutations in the neurobeachin-like 2 gene, *NBEAL2* (Albers et al. 2011; Gunay-Aygun et al. 2011; Kahr et al. 2011). Although the function of NBEAL2 is not completely understood, it is likely involved in vesicular trafficking and granule biogenesis, causing inability to properly package alpha-granules that results in both a quantitative and qualitative platelet disorder (Hinckley and Di Paola 2014).

11.3.6 MYH9-Related Thrombocytopenias

MYH9-related diseases are a collection of autosomal dominant inherited thrombocytopenia disorders that demonstrate macrothrombocytopenia but also may be associated with progressive sensorineural deafness, kidney disease, and neutrophil inclusions.(Seri et al. 2003) In the past these thrombocytopenias were described as May-Hegglin anomaly, Fechtner syndrome, Epstein syndrome, and Sebastian syndrome. However, more recently, mutations in the *MYH9* gene located on chromosome 22 were reported to cause all these disorders (Seri et al. 2000). These mutations result in abnormal non-muscle myosin production that impacts platelet cytoskeleton structure. Peripheral blood smear often demonstrates giant platelets and cytoplasmic aggregates in leukocytes, however, confirmatory diagnosis is often made through *MYH9* gene sequencing. As with several of these platelet disorders the degree of thrombocytopenia is variable and patients may exhibit a mild qualitative platelet disorder. However, the bleeding tendency is often mild and can be managed with supportive care including antifibrinolytics and platelet transfusions.

11.3.7 Bernard-Soulier Syndrome

Bernard-Soulier syndrome (BSS) is an autosomal recessive inherited thrombocytopenia disorder associated with macrothrombocytopenia. First described by Jean Bernard and Jean Pierre Soulier in 1948, its prevalence is thought to be approximately 1:1,000,000 (Bernard and Soulier 1948). Patients with BSS have platelets with severely reduced or functionally impaired surface glycoprotein Ib-IX-V (GPIb-IX-V) complex, which is the main platelet receptor for von Willebrand factor (VWF). Mutations in the genes *GP1BA*, *GP1BB*, and *GP9* (located on chromosomes 17, 22, and 3, respectively) result in defective GPIb-IX-V complex structure, which impacts not only platelet function but also megakaryocytes causing thrombocytopenia (Gothwal et al. 2014).

Flow cytometry or platelet aggregometry can be used to diagnose BSS as the assay reveals severely impaired agglutination after stimulation with the agonist ristocetin. Supportive care measures including antifibrinolytics and DDAVP are used for minor bleeding, whereas recombinant factor VIIA and platelet transfusions may be required for more severe bleeds.

Autosomal dominant Mediterranean macrothrombocytopenia and velocardiofacial syndromes are rare disorders in which only a single allele of a component of the GPIb-IX-V complex is mutated. Unlike BSS, these syndromes are characterized by larger than normal but not giant platelets and mild bleeding symptoms. Genetic analysis of several families with autosomal dominant Mediterranean macrothrombocytopenia syndrome led to the identification of a heterozygous missense mutation (Ala156Val) of GPIbα as the cause of the thrombocytopenia in 10 of 12 pedigrees analyzed (Savoia et al. 2001). Heterozygous absence of a component of the GPIb-IX-V complex also accounts for the thrombocytopenia observed in approximately 40% of patients with velocardiofacial syndrome (22q11), often referred to as DiGeorge syndrome (Van Geet et al. 1998; Kato et al. 2003). The *GP1B* gene that encodes for GPIbβ is located within the commonly deleted region. Interestingly, only 60% of patients heterozygous for the absence of the GPIb-IX-V complex exhibit macrothrombocytopenia. Accordingly, the manifestations of the heterozygote carriers of mutations known to cause BSS are quite variable.

Platelet-type VWD also known as pseudo-VWD is an autosomal dominant disorder characterized by mild to moderate mucocutaneous bleeding, mild thrombocytopenia, and decreased plasma levels of the VWF high molecular weight multimers (Miller and Castella 1982). Gain-of-function mutations within the VWF binding domain of GPIbα have been identified in patients with platelet-type VWD (Lopez et al. 1998, Othman et al. 2005). As a result, GPIb demonstrates increased affinity for VWF, and thrombocytopenia is noted presumably due of the increased clearance of VWF/platelet complexes.

11.3.8 ANKRD 26 Thrombocytopenia

Thrombocytopenia 2 (THC2), an autosomal dominant form of thrombocytopenia, was initially mapped to chromosome 10p11.2–12 in two large unrelated Caucasian kindreds from Italy and the United States (Savoia et al. 1999; Drachman et al. 2000). Sequencing of 32 regional candidate genes identified 6 mutations in a conserved 19-base pair (bp) region of the 5′-untranslated region (UTR) of *ANKRD26* in 9 Italian families. Further sequence analysis identified a total of 12 candidate mutations confined to a 22 bp region of the 5′-UTR in 21 of 210 families with inherited thrombocytopenias of unknown cause (Noris et al. 2011). Interestingly, *ANKRD26* 5'-UTR mutations have also been associated with a predisposition for myeloid malignancies in conjunction with familial thrombocytopenia (Noris et al. 2013; Marquez et al. 2014). The role of *ANKRD26* in megakaryopoiesis remains unclear. However, it was recently proposed that thrombocytopenia 2 might be caused by abnormal MAP kinase signaling, where 5'-UTR mutations in *ANKRD26* result in loss of RUNX1 and FLI1 protein binding, both transcription factors previously implicated in inherited thrombocytopenia (Bluteau et al. 2014).

11.3.9 ETV6 Thrombocytopenia

Several families with germline mutations in *ETV6* leading to autosomal dominant thrombocytopenia, red cell macrocytosis, and predisposition to leukemia were recently described (Noetzli et al.

2015; Zhang et al. 2015). *ETV6* encodes an E26 transformation-specific (Ets) family transcription repressor (variant 6), which exerts its activity by binding a consensus sequence in the promoter regions of DNA, and has been shown to play a key role in hematopoiesis. The bone marrow of affected individuals shows hyperplasia of small, hypolobulated immature megakaryocytes suggesting a differentiation arrest. This discovery led to subsequent studies that confirmed the findings (Topka et al. 2015) and to additional larger studies that demonstrated a 1% frequency of germline *ETV6* mutations among 4405 individuals with acute lymphoblastic leukemia (Moriyama et al. 2015). Additionally, a 4.5% prevalence of *ETV6* germline mutations was reported in families with inherited thrombocytopenia (Melazzini et al. 2016). More importantly, while only a fraction of individuals with *ETV6* germline mutations develop leukemia or other malignancies, the penetrance for thrombocytopenia is close to 100%.

Conclusion

The accurate and timely diagnosis of inherited thrombocytopenia disorders is critical to determine the correct clinical treatment and management of symptomatic patients. There have been great advances in the methods of diagnosis and the identification of causative genetic mutations, which has furthered our understanding of megakaryopoiesis and thrombopoiesis. However, a genetic cause is not found in many individuals, and clinical suspicion is required to initiate the appropriate investigation and treatment plan. A thorough family history and physical exam combined with molecular analysis can now lead to rapid diagnosis and improved clinical outcomes.

References

Al Kaissi A, Girsch W, Kenis V, Melchenko E, Ben Ghachem M, Pospischill R, Klaushofer K, Grill F, Ganger R (2015) Reconstruction of limb deformities in patients with thrombocytopenia-absent radius syndrome. Orthop Surg 7(1):50–56

Al-Ahmari A, Ayas M, Al-Jefri A, Al-Mahr M, Rifai S, El-Solh H (2004) Allogeneic stem cell transplantation for patients with congenital amegakaryocytic thrombocytopenia (CAT). Bone Marrow Transplant 33(8):829–831

Albers CA, Cvejic A, Favier R, Bouwmans EE, Alessi MC, Bertone P, Jordan G, Kettleborough RN, Kiddle G, Kostadima M, Read RJ, Sipos B, Sivapalaratnam S, Smethurst PA, Stephens J, Voss K, Nurden A, Rendon A, Nurden P, Ouwehand WH (2011) Exome sequencing identifies NBEAL2 as the causative gene for gray platelet syndrome. Nat Genet 43(8):735–737

Albers CA, Newbury-Ecob R, Ouwehand WH, Ghevaert C (2013) New insights into the genetic basis of TAR (thrombocytopenia-absent radii) syndrome. Curr Opin Genet Dev 23(3):316–323

Alexander WS, Roberts AW, Maurer AB, Nicola NA, Dunn AR, Metcalf D (1996a) Studies of the c-Mpl thrombopoietin receptor through gene disruption and activation. Stem Cells 14(Suppl 1):124–132

Alexander WS, Roberts AW, Nicola NA, Li R, Metcalf D (1996b) Deficiencies in progenitor cells of multiple hematopoietic lineages and defective megakaryocytopoiesis in mice lacking the thrombopoietic receptor c-Mpl. Blood 87(6):2162–2170

Alter BP (1992) Arm anomalies and bone marrow failure may go hand in hand. J Hand Surg Am 17(3): 566–571

Alter BP (2002) Bone marrow failure syndromes in children. Pediatr Clin N Am 49(5):973–988

Ballmaier M, Germeshausen M, Schulze H, Cherkaoui K, Lang S, Gaudig A, Krukemeier S, Eilers M, Strauss G, Welte K (2001) c-mpl mutations are the cause of congenital amegakaryocytic thrombocytopenia. Blood 97(1):139–146

Bernard J, Soulier JP (1948) Sur une nouvelle variete de dystrophie thrombocytaire-hemorragipare congenitale. Sem Hop 24(Spec. No.):3217–3223

Bluteau D, Glembotsky AC, Raimbault A, Balayn N, Gilles L, Rameau P, Nurden P, Alessi MC, Debili N, Vainchenker W, Heller PG, Favier R, Raslova H (2012) Dysmegakaryopoiesis of FPD/AML pedigrees with constitutional RUNX1 mutations is linked to myosin II deregulated expression. Blood 120(13):2708–2718

Bluteau D, Balduini A, Balayn N, Currao M, Nurden P, Deswarte C, Leverger G, Noris P, Perrotta S, Solary E, Vainchenker W, Debili N, Favier R, Raslova H (2014) Thrombocytopenia-associated mutations in the ANKRD26 regulatory region induce MAPK hyperactivation. J Clin Invest 124(2):580–591

Bottillo I, Castori M, De Bernardo C, Fabbri R, Grammatico B, Preziosi N, Scassellati GS, Silvestri E, Spagnuolo A, Laino L, Grammatico P (2013) Prenatal diagnosis and post-mortem examination in a fetus with thrombocytopenia-absent radius (TAR) syndrome due to compound heterozygosity for a 1q21.1 microdeletion and a RBM8A hypomorphic allele: a case report. BMC Res Notes 6:376

Camitta BM, Rock A (1993) Acute lymphoidic leukemia in a patient with thrombocytopenia/absent radii (Tar) syndrome. Am J Pediatr Hematol Oncol 15(3):335–337

Chen J, Herceg-Harjacek L, Groopman JE, Grabarek J (1995) Regulation of platelet activation in vitro by the c-Mpl ligand, thrombopoietin. Blood 86(11):4054–4062

Cheng Y, Wu W, Kumar SA, Yu D, Deng W, Tripic T, King DC, Chen KB, Zhang Y, Drautz D, Giardine B, Schuster SC, Miller W, Chiaromonte F, Zhang Y, Blobel GA, Weiss MJ, Hardison RC (2009) Erythroid GATA1 function revealed by genome-wide analysis of transcription factor occupancy, histone modifications, and mRNA expression. Genome Res 19(12):2172–2184

Cines DB, Bussel JB, McMillan RB, Zehnder JL (2004) Congenital and acquired thrombocytopenia. Hematology Am Soc Hematol Educ Program: 390–406

Ciovacco WA, Raskind WH, Kacena MA (2008) Human phenotypes associated with GATA-1 mutations. Gene 427(1–2):1–6

Cocault L, Bouscary D, Le Bousse Kerdiles C, Clay D, Picard F, Gisselbrecht S, Souyri M (1996) Ectopic expression of murine TPO receptor (c-mpl) in mice is pathogenic and induces erythroblastic proliferation. Blood 88(5):1656–1665

Coccia P, Ruggiero A, Mastrangelo S, Attina G, Scalzone M, Pittiruti M, Zampino G, Maurizi P, Riccardi R (2012) Management of children with thrombocytopenia-absent radius syndrome: an institutional experience. J Paediatr Child Health 48(2):166–169

Di Paola J (2015) Paris-Trousseau: evidence keeps pointing to FLI1. Blood 126(17):1973–1974

Di Paola J, Johnson J (2011) Thrombocytopenias due to gray platelet syndrome or THC2 mutations. Semin Thromb Hemost 37(6):690–697

Drachman JG, Jarvik GP, Mehaffey MG (2000) Autosomal dominant thrombocytopenia: incomplete megakaryocyte differentiation and linkage to human chromosome 10. Blood 96(1):118–125

Dreyfus M, Tchernia G (2000) Thrombocytopenia with absent radii (TAR syndrome): new advances in the mechanism of thrombocytopenia. Pediatr Hematol Oncol 17(7):521–522

Ezumi Y, Takayama H, Okuma M (1995) Thrombopoietin, c-Mpl ligand, induces tyrosine phosphorylation of Tyk2, JAK2, and STAT3, and enhances agonists-induced aggregation in platelets in vitro. FEBS Lett 374(1): 48–52

Fadoo Z, Naqvi SM (2002) Acute myeloid leukemia in a patient with thrombocytopenia with absent radii syndrome. J Pediatr Hematol Oncol 24(2):134–135

Foudi A, Kramer DJ, Qin J, Ye D, Behlich AS, Mordecai S, Preffer FI, Amzallag A, Ramaswamy S, Hochedlinger K, Orkin SH, Hock H (2014) Distinct, strict requirements for Gfi-1b in adult bone marrow red cell and platelet generation. J Exp Med 211(5):909–927

Fox NE, Lim J, Chen R, Geddis AE (2010) F104S c-Mpl responds to a transmembrane domain-binding thrombopoietin receptor agonist: proof of concept that selected receptor mutations in congenital amegakaryocytic thrombocytopenia can be stimulated with alternative thrombopoietic agents. Exp Hematol 38(5):384–391

Frangoul H, Keates-Baleeiro J, Calder C, Manes B, Crossno C, Castaneda VL, Domm J (2010) Unrelated bone marrow transplant for congenital amegakaryocytic thrombocytopenia: report of two cases and review of the literature. Pediatr Transplant 14(4):E42–E45

Freson K, Wijgaerts A, van Geet C (2014) Update on the causes of platelet disorders and functional consequences. Int J Lab Hematol 36(3):313–325

Geddis AE (2009) Congenital amegakaryocytic thrombocytopenia and thrombocytopenia with absent radii. Hematol Oncol Clin North Am 23(2):321–331

Geddis AE (2011) Congenital amegakaryocytic thrombocytopenia. Pediatr Blood Cancer 57(2):199–203

Geddis AE (2013) Inherited thrombocytopenias: an approach to diagnosis and management. Int J Lab Hematol 35(1):14–25

Germeshausen M, Ballmaier M, Welte K (2006) MPL mutations in 23 patients suffering from congenital amegakaryocytic thrombocytopenia: the type of mutation predicts the course of the disease. Hum Mutat 27(3):296

Goldfarb CA, Wustrack R, Pratt JA, Mender A, Manske PR (2007) Thumb function and appearance in thrombocytopenia: absent radius syndrome. J Hand Surg Am 32(2):157–161

Gothwal M, Sandrock-Lang K, Zieger B (2014) Genetics of inherited platelet disorders. Hamostaseologie 34(2):133–141

Greenhalgh KL, Howell RT, Bottani A, Ancliff PJ, Brunner HG, Verschuuren-Bemelmans CC, Vernon E, Brown KW, Newbury-Ecob RA (2002) Thrombocytopenia-absent radius syndrome: a clinical genetic study. J Med Genet 39(12):876–881

Greenwald HM, Sherman I (1929) Congenital essential thrombocytopenia. Am J Dis Child 38:1245–1251

Grozovsky R, Begonja AJ, Liu K, Visner G, Hartwig JH, Falet H, Hoffmeister KM (2015) The Ashwell-Morell receptor regulates hepatic thrombopoietin production via JAK2-STAT3 signaling. Nat Med 21(1):47–54

Guinan EC, Lee YS, Lopez KD, Kohler S, Oette DH, Bruno E, Kozakewich H, Nathan DG, Hoffman R (1993) Effects of interleukin-3 and granulocyte-macrophage colony-stimulating factor on thrombopoiesis in congenital amegakaryocytic thrombocytopenia. Blood 81(7):1691–1698

Gunay-Aygun M, Zivony-Elboum Y, Gumruk F, Geiger D, Cetin M, Khayat M, Kleta R, Kfir N, Anikster Y, Chezar J, Arcos-Burgos M, Shalata A, Stanescu H, Manaster J, Arat M, Edwards H, Freiberg AS, Hart PS, Riney LC, Patzel K, Tanpaiboon P, Markello T, Huizing M, Maric I, Horne M, Kehrel BE, Jurk K, Hansen NF, Cherukuri PF, Jones M, Cruz P, Mullikin JC, Nurden A, White JG, Gahl WA, Falik-Zaccai T (2010) Gray platelet syndrome: natural history of a large patient cohort and locus assignment to chromosome 3p. Blood 116(23):4990–5001

Gunay-Aygun M, Falik-Zaccai TC, Vilboux T, Zivony-Elboum Y, Gumruk F, Cetin M, Khayat M, Boerkoel

CF, Kfir N, Huang Y, Maynard D, Dorward H, Berger K, Kleta R, Anikster Y, Arat M, Freiberg AS, Kehrel BE, Jurk K, Cruz P, Mullikin JC, White JG, Huizing M, Gahl WA (2011) NBEAL2 is mutated in gray platelet syndrome and is required for biogenesis of platelet alpha-granules. Nat Genet 43(8):732–734

Hall JG (1987) Thrombocytopenia and absent radius (TAR) syndrome. J Med Genet 24(2):79–83

Hall JG, Levin J, Kuhn JP, Ottenheimer EJ, van Berkum KA, McKusick VA (1969) Thrombocytopenia with absent radius (TAR). Medicine (Baltimore) 48(6):411–439

Hart A, Melet F, Grossfeld P, Chien K, Jones C, Tunnacliffe A, Favier R, Bernstein A (2000) Fli-1 is required for murine vascular and megakaryocytic development and is hemizygously deleted in patients with thrombocytopenia. Immunity 13(2):167–177

Hedberg VA, Lipton JM (1988) Thrombocytopenia with absent radii. A review of 100 cases. Am J Pediatr Hematol Oncol 10(1):51–64

Henter JI, Winiarski J, Ljungman P, Ringden O, Ost A (1995) Bone marrow transplantation in two children with congenital amegakaryocytic thrombocytopenia. Bone Marrow Transplant 15(5):799–801

Hinckley J, Di Paola J (2014) Genetic basis of congenital platelet disorders. Hematology Am Soc Hematol Educ Program 2014(1):337–342

Houeijeh A, Andrieux J, Saugier-Veber P, David A, Goldenberg A, Bonneau D, Fouassier M, Journel H, Martinovic J, Escande F, Devisme L, Bisiaux S, Chaffiotte C, Baux M, Kerckaert JP, Holder-Espinasse M, Manouvrier-Hanu S (2011) Thrombocytopenia-absent radius (TAR) syndrome: a clinical genetic series of 14 further cases. impact of the associated 1q21.1 deletion on the genetic counselling. Eur J Med Genet 54(5):e471–e477

Ihara K, Ishii E, Eguchi M, Takada H, Suminoe A, Good RA, Hara T (1999) Identification of mutations in the c-mpl gene in congenital amegakaryocytic thrombocytopenia. Proc Natl Acad Sci U S A 96(6):3132–3136

Jalagadugula G, Mao G, Kaur G, Goldfinger LE, Dhanasekaran DN, Rao AK (2010) Regulation of platelet myosin light chain (MYL9) by RUNX1: implications for thrombocytopenia and platelet dysfunction in RUNX1 haplodeficiency. Blood 116(26):6037–6045

Kahr WH, Hinckley J, Li L, Schwertz H, Christensen H, Rowley JW, Pluthero FG, Urban D, Fabbro S, Nixon B, Gadzinski R, Storck M, Wang K, Ryu GY, Jobe SM, Schutte BC, Moseley J, Loughran NB, Parkinson J, Weyrich AS, Di Paola J (2011) Mutations in NBEAL2, encoding a BEACH protein, cause gray platelet syndrome. Nat Genet 43(8):738–740

Kato T, Kosaka K, Kimura M, Imamura S, Yamada O, Iwai K, Ando M, Joh-o K, Kuroe K, Ohtake A, Takao A, Momma K, Matsuoka R (2003) Thrombocytopenia in patients with 22q11.2 deletion syndrome and its association with glycoprotein Ib-beta. Genet Med 5(2):113–119

Kaushansky K (2008) Historical review: megakaryopoiesis and thrombopoiesis. Blood 111(3):981–986

Kerenyi MA, Orkin SH (2010) Networking erythropoiesis. J Exp Med 207(12):2537–2541

Khincha PP, Savage SA (2013) Genomic characterization of the inherited bone marrow failure syndromes. Semin Hematol 50(4):333–347

King S, Germeshausen M, Strauss G, Welte K, Ballmaier M (2005) Congenital amegakaryocytic thrombocytopenia: a retrospective clinical analysis of 20 patients. Br J Haematol 131(5):636–644

Klopocki E, Schulze H, Strauss G, Ott CE, Hall J, Trotier F, Fleischhauer S, Greenhalgh L, Newbury-Ecob RA, Neumann LM, Habenicht R, Konig R, Seemanova E, Megarbane A, Ropers HH, Ullmann R, Horn D, Mundlos S (2007) Complex inheritance pattern resembling autosomal recessive inheritance involving a microdeletion in thrombocytopenia-absent radius syndrome. Am J Hum Genet 80(2):232–240

Liew E, Owen C (2011) Familial myelodysplastic syndromes: a review of the literature. Haematologica 96(10):1536–1542

Lopez JA, Andrews RK, Afshar-Kharghan V, Berndt MC (1998) Bernard-Soulier syndrome. Blood 91(12):4397–4418

Lordier L, Bluteau D, Jalil A, Legrand C, Pan J, Rameau P, Jouni D, Bluteau O, Mercher T, Leon C, Gachet C, Debili N, Vainchenker W, Raslova H, Chang Y (2012) RUNX1-induced silencing of non-muscle myosin heavy chain IIB contributes to megakaryocyte polyploidization. Nat Commun 3:717

Machlus KR, Italiano JE Jr (2013) The incredible journey: from megakaryocyte development to platelet formation. J Cell Biol 201(6):785–796

Marquez R, Hantel A, Lorenz R, Neistadt B, Wong J, Churpek JE, Mardini NA, Shaukat I, Gurbuxani S, Miller JL, Godley LA (2014) A new family with a germline ANKRD26 mutation and predisposition to myeloid malignancies. Leuk Lymphoma 55(12):2945–2946

Martinez-Frias ML, Bermejo Sanchez E, Garcia Garcia A, Perez Fernandez JL, Cucalon Manzanos F, Calvo Aguilar MJ, Ripalda Crespo MJ (1998) An epidemiological study of the thrombocytopenia with radial aplasia syndrome (TAR) in Spain. An Esp Pediatr 49(6):619–623

Maserati E, Panarello C, Morerio C, Valli R, Pressato B, Patitucci F, Tassano E, Di Cesare-Merlone A, Cugno C, Balduini CL, Lo Curto F, Dufour C, Locatelli F, Pasquali F (2008) Clonal chromosome anomalies and propensity to myeloid malignancies in congenital amegakaryocytic thrombocytopenia (OMIM 604498). Haematologica 93(8):1271–1273

Melazzini F, Palombo F, Balduini A, De Rocco D, Marconi C, Noris P, Gnan C, Pippucci T, Bozzi V, Faleschini M, Barozzi S, Doubek M, Di Buduo CA, Stano Kozubik K, Radova L, Loffredo G, Pospisilova S, Alfano C, Seri M, Balduini CL, Pecci A, Savoia A (2016) Clinical and pathogenetic features of ETV6 related thrombocytopenia with predisposition to acute lymphoblastic leukemia. Haematologica 101(11): 1333–1342

Miller JL, Castella A (1982) Platelet-type von Willebrand's disease: characterization of a new bleeding disorder. Blood 60(3):790–794

Moliterno AR, Williams DM, Gutierrez-Alamillo LI, Salvatori R, Ingersoll RG, Spivak JL (2004) Mpl Baltimore: a thrombopoietin receptor polymorphism associated with thrombocytosis. Proc Natl Acad Sci U S A 101(31):11444–11447

Monteferrario D, Bolar NA, Marneth AE, Hebeda KM, Bergevoet SM, Veenstra H, Laros-van Gorkom BA, MacKenzie MA, Khandanpour C, Botezatu L, Fransen E, Van Camp G, Duijnhouwer AL, Salemink S, Willemsen B, Huls G, Preijers F, Van Heerde W, Jansen JH, Kempers MJ, Loeys BL, Van Laer L, Van der Reijden BA (2014) A dominant-negative GFI1B mutation in the gray platelet syndrome. N Engl J Med 370(3):245–253

Moriyama T, Metzger ML, Wu G, Nishii R, Qian M, Devidas M, Yang W, Cheng C, Cao X, Quinn E, Raimondi S, Gastier-Foster JM, Raetz E, Larsen E, Martin PL, Bowman WP, Winick N, Komada Y, Wang S, Edmonson M, Xu H, Mardis E, Fulton R, Pui CH, Mullighan C, Evans WE, Zhang J, Hunger SP, Relling MV, Nichols KE, Loh ML, Yang JJ (2015) Germline genetic variation in ETV6 and risk of childhood acute lymphoblastic leukaemia: a systematic genetic study. Lancet Oncol 16(16):1659–1666

Muraoka K, Ishii E, Tsuji K, Yamamoto S, Yamaguchi H, Hara T, Koga H, Nakahata T, Miyazaki S (1997) Defective response to thrombopoietin and impaired expression of c-mpl mRNA of bone marrow cells in congenital amegakaryocytic thrombocytopenia. Br J Haematol 96(2):287–292

Myers KC, Davies SM (2009) Hematopoietic stem cell transplantation for bone marrow failure syndromes in children. Biol Blood Marrow Transplant 15(3):279–292

Nicchia E, Giordano P, Greco C, De Rocco D, Savoia A (2016) Molecular diagnosis of thrombocytopenia-absent radius syndrome using next-generation sequencing. Int J Lab Hematol 38(4):412–418

Nichols KE, Crispino JD, Poncz M, White JG, Orkin SH, Maris JM, Weiss MJ (2000) Familial dyserythropoietic anaemia and thrombocytopenia due to an inherited mutation in GATA1. Nat Genet 24(3):266–270

Niihori T, Ouchi-Uchiyama M, Sasahara Y, Kaneko T, Hashii Y, Irie M, Sato A, Saito-Nanjo Y, Funayama R, Nagashima T, Inoue S, Nakayama K, Ozono K, Kure S, Matsubara Y, Imaizumi M, Aoki Y (2015) Mutations in MECOM, encoding oncoprotein EVI1, cause radioulnar synostosis with amegakaryocytic thrombocytopenia. Am J Hum Genet 97(6):848–854

Noetzli L, Lo RW, Lee-Sherick AB, Callaghan M, Noris P, Savoia A, Rajpurkar M, Jones K, Gowan K, Balduini CL, Pecci A, Gnan C, De Rocco D, Doubek M, Li L, Lu L, Leung R, Landolt-Marticorena C, Hunger S, Heller P, Gutierrez-Hartmann A, Xiayuan L, Pluthero FG, Rowley JW, Weyrich AS, Kahr WH, Porter CC, Di Paola J (2015) Germline mutations in ETV6 are associated with thrombocytopenia, red cell macrocytosis and predisposition to lymphoblastic leukemia. Nat Genet 47(5):535–538

Noris P, Perrotta S, Seri M, Pecci A, Gnan C, Loffredo G, Pujol-Moix N, Zecca M, Scognamiglio F, De Rocco D, Punzo F, Melazzini F, Scianguetta S, Casale M, Marconi C, Pippucci T, Amendola G, Notarangelo LD, Klersy C, Civaschi E, Balduini CL, Savoia A (2011) Mutations in ANKRD26 are responsible for a frequent form of inherited thrombocytopenia: analysis of 78 patients from 21 families. Blood 117(24):6673–6680

Noris P, Favier R, Alessi MC, Geddis AE, Kunishima S, Heller PG, Giordano P, Niederhoffer KY, Bussel JB, Podda GM, Vianelli N, Kersseboom R, Pecci A, Gnan C, Marconi C, Auvrignon A, Cohen W, Yu JC, Iguchi A, Miller Imahiyerobo A, Boehlen F, Ghalloussi D, De Rocco D, Magini P, Civaschi E, Biino G, Seri M, Savoia A, Balduini CL (2013) ANKRD26-related thrombocytopenia and myeloid malignancies. Blood 122(11):1987–1989

Othman M, Notley C, Lavender FL, White H, Byrne CD, Lillicrap D, O'Shaughnessy DF (2005) Identification and functional characterization of a novel 27-bp deletion in the macroglycopeptide-coding region of the GPIBA gene resulting in platelet-type von Willebrand disease. Blood 105(11):4330–4336

Pikman Y, Lee BH, Mercher T, McDowell E, Ebert BL, Gozo M, Cuker A, Wernig G, Moore S, Galinsky I, DeAngelo DJ, Clark JJ, Lee SJ, Golub TR, Wadleigh M, Gilliland DG, Levine RL (2006) MPLW515L is a novel somatic activating mutation in myelofibrosis with myeloid metaplasia. PLoS Med 3(7):e270

Raslova H, Komura E, Le Couedic JP, Larbret F, Debili N, Feunteun J, Danos O, Albagli O, Vainchenker W, Favier R (2004) FLI1 monoallelic expression combined with its hemizygous loss underlies Paris-Trousseau/Jacobsen thrombopenia. J Clin Invest 114(1):77–84

Richard RE, Blau CA (2003) Small-molecule-directed mpl signaling can complement growth factors to selectively expand genetically modified cord blood cells. Stem Cells 21(1):71–78

Savoia A, Del Vecchio M, Totaro A, Perrotta S, Amendola G, Moretti A, Zelante L, Iolascon A (1999) An autosomal dominant thrombocytopenia gene maps to chromosomal region 10p. Am J Hum Genet 65(5):1401–1405

Savoia A, Balduini CL, Savino M, Noris P, Del Vecchio M, Perrotta S, Belletti S, Poggi, Iolascon A (2001) Autosomal dominant macrothrombocytopenia in Italy is most frequently a type of heterozygous Bernard-Soulier syndrome. Blood 97(5):1330–1335

Savoia A, Dufour C, Locatelli F, Noris P, Ambaglio C, Rosti V, Zecca M, Ferrari S, di Bari F, Corcione A, Di Stazio M, Seri M, Balduini CL (2007) Congenital amegakaryocytic thrombocytopenia: clinical and biological consequences of five novel mutations. Haematologica 92(9):1186–1193

Seri M, Cusano R, Gangarossa S, Caridi G, Bordo D, Lo Nigro C, Ghiggeri GM, Ravazzolo R, Savino M, Del Vecchio M, d'Apolito M, Iolascon A, Zelante LL,

Savoia A, Balduini CL, Noris P, Magrini U, Belletti S, Heath KE, Babcock M, Glucksman MJ, Aliprandis E, Bizzaro N, Desnick RJ, Martignetti JA (2000) Mutations in MYH9 result in the May-Hegglin anomaly, and Fechtner and Sebastian syndromes. The May-Heggllin/Fechtner Syndrome Consortium. Nat Genet 26(1):103–105

Seri M, Pecci A, Di Bari F, Cusano R, Savino M, Panza E, Nigro A, Noris P, Gangarossa S, Rocca B, Gresele P, Bizzaro N, Malatesta P, Koivisto PA, Longo I, Musso R, Pecoraro C, Iolascon A, Magrini U, Rodriguez Soriano J, Renieri A, Ghiggeri GM, Ravazzolo R, Balduini CL, Savoia A (2003) MYH9-related disease: May-Hegglin anomaly, Sebastian syndrome, Fechtner syndrome, and Epstein syndrome are not distinct entities but represent a variable expression of a single illness. Medicine (Baltimore) 82(3):203–215

Song WJ, Sullivan MG, Legare RD, Hutchings S, Tan X, Kufrin D, Ratajczak J, Resende IC, Haworth C, Hock R, Loh M, Felix C, Roy DC, Busque L, Kurnit D, Willman C, Gewirtz AM, Speck NA, Bushweller JH, Li FP, Gardiner K, Poncz M, Maris JM, Gilliland DG (1999) Haploinsufficiency of CBFA2 causes familial thrombocytopenia with propensity to develop acute myelogenous leukaemia. Nat Genet 23(2): 166–175

Steinberg O, Gilad G, Dgany O, Krasnov T, Zoldan M, Laor R, Kapelushnik J, Gabriel H, Churi C, Stein J, Yaniv I, Tamary H (2007) Congenital amegakaryocytic thrombocytopenia-3 novel c-MPL mutations and their phenotypic correlations. J Pediatr Hematol Oncol 29(12):822–825

Stevenson WS, Rabbolini DJ, Beutler L, Chen Q, Gabrielli S, Mackay JP, Brighton TA, Ward CM, Morel-Kopp MC (2015) Paris-Trousseau thrombocytopenia is phenocopied by the autosomal recessive inheritance of a DNA-binding domain mutation in FLI1. Blood 126(17):2027–2030

Stockley J, Morgan NV, Bem D, Lowe GC, Lordkipanidze M, Dawood B, Simpson MA, Macfarlane K, Horner K, Leo VC, Talks K, Motwani J, Wilde JT, Collins PW, Makris M, Watson SP, Daly ME, U. K. Genotyping and G. Phenotyping of Platelets Study (2013) Enrichment of FLI1 and RUNX1 mutations in families with excessive bleeding and platelet dense granule secretion defects. Blood 122(25):4090–4093

Strippoli P, Savoia A, Iolascon A, Tonelli R, Savino M, Giordano P, D'Avanzo M, Massolo F, Locatelli F, Borgna C, De Mattia D, Zelante L, Paolucci G, Bagnara GP (1998) Mutational screening of thrombopoietin receptor gene (c-mpl) in patients with congenital thrombocytopenia and absent radii (TAR). Br J Haematol 103(2):311–314

Symonds RP, Clark BJ, George WD, Bryant PE, Liu N, Connor JM (1995) Thrombocytopenia with absent radii (TAR) syndrome: a new increased cellular radiosensitivity syndrome. Clin Oncol (R Coll Radiol) 7(1):56–58

Tarek N, Kernan NA, Prockop SE, Scaradavou A, Small TN, O'Reilly RJ, Boulad F (2012) T-cell-depleted hematopoietic SCT from unrelated donors for the treatment of congenital amegakaryocytic thrombocytopenia. Bone Marrow Transplant 47(5):744–746

Thompson AA, Nguyen LT (2000) Amegakaryocytic thrombocytopenia and radio-ulnar synostosis are associated with HOXA11 mutation. Nat Genet 26(4):397–398

Thompson AA, Woodruff K, Feig SA, Nguyen LT, Schanen NC (2001) Congenital thrombocytopenia and radio-ulnar synostosis: a new familial syndrome. Br J Haematol 113(4):866–870

Thon JN, Italiano JE (2010) Platelet formation. Semin Hematol 47(3):220–226

Thon JN, Montalvo A, Patel-Hett S, Devine MT, Richardson JL, Ehrlicher A, Larson MK, Hoffmeister K, Hartwig JH, Italiano JE Jr (2010) Cytoskeletal mechanics of proplatelet maturation and platelet release. J Cell Biol 191(4):861–874

Topka S, Vijai J, Walsh MF, Jacobs L, Maria A, Villano D, Gaddam P, Wu G, McGee RB, Quinn E, Inaba H, Hartford C, Pui CH, Pappo A, Edmonson M, Zhang MY, Stepensky P, Steinherz P, Schrader K, Lincoln A, Bussel J, Lipkin SM, Goldgur Y, Harit M, Stadler ZK, Mullighan C, Weintraub M, Shimamura A, Zhang J, Downing JR, Nichols KE, Offit K (2015) Germline ETV6 mutations confer susceptibility to acute lymphoblastic leukemia and thrombocytopenia. PLoS Genet 11(6):e1005262

Toriello HV (1993) Thrombocytopenia absent radius syndrome. In: Pagon RA, Adam MP, Ardinger HH et al (eds) GeneReviews®. University of Washington, Seattle, WA

Toriello HV (2011) Thrombocytopenia-absent radius syndrome. Semin Thromb Hemost 37(6):707–712

Van Geet C, Devriendt K, Eyskens B, Vermylen J, Hoylaerts MF (1998) Velocardiofacial syndrome patients with a heterozygous chromosome 22q11 deletion have giant platelets. Pediatr Res 44(4):607–611

Wicke DC, Meyer J, Buesche G, Heckl D, Kreipe H, Li Z, Welte KH, Ballmaier M, Baum C, Modlich U (2010) Gene therapy of MPL deficiency: challenging balance between leukemia and pancytopenia. Mol Ther 18(2):343–352

Woods G, Bajwa RP, Rose MJ (2014) Reduced intensity transplantation for congenital amegakaryocytic thrombocytopenia: report of a case and review of the literature. Pediatr Transplant 18(1):E31–E34

Zhang MY, Churpek JE, Keel SB, Walsh T, Lee MK, Loeb KR, Gulsuner S, Pritchard CC, Sanchez-Bonilla M, Delrow JJ, Basom RS, Forouhar M, Gyurkocza B, Schwartz BS, Neistadt B, Marquez R, Mariani CJ, Coats SA, Hofmann I, Lindsley RC, Williams DA, Abkowitz JL, Horwitz MS, King MC, Godley LA, Shimamura A (2015) Germline ETV6 mutations in familial thrombocytopenia and hematologic malignancy. Nat Genet 47(2):180–185

MIX
Papier aus verantwortungsvollen Quellen
Paper from responsible sources
FSC® C105338

If you have any concerns about our products,
you can contact us on
ProductSafety@springernature.com

In case Publisher is established outside the EU,
the EU authorized representative is:
Springer Nature Customer Service Center GmbH
Europaplatz 3, 69115 Heidelberg, Germany

Printed by Libri Plureos GmbH
in Hamburg, Germany